THE PATIENT AS PERSON

The Institution for Social and Policy Studies
at Yale University

The Yale ISPS Series

THE PATIENT AS PERSON

Explorations in Medical Ethics

Second Edition

by Paul Ramsey

with a new foreword by Margaret A. Farley
and essays by Albert R. Jonsen and William F. May

Yale University Press   New Haven and London

Second edition first published by Yale University Press in 2002.
First edition published by Yale University Press in 1970.
Originally presented, with the exception of the Preface,
as the Lyman Beecher Lectures at Yale University, 1969.

Foreword, "The Structure of an Ethical Revolution,"
and "The Patient as Person: Beyond Ramsey's Beecher Lectures"
copyright © 2002 by Yale University.
Copyright © 1970 by Yale University.

Originally published with assistance from the foundation
established in memory of Philip Hamilton McMillan
of the Class of 1894, Yale College.

Printed in the United States of America

Library of Congress Control Number: 2001099040

ISBN 0-300-09396-9 (pbk. : alk. paper)

A catalogue record for this book is available from the
British Library.

10 9 8 7 6 5 4 3 2 1

For

Jenifer Ramsey,

nurse

As a stream cannot rise above its source, so a code cannot change a low-grade man into a high-grade doctor, but it can help a good man to be a better man and a more enlightened doctor. It can quicken and inform a conscience, but not create one.

International Code of Medical Ethics,
adopted by the General Assembly of the
World Medical Association, London, 1949

Medical art and science rest like others on a legitimate use of the possibilities given to man. If the history of medicine has been as little free from error, negligence, one-sidedness and exaggeration as any other science, in its main development it has been and still is, to lay eyes at least, as impressive, honourable and promising as, for instance, theology.

Karl Barth, *Church Dogmatics*, III/4, p. 362

Contents

Foreword

Thirty-two years ago an extraordinary event took place. Out of it came the beginnings of a new and astoundingly influential scholarly and practical discipline. The event was a conference that brought together theologians, philosophers, scientists, physicians, legal scholars, representatives of the clergy, and many others. Its purpose was to probe and debate key ethical questions emerging in the context of medical care and research. The conference took place in the spring of 1969 at Yale University, under the sponsorship of Yale Divinity School and the Yale School of Medicine. Its inspiration came from ethicist James M. Gustafson, longtime faculty member of the Divinity School and the first chair of the Department of Religious Studies. Gustafson recognized that the issues facing medical practitioners, religious traditions, and Western society as a whole could not be addressed by one discipline or one profession alone. They required interdisciplinary (and interreligious, interprofessional, cross-cultural) attention of the most rigorous and wide-ranging kind. Hence, while the occasion for the conference was the Divinity School's 1969 Lyman Beecher Lecture Series, the ordinary format of the lectures was quickly broadened to include multidisciplinary responses and numerous satellite seminars in which a wide range of academic and professional experience could be represented.

The catalyst for the conference was Paul Ramsey, the nationally recognized ethicist from Princeton University, and Beecher Lecturer for that year. Ramsey was not new to heated public debate and interdisciplinary discernment, but he was relatively new to issues of medical practice and research. He prepared to address these issues with a year of clinical experience, and then plunged in with his usual vigorous analysis and strong proposals. The discussion that ensued was electric, and debates raged during the week-long series of lectures and responses. Thus was launched a new phase of medical ethical concern and a largely new method of moral discernment. This conference and Ramsey's lectures were not the only progenitors of the contemporary discipline of medical ethics (which later modulated

xi

into the wider concerns of the discipline of bioethics), but they were among the most important. Not only did they help to jump-start a new discipline, but they significantly shaped it for years to come.

It seemed fitting, then, on the thirtieth anniversary of the lectures, to do something to mark once again the milestone they had clearly provided. At the suggestion of Albert Jonsen, the first Bioethicist-in-Residence for the newly organized Yale Interdisciplinary Bioethics Project, a symposium was planned for October 2000. It would mark the three decades since the 1969 lectures and their 1970 publication in *The Patient as Person*. Although this would be a small event compared with the massive 1969 conference, it would allow both retrospective and prospective assessments of the significance of *The Patient as Person*. Like the original conference, the symposium would bring together students and faculty (especially those active in the Yale Bioethics Project) from many disciplines and professions. Lectures would be offered by Jonsen and William F. May (the second Yale Bioethicist-in-Residence). Responses and discussions would engage the many disciplines and perspectives of the participants—representing not only diverse areas of scholarship and practice, but (as in the 1969 conference) diverse religious and cultural perspectives as well.

This new edition of *The Patient as Person* represents a consensus that Paul Ramsey's lectures continue to contribute significantly to the concerns of medical ethics and bioethics in the twenty-first century. Jonsen's and May's symposium lectures are included as introductory essays in this edition. As such, they situate *The Patient as Person* in our present processes of discernment and debate. Jonsen's essay provides insights into Ramsey himself as a scholar and an "argumentative talker." These characteristics, Jonsen insists, are what made the Beecher Lectures so powerful, and what allowed Ramsey (whether or not he would have named his own work this way) to inaugurate a "revolution in ethical analysis." According to Jonsen's interpretation, this revolution is a shift from what might be called "armchair" ethics, where debate is among scholars of ethics, to interdisciplinary ethics, where the debate includes representatives of other disciplines as well as vital contact with public discourse. Under both paradigms, the discipline is marked by careful use of language, logical coherence, and rationally defensible justification. But ethics in its revolutionary form necessarily involves attention to concrete cases, a sustained conversation with scientists, physicians, lawyers, and other scholars and practitioners, and interaction with policy-makers, the media, and others engaged in public ethical discourse.

William May, in contrast, is reluctant to describe Ramsey's work in revolutionary terms. He thinks Ramsey primarily wanted to sustain and advance the conversation, and—for all his grandiloquence—to end with rather smaller claims than those of a revolutionary. Yet May, too, describes Paul Ramsey's lectures (and his work beyond them) as being on the frontier of "applied ethics." Ramsey was, says May, a pioneer in turning to concrete cases and in sparking public debate. Like Jonsen, May offers us insight into Ramsey the person. He goes on to consider the relation of *The Patient as Person* to the whole of Ramsey's work and, beyond this, to its significance in the larger context of medical ethics as a discipline. Here May notes the emergence of contemporary questions about the relative importance of a principled approach to ethics (like Ramsey's) and an approach that takes into account the development of moral character (or a theory of virtue). He also raises current issues regarding the structure of health care delivery—issues of medical education and of the general economics of health care. While Ramsey had basically demurred when it came to proposals for health care reform, May argues that ethicists can no longer ignore this major set of questions. Although they lead into questions of political and social ethics, these are precisely areas that medical ethics must address.

Both Jonsen and May emphasize Ramsey's concern with bringing a distinctively Christian perspective to medical ethics. For Paul Ramsey, the heart of a Christian medical ethics should focus on biblical notions of covenant, and therefore on canons of loyalty for the faithful keeping of covenants. Although the theme of covenant recedes after the first part of *The Patient as Person*, it nonetheless remains a thread to be pulled through the fabric of the whole. Along with it are the values and action guides derived from perceptions of the sanctity of life and the obligations of faithfulness to committed relationships, including the relationship between medical caregivers and patients. And perhaps above all, whether so intended or not, *The Patient as Person* has proved to be a major force in the focus on informed consent, on the autonomy of the patient, that has held sway in medical ethics, law, and the practice of medicine for thirty years.

Whether or not one agrees with Ramsey's particular articulation of Christian duties in clinical and research contexts, his clear and forthright proposals in this regard stand as a model for the doing of religious medical ethics and bioethics. At the same time, Ramsey's model is intelligible in secular contexts and hence accessible to those whose task of discernment takes them into the public forum. *The Patient as Person*'s treatments of such issues as research on children, care of the dying, organ harvesting from the dead for transplantation, research adventures involving human subjects, and the allocation of scarce medical resources, remain relevant to the ongoing debates on these and other issues. Questions, for example, of whether to prolong living or dying can still become urgent in the clinical setting (even though they appear to have lost their edge for the theorists who consider them settled). If, by and large, medical personnel no longer unreasonably insist on the use of sophisticated medical technology to keep the "signs of life" going, frequently families still do. Questions surrounding organ transplantation have expanded, not disappeared, since Ramsey's work was first published. And the issues of research on human subjects are now just as urgent as when Ramsey was writing his Beecher Lectures—although the concerns are now likely to be for subjects in relatively less developed nations.

Through all these and other issues remains Paul Ramsey's central question: What threatens the human person as a person? Today Ramsey might well see himself as having to take on questions he once thought intractable (such as the macroallocation of scarce medical resources and the health care delivery financing environment). He might qualify his central insistence on respect for the consent (or refusal) of patients and research subjects—not by weakening concern for their autonomy but by addressing it in new contexts. Ramsey's work thirty years ago still constitutes a challenge to new and urgent efforts to hold together patient freedom, well-being, and the common good. Threats to human personhood may have changed, but they have hardly diminished since Paul Ramsey shaped our understandings of why and how they must be addressed.

Those of us involved in the Yale Interdisciplinary Bioethics Project are grateful to Albert Jonsen and William F. May, as well as to all the

participants in the symposium of 2000. We are indebted to the major
support received from Donald P. Green and the Institution for Social
and Policy Studies at Yale. We also acknowledge with gratitude the
able work of Carol Pollard and Christiana Zenner in shepherding
this new edition of *The Patient as Person* to publication. Finally, our
thanks go to Jean Black, our editor at Yale University Press, for her
enthusiasm and her patience, and above all for her recognition that
such classics as *The Patient as Person* remain visionary even in new
times and places.

Margaret A. Farley
Yale University, 2001

The Structure of an Ethical Revolution:
Paul Ramsey, the Beecher Lectures,
and the Birth of Bioethics

The first edition of *The Patient as Person* appeared in 1970. The book was the published form of the Lyman Beecher Lectures at Yale University, delivered by Professor Paul Ramsey of Princeton University in April 1969. Those lectures and the book that resulted from them can rightly be called the founding preaching and scriptures of the field of bioethics. Bioethics did not exist when Paul Ramsey stepped to the podium on April 14, 1969. The word itself first appeared a year later in an article by Dr. Van Rensselaer Potter entitled "Bioethics: The Science of Survival."[1] However, the topics that Ramsey addressed in his lectures—the definition of death, care for the dying, organ transplantation, and research with human subjects—were beginning to be discussed and debated, mostly in obscure scientific gatherings but occasionally in public places, such as congressional hearing rooms. In 1962 the Ciba Foundation in Great Britain sponsored one of those obscure scientific conferences that gathered some not-so-obscure figures of science to discuss "Man and His Future." For several days, Nobel Prize winners in medicine and molecular biology, along with many leading physicians and scientists and a few (very few) humanists, reflected on the prospects for genetics, the neurosciences, and behavioral modification by drugs and surgery. The savants reached no conclusions but expressed concern that scientific progress, desirable as it might be, could lead humankind in unexpected directions, where technical achievement might outstrip moral wisdom. In 1968, in the more public setting of a congressional hearing called by Senator Walter Mondale, the social implications of advances in medicine and the biosciences were reviewed over eight days of hearings. Organ transplantation and genetic research took center stage, with prominent scientists extolling progress and occa-

1. Van Rensselaer Potter, *Perspectives in Biology and Medicine* 14 (1970): 127–153.

sionally, together with a few humanists, calling attention to the paradoxical consequences of many advances. Mondale and his fellow senators asked whether some form of public oversight might be advisable. With few exceptions, the scientists and physicians repudiated this idea, with Dr. Owen Wangansteen, one of the nation's senior surgeons and himself a professor at Mondale's own University of Minnesota, disdainfully saying, "If you are thinking of theologians, lawyers, philosophers and others to give some direction. . . . I cannot see how they could help. . . . The fellow who holds the apple can peel it best."[2] So when Paul Ramsey took up the general topic of medical ethics in an era of rapid technological advances, he was addressing an audience that had heard rumors of problems. No one had yet attempted to articulate these problems in a systematic and comprehensive fashion. Ramsey, then, was not the first to speak of these questions as ethical, but he was the first to take a synoptic view.

The Lyman Beecher Lectures were a strange venue for this expression. Established in 1873 to honor a Yale graduate of 1797, the lectures had usually expounded on a theological topic, often on the work of the Christian ministry, before a Divinity School audience. In the past, distinguished speakers, usually from the ecclesiastical world, had delivered impressive lectures from the pulpit of the Divinity School chapel. The 1969 lectures, however, were jointly sponsored by Yale Divinity School and the Yale School of Medicine and were organized as never before. Professor Ramsey lectured four times in the Harkness Auditorium of the Sterling Hall of Medicine. Each lecture was followed by panels in which commentators from medicine, law, theology, philosophy, and elsewhere, responded to Ramsey's points. Also, each day, seminars were led by prominent scholars from many fields and theologians from the major denominations to expand on the issues Ramsey raised. Thus, the Beecher Lectures were transformed from a solo performance by a prominent church figure to a week of active debate across disciplinary and denominational lines. All of this was a response to a series of questions that were quite novel and unfamiliar to many of the participants.

Paul Ramsey held the post of Harrington Spear Paine Professor of

2. Albert R. Jonsen, *The Birth of Bioethics* (New York: Oxford University Press, 1998), p. 93.

Religion at Princeton University. He received his divinity degree and doctorate at Yale in the early 1940s and had been at Princeton since 1944. Having achieved preeminence in the field of Christian ethics, he wrote extensively about moral philosophy and moral theology in traditions beyond his native Protestantism. He had devoted three books to the moral problem of warfare, a topic that in the 1960s was, to put it mildly, hot. In the mid-1960s, Ramsey was frequently invited to conferences devoted to ethical quandaries in the biosciences, where he spoke cogently and somewhat acerbically about the shallowness of scientists' moral thinking about abortion and genetics. So when he arrived at Yale for the Beecher Lectures, he was not only a name in theological ethics; he was one of the few proper ethicists who had addressed these questions. The other few were Joseph Fletcher, then Professor of Moral Theology at Episcopal School of Theology in Cambridge, Massachusetts, who had enunciated liberal positions on such topics as abortion, euthanasia, and reproductive technology,[3] and Professor James Gustafson, then Chairman of Yale's new Department of Religious Studies. Gustafson had written, just a year before Ramsey's Beecher Lectures, a comment on the growing number of conferences on moral questions in the biosciences: "Such conferences and the papers that are published from them are important at this stage of the discussion . . . but one hopes we can move beyond the conference procedure to a more disciplined, careful, long range way of working in which areas of disagreement can not only be defined but in part at least overcome. What is needed, it seems to me, is interdisciplinary work within universities or centers that have personnel and resources for the arduous tasks of intensive and long-term work."[4]

Gustafson initiated the invitation to Ramsey. He intended to use the setting of the Beecher Lectures as the beginning of the "interdisciplinary work within universities" that, in his opinion, would come to grips with these looming issues in a systematic way. Gustafson and Ramsey had a long collegial association, and Gustafson, who had himself recently become interested in the ethical questions associated with advances in bioscience, knew that Ramsey had begun to

    3. Joseph Fletcher, *Morals and Medicine* (Princeton: Princeton University Press, 1954).
    4. James Gustafson, "Review of *Life or Death: Ethics and Options*," *Commonweal* 89 (1968): 27–30.

address these issues. Gustafson suggested that the staid Beecher Lectures be transformed into a week of seminars and discussions, involving participants from Yale's schools of medicine, law, and the arts, and including distinguished scholars from other institutions. He proposed that Catholic theologians and Jewish rabbis, at that time not present in the world of Ivy League scholarship, be invited to participate. Out of these ideas, a unique event emerged: interdisciplinary, interdenominational, interuniversity, designed to begin, even in temporary and transitory fashion, "the arduous tasks of intensive and long-term work" that would bring into the desultory discussions both a disciplined and principled analysis and an informed discourse.

Paul Ramsey not only presided over this unusual event, he had prepared himself for it in an unusual fashion. After receiving the invitation to present the Beecher Lectures, Ramsey determined to speak of these novel topics, not from a speculative viewpoint, but out of an experience of joining scientists and physicians as they actually confront the problems he wished to elucidate. With the cooperation of Dr. Andre Hellegers of Georgetown University School of Medicine, he approached the Joseph P. Kennedy Foundation with a request to support a year of residency as Visiting Professor of Genetic Ethics. During the spring semesters of 1968 and 1969, this Princeton theologian joined Georgetown internists, transplant surgeons, obstetricians, and geneticists on their ward rounds and in their conferences. Special conferences were arranged in which medical faculty presented cases for discussion and where Ramsey could both learn the nature of the issues in a practical way, and begin to formulate responses that reflected the mind of a scholarly theological ethicist. As he wrote in the preface to *The Patient as Person,* "I could put my questions to experts in many fields of medicine, overhear discussions among them, and begin to learn how teachers of medicine, researchers, and practitioners themselves understand the moral aspects of their practice."[5]

Paul Ramsey was a scholar and a talker. As scholar, he possessed a capacious intelligence and acute analytic skills. He was widely read within and without his tradition. He wrote with eloquence, though

---

5. Paul Ramsey, *The Patient as Person* (New Haven: Yale University Press, 1970), p. xx.

some might say, with grandiloquence. As talker, he was articulate and, some might say, incessant. But above all, as talker, he argued. He loved to tear a thesis to tatters, puncture a careless proposition, and reveal the weaknesses in an opponent's strong points. Although some found him ruthless and intimidating, they frequently followed his line to a sharper, sounder opinion of their own. Some of his fiercest opponents became his closest friends, and many students who cringed under his criticism came away more confident. These qualifications, of scholar and argumentative talker, fit the bill for the Beecher Lecturers as Gustafson conceived them. They also inaugurated a revolution in ethical analysis.

Ramsey chose four topics for his four lectures: "Updating Death," "Caring for the Dying," "Giving and Taking Organs for Transplantation," and "Consent in Medical Experimentation." A fifth lecture, "Choosing Patients for Sparse Medical Resources," was prepared but not given, although it is included in *The Patient as Person*. These topics covered the ground of contentious issues in medical ethics, with the exception of issues related to reproduction and genetics. In each lecture Ramsey reviewed the current state of scientific discussion, stated the moral problems at issue, carefully dissected those issues, and made proposals for structuring a moral argument. As scholar, Ramsey moved beyond a description of the problems to the construction of a moral argument built on certain fundamental concepts and principles and following certain logically dictated steps.

Ramsey opens this project by alluding to a fundamental notion of Judeo-Christian belief: God makes a covenant with humanity, offering steadfast love and fidelity and asking in return that humans manifest to each other the care that mirrors that divine fidelity. That covenant comes to each human, constituting each one as sacred. He says, the "chief aim of [these lectures] is . . . simply to explore the meaning of *care*, to find the actions and abstentions that come from adherence to *covenant*, to ask the meaning of the *sanctity* of life, to articulate the requirements of steadfast *faithfulness* to a fellow man. We shall ask, What are the moral claims upon us in crucial medical situations and human relations in which some decision must be made about how to show respect for, protect, preserve, and honor the life of fellow man?"[6] These words appear in the preface of the published

---

6. Ibid., p. xiii.

edition of the lectures. Despite an assiduous search, I have not been able to locate the actual text of the lectures as delivered, so I do not know how Ramsey introduced these fundamental ideas. The actual chapters open not with the first lecture, on defining death, but with the concluding one, on consent as a canon of loyalty in medical research. That chapter begins with a brief allusion to consent as the expression of a bond of fidelity between persons: fidelity, as Ramsey says, is "normative for all the covenants or moral bonds of life with life."[7] However, throughout the lengthy text of each chapter, and presumably of each lecture, little more is said about covenant itself. This profound theological notion disappears into a moral analysis that is accessible to readers who might not share or understand its deep implications for human relationships. It disappears but is not gone, for the ideas of both the sacredness of each individual, specifically as individual, and that humans must not only respect that sacredness but care for each one who suffers, needs, or is threatened or diminished, sustain the moral analysis of each topic. This insistence on the sacredness of each individual repudiates the counterpoint utilitarian thesis—that individuals may be subordinated to social uses and communal purposes—which Ramsey contends has crept into medical ethics under the pressure of technological advance.

The Patient as Person exhibits the sharp mind of a thinker who has read the literature in moral philosophy and moral theology, reflected on complex methods of ethical argumentation, and applied them to real moral perplexities. In the years preceding the Beecher lectures, he had taken a step, unusual for Protestant theologians of his day, into the arcane but highly developed world of Roman Catholic moral theology. Such concepts as natural law, the principle of double effect, and the techniques of casuistry (or moral analysis in "the prism of the case," as Ramsey puts it) had been incorporated, in his own idiosyncratic way, into Ramsey's mode of moral analysis. In particular, he formulated a tightly reasoned thesis that some ethical principles were "exceptionless," that is, had an absolute status in moral argument that did not allow for any relaxation.[8] This essay is not the place to follow Paul Ramsey's ethical theory: suffice to say

7. Ibid., p. 5.
8. "The Case of the Curious Exception," in G. Outka and P. Ramsey (eds.), *Norm and Context in Christian Ethics* (New York: Scribner's and Sons, 1968), pp. 67–135.

that he approached medical ethics as a Christian believer with a refined concept of the way Christian belief viewed the moral life and a
thesis that the central notions of Christian morality could be applied
beyond the doctrinal limits to the moral life of humankind. What the
Christian could understand as fidelity to God's covenant, any human
open to honest moral reflection could see as canons of faithfulness
between persons in need of each other. Further, Ramsey the Christian ethicist brought to medical ethics a set of finely and firmly argued principles and methods for moral analysis. As he said in the
preface to *The Patient as Person,* "medical ethics cannot remain at the
level of surface intuitions or in an impasse of conversation stoppers.
At this point there can be no other resort than to ethical theory."[9]

Using these talents, Paul Ramsey worked out the first explicit reasoning on several much-discussed questions. He prefaces his particular topics with the assertion that "medical ethics today must indeed
be 'casuistry'; it must deal as competently and exhaustively as possible with the concrete features of actual moral decisions of life and
death and medical care."[10] Each lecture then addresses several actual cases, subjects the moral propositions about them to criticism,
and emerges with a reasoned critique. Ramsey offers a sustained
commentary on the efforts to update the definition of death, uncovering major confusions between death, immanent dying, and permanent coma in such prestigious proposals as the Harvard Report
on the Definition of Death, which had been issued two years before.
He provides the first detailed argumentation about discontinuing
life support, expanding with exquisite refinement the traditional
Roman Catholic doctrine of ordinary versus extraordinary means of
sustaining life. He refutes utilitarian justifications of taking human
organs for transplantation without consent of the source of those organs. He erects a monumental argument that research involving human beings can be ethical only with the consent of the experimental
subject and can never be justified only by contributions to the common good. In this latter argument he encounters one of his "excep-

9. *Patient as Person,* p. xv; see also James Johnson and David Smith (eds.), *Love and So-
ciety: Essays in the Ethics of Paul Ramsey* (Missoula: Scholars Press, 1974); David Smith, "On
Paul Ramsey: A Covenant Centered Ethic for Medicine," in Allen Verhey and Stephen
Lammers (eds.), *Theological Voices in Medical Ethics* (Grand Rapids: Eerdmans, 1993).

10. *The Patient as Person,* p. xvii.

tionless rules," namely that proxy consent for research interventions can never be ethically justified, thus ruling out, without exception, research on all who cannot give consent, including children.

The work of an ethicist is to articulate structured arguments of principles, facts, and conclusions, and apply these to particular topics that arise in the moral life of individuals and society. Ramsey's Beecher Lectures did this for the novel topics posed by the advancing biomedical sciences. In so doing, he began to create a discipline. An academic discipline is a recognized body of theory, principles, and methods relevant to a subject matter, which can be taught to students and elaborated by colleagues. Disciplines appear around inquiry, merge as inquiry grows more complex, and fade as inquiry moves into different paths. Ramsey was a scholar in one such teachable body of fact, theory, and method, that is, theological ethics (some would say, of course, that theology has no facts, but leave that aside). When Ramsey began the Beecher Lectures there was no discipline of bioethics, or even medical ethics. When he finished, there was the inkling of a new discipline. Inkling only, for as others followed Ramsey, and as Ramsey himself continued on, the theories, principles, and methods took different shapes. Different approaches were tried over the next decade, but clearly, the move to formulate a discipline that could comprehend the moral issues of medicine and the biosciences was under way. When Dan Callahan wrote his essay "Bioethics as a Discipline" in 1973, he assumed that a discipline was emerging from the discussions and debates, and when James Childress and Tom Beauchamp wrote *Principles of Biomedical Ethics* in 1979, all the apparatus of a discipline was in place.[11]

By that time, there was not much left of Ramsey's theory of covenant. His reliance on the "sanctity of the individual" was converted, or diluted, he would say, into the more secular respect for the dignity of persons. His rich canon of fidelity was reduced to the bare concept of informed consent. His casuistic method remained an integral piece of bioethical discourse. His arguments about "only caring for the dying" and discontinuing life support for the imminently dying remained and were worked over by many subsequent contribu-

11. Daniel Callahan, "Bioethics as a Discipline," *Hastings Center Studies* 1 (1973): 66–73; Tom Beauchamp and James Childress, *Principles of Biomedical Ethics* (New York: Oxford University Press, 1979).

tors. His thesis about the gifting of organs as distinguished from
harvesting without consent had become public policy. His view of experimentation as "joint venturing in the common cause of cure," in
which the venturers—investigator and subject—are bound by a consensual bond remained an ideal only feebly translated into practice
by federal regulations requiring peer review and informed consent
to perform research with human subjects.[12] What Ramsey spoke
about in 1969 had become, by 1979, the subject matter of an evolv-
ing discipline that by the mid-1970s was commonly designated "bioethics."

Ramsey was not only scholar but talker. He had prepared for the
Beecher Lectures by taking the unusual course of spending two full
semesters talking with doctors and scientists at Georgetown University School of Medicine. Although titled professor, he made himself
a student who asked questions and ventured answers at the "biweekly
conferences arranged for his instruction."[13] The Beecher Lectures
allowed him an hour on four successive days to talk in the scholarly
mode of a formal lecture. During that hour, he could lay down the
framework of a disciplinary analysis by stating principles, arguing
cases, and drawing conclusions. Then he had to enter into debate
with other scholars on responder's panels. Ramsey's words about the
definition of death had to meet the words of Harvard University's Dr.
Henry Beecher, who had composed the Harvard Definition of Death
document. His comments about organ transplantation faced those
of Rabbi Seymour Siegel of the Jewish Theological Seminary, representing a tradition that repudiated autopsy. His arguments about allowing the dying to die confronted the deep convictions about personal autonomy associated with Dr. Jay Katz of Yale Law School.
There is no way to know what was actually said in those post-lecture
comments: no record exists. But given Ramsey's propensity for
strong argument and the reputations of the responders, we can
imagine that the discussions were vigorous.

Among the respondents was Father Richard McCormick, a Jesuit
moral theologian of rising provenance. McCormick heard Ramsey
defend the thesis that children could never be the subjects of experimentation. What the Catholic scholar said on that occasion, we can-

12. *The Patient as Person*, pp. 5–6.
13. Ibid., p. xx.

not know. (Father McCormick died in early 2000.) However, six years after the Beecher Lectures, McCormick debated Ramsey on this issue before the National Commission for Protection of Human Subjects of Biomedical and Behavioral Research, where the Protestant and the Catholic ethicists formulated opposing views, with clearly articulated arguments to support them. This allowed the commission, of which I was a member, to evaluate this most difficult problem and carefully formulate a public policy response that respected essential values, although it rejected Ramsey's contention of an exceptionless rule in this matter.

The debate before the National Commission was one manifestation of a second contribution to bioethics that Ramsey's Beecher Lectures inaugurated. As we noted above, an array of discussions and debates took place around Ramsey's magisterial lectures. Not only were there three respondents to each lecture but also, on three days, seminars were held from 10 A.M. to 4 P.M. at both the Divinity School and the School of Medicine on the topics of medical ethics. Again, distinguished scholars met with students in law, medicine, and divinity to explore the issues. Callahan's essay, "Bioethics as a Discipline," had suggested that this new discipline should consist not only of logic, consistency, careful use of terms, and rational justification—the standard stuff of disciplinary thought—but also of a rich and wide-ranging discussion, "a continuing, tension ridden dialectic . . . kept alive by a continued exposure to specific cases in all their human dimensions."[14] The very structure of the Beecher Lectures of 1969, as devised by Professor James Gustafson, fostered that discussion across disciplines. Never before had the staid Beecher Lectures been so structured; never before had the measured eloquence of the famed speakers been thrown into the turmoil of debate. But bioethics began as discussion and debate, in many small circles, and gradually widened into a discourse in which many persons participated. During the 1970s, governmental commissions were established to debate certain issues and recommend public policy. Committees were appointed in research institutions to review protocols that recruited human subjects. Hospitals initiated ethics committees to clarify policy on life support. Courts heard arguments on life-and-

14. Callahan, p. 73.

death cases. Courses were offered in many schools of medicine and schools of nursing, in some law schools, and even in undergraduate colleges. The media began to notice these discussions and, more and more frequently, articles appeared in the press and stories on television. Legislatures voted on bills about research, death, and genetics, and electorates were offered initiatives about life and death. A discourse was under way in corners where the proprieties of academic disciplines gave way to more impassioned debate.

At the same time, this wider discourse has been well informed by the discipline. The commissions and committees produce documents and regulations formulated with the principles of the discipline in the background. The courses use texts written by scholars in bioethics. Even the courts echo disciplinary conclusions in their obiter dicta. The media, undisciplined as it is, invites disciplinary scholars to comment, and the "ethicist" has become an obligatory face or voice on page and screen. The discourse about bioethics runs alongside, and sometimes overtakes, the discipline of bioethics. The Beecher Lectures of 1969 previsioned this dual development, and the lost words of the commentators and the seminar attendees are as important as the preserved words of the lecturer published in *The Patient as Person.*

I titled this essay "The Structure of an Ethical Revolution." A few years before the Beecher Lectures, Thomas Kuhn published an epochal book with an analogous title and a contentious thesis about the ways science advances from paradigm to paradigm.[15] I abstract from Kuhn's thesis and allude to his title only to make one point: the paradigm of doing ethics was changed radically by Ramsey's Beecher Lectures. The previous paradigm, in place from time immemorial in Western culture, had been the thoughtful person observing the moral life of his or her society, and elucidating a series of reasoned propositions about the ways in which the moral life should be conceived and lived. Of course, also from time immemorial, persons have argued among themselves in church meetings, in legislative halls and in saloons, about the strictures and ideals of the moral life. Still, the creation of a discipline of ethics has not generally been in close contact with the public discourse about morality. Bioethics

15. Thomas Kuhn, *The Structure of Scientific Revolutions* (Chicago: University of Chicago Press, 1962).

must touch the emotional and affective sources of moral dilemmas as well as elucidate the rational and intellectual facets of problems. It must also work with the accurate data of science and the factual features of events and institutions, as well as with theory and principle. Bioethics is, and must be, both discipline and discourse, and the Beecher Lectures, in their intellectual content and in their programmatic structure, set the direction.

Paul Ramsey died in 1988. What if his imposing figure were standing here today, thirty years after he mounted the podium in the Harkness Auditorium? What might he say about bioethics, the discipline and discourse to whose inauguration he contributed? During the years after the Beecher Lectures, Ramsey wrote much about bioethics, touching on many of its topics with cogent remarks. He took stands against involuntary euthanasia, particularly of the severely ill newborn. He continued to oppose research with children. He reiterated his opposition to certain forms of genetic engineering and reproductive technology. But, if he examined the vital field of bioethics today, he would be dismayed to see that it remains conflicted about its ethical foundations. He would decry the wavering about principle and cases, a problem that he probably felt he settled in his 1976 treatise, *Deeds and Rules in Christian Ethics.*[16] He would be appalled to see the intricate structure of ethical argument, with its exceptionless principles, collapse into a principle of autonomy, which, as he once said, merely "enthrones arbitrary freedom."[17] He might be amused and somewhat sardonic about the scramble to collect arguments against human cloning, an issue he put to rest when cloning was merely a dream.[18] He would probably be sad to discover that the strong religious voices of early bioethics are now drowned out in an essentially secular discourse.

Ramsey resuscitated might utter a harsh judgment about bioethics as a discipline, but it is certain that, were he here, he would plunge into bioethics as a discourse. Ramsey the talker would have something cogent to say about stem cell research, fetal cell transplan-

16. Paul Ramsey, *Deeds and Rules in Christian Ethics* (New York: Scribner's and Sons, 1965).

17. Paul Ramsey, *Ethics at the Edges of Life* (New Haven: Yale University Press, 1968), p. 157.

18. Paul Ramsey, *Fabricated Man: The Ethics of Genetic Control* (New Haven: Yale University Press, 1970).

tation, genetic testing and therapy, physician-assisted suicide, and random clinical trials in third-world countries. He would find it exhilarating to plunge into the new territories open to bioethics, those issues of environmental health and safety, genetically engineered foods, and ecological protection that move bioethics from the medical world into the wider world of the relation between humans and the biosphere. He would certainly relish participation in the debates about evolutionary psychology, sociobiology and psychoneurology.

Paul Ramsey would be pleased to see that Yale University has initiated an Interdisciplinary Bioethics Project to pursue all these questions in an interdisciplinary manner. He would echo today what he said in the preface to the Beecher Lectures, "[These lectures are] a plea for fundamental dialogue about the urgent moral issues arising in medical practice. . . . To take up the questions of medical ethics for probing, to try to enter into the heart of these problems with reasonable and compassionate moral reflection, is to engage in the greatest of joint ventures: the moral becoming of man. This is to see in the prism of medical cases the claims of any man to be honored and respected. So might we enter thoughtfully and actively into the moral history of mankind's fidelity to covenants. In this everyone is engaged."[19]

Albert R. Jonsen
2001

19. *The Patient as Person,* p. xviii.

The Patient as Person:
Beyond Ramsey's Beecher Lectures

In reading Albert Jonsen's historical account *The Birth of Bioethics,*[1] I realized that he met Paul Ramsey at a very different point in their respective lives than my first contacts with the Princeton professor. When they met in the 1970s, Ramsey was already a leading figure in Protestant ethics, a player to be reckoned with across disciplinary lines in the neonatal field of bioethics. Jonsen himself had a Ph.D. and developing interests in the field.

I met Ramsey almost thirty years earlier, in the summer of 1945, when I was a seventeen-year-old sophomore at Princeton University, still in the midst of those chirping "who am I questions," which Ramsey, a young assistant professor just finishing his own sophomore year as a teacher at the university, was provoking in undergraduates. I recall, after one class session, Galway Kinnell—eventually a distinguished American poet—shaking his head over one of Paul's particularly convoluted lectures about neighbor-regarding duties to oneself (as opposed to self-regarding duties to oneself). Kinnell said, "It looks as though you have to be very smart to be a Christian." Considering Jesus' disciples, I wasn't sure about that. But I thought that you certainly had to be smart to get a good grade in the course.

Ramsey made a deep impression on a substantial following of undergraduates each year. Students responded partly to his manner and style. Compared with the polished, seamless delivery of other professors in Ivy League attire, Ramsey came across as a theological calliope—full of snorts and harrumphs, throat clearings and chortles, bolts of laughter, and a constant reliance on a reiterated "You see, you see," as he gathered intellectual steam. And outside the lecture hall, in the more intimate setting of a precept, his energy still flowed, along with the vesuvial curl of smoke from his pipe.

Style was surely part of it. At his retirement banquet more than forty years later, I remarked to those gathered in Princeton that Paul

1. Jonsen, Albert R., *The Birth of Bioethics* (New York: Oxford University Press, 1998).

had published 183 articles—all of them first drafts. His work was a triumph of substance over style.

Actually, Ramsey was rather sensitive about his writing. Scouring his reviews, he managed to find one sentence from a critic who complimented him on his prose. He clipped it, had it laminated, and whipped it out, like a cross, whenever one of his dracular critics attacked him for writing clumsily. But maybe the lone defender of his style was correct. In retrospect, a remarkable number of vivid, forcefully expressed, and even memorable sentences stand out in the midst of all the ungainliness. Some of them will endure in the literature long after most of the conventionally crafted set-pieces in bioethics have faded.

Paul Ramsey also made a powerful impression on his students morally. I couldn't have named it then, but ethically, Ramsey was what the philosophers call a deontologist, a duty-based ethicist—an ancient Roman in spirit, a Roman shaped by duty; a Christian centurion, if you will; a Methodist in a toga. Much later, I came to realize just how powerful his personal sense of duty was.

And in the classroom, a sovereign duty to press for the truth drove him. He treated the authors we read as partners in the quest for the best possible perspective on an issue. Ramsey's opponents were as important to him as his supporters, although he sometimes reminded one of a Rottweiler sinking his teeth into a body and shaking it for what it would yield: maybe not final truth, but something better than what was available before the encounter.

In preparing his Beecher Lectures, Ramsey spent two springs in residence as Visiting Professor of Genetic Ethics at the Georgetown University School of Medicine. That in itself was a bold move. In an age dominated by metaethics and a highly theoretical analysis of moral language removed from the fray of decision making, Ramsey put himself in the midst of researchers and practitioners in the field. He was a pioneer in applied ethics. Until recent decades, applied ethicists occupied a kind of no-person's land. They faced disdain both from theoreticians, who criticized them as engaged in a derivative enterprise dependent upon the foundational work of others, and from practitioners, who complained that ethicists were too little acquainted with decisions on the firing lines. Applied ethicists were in the somewhat comical position of carrying water from wells that they had not dug to fight fires they couldn't quite find. Ramsey's work helped demonstrate that applied ethics, at its best, does not merely package what is already known, but shows sources in a new light even as it illuminates a field of practice.

Ramsey announces in the preface to his book that the biblical notion of covenant fidelity serves as his chief source. He writes unabashedly as a Christian ethicist. Covenant fidelity, a phrase he converts into a canon of loyalty to the patient as person, defines the ruling principle in his pioneering work. He rigorously applies this principle of fidelity to the patient and inveighs against a "technological triumphalism" that tempted some researchers and physicians into a series of wrongs:

- experimenting on human subjects and extracting organs for transplants without securing patient consent;
- bombarding the dying with ingenious technical strategies in order to keep them alive when simply caring for them would be more appropriate;
- redefining death for the inadmissible reason of gaining access to organs for transplants;
- or selecting patients for treatment with scarce life-saving resources on the basis of their social utility.

In the jargon of the trade of ethics, Ramsey wrote as an obligation, rather than a virtue, theorist. He was less interested in giving us a portrait of the virtuous physician or patient than in spelling out the duties that should shape and restrain medical practice. Faith in a promise-keeping God converts into a general canon of loyalty to persons and into the correlative, limiting principle of the sacredness of life.

Taken together, the two principles he derives from biblical faith make a huge difference. They distinguish Ramsey's work on treating the patient as person from the libertarians who hoisted the flag of patient autonomy. In a sense, the second principle of the sacredness of life grounds the first. Physicians must not ride roughshod over patients in the pursuit of research and other goals *because* patients' lives are sacred. That sacredness derives from God who bestows it and not from human accomplishment or status. This transcendent bestowal forbids professionals from making instrumental judgments about the relative worth of their patients. Further, the principle of the sacredness of life also constrains the decision making of patients—with critical implications, Ramsey draws out later—regarding decisions on abortion, in-vitro fertilization, genetic engineering, and cloning.

We do not have to agree with Ramsey's judgments on each of these particular issues in order to appreciate that at least by engaging in debate on these problems he imputes to patients a moral dignity. Their decisions matter to him morally. Libertarians seem to bestow a greater moral significance on patients as they emphasize patient autonomy to the exclusion of all other considerations. However, if one affirms no more than an indeterminate liberty over which the patient presides, one may, in fact, diminish the patient. The patient tends to evaporate morally. It suffices merely that the patient makes her own decisions. This apparent respect for autonomy eventually marginalizes the patient. Marginalized groups (such as patients, minorities, women, children, and the elderly) take a first step back into moral community when others treat them as more than mere bundles of morally indifferent wants and interests. While paternalists surely fail to respect others when they preempt their liberty, autonomists also fail to respect others when they patronize any and all forms of its exercise.

In his next book, *Fabricated Man,* Ramsey deals with the threat to persons he foresees in the practices of genetic control, cloning, and artificial donor insemination. He worries there chiefly about a downward moral slide from parenting into manufacturing. Separating generation from sexuality, he fears, will move us from procreation to reproduction, from home to laboratory, from love to labor, from what Leon Kass described as the darkness of the womb to the fluorescent light of the lab, from begetting to decanting. Further, the reduction of humans to fabricated products will increase, he fears, when the ideology of positive eugenics drives the technology.[2] I happen to disagree with Ramsey's charge that the in-vitro use of a donated egg or semen shifts parenting into manufacturing. But the sound of alarm strikes a deep chord in a culture such as ours, which,

2. Ramsey, Paul, *Fabricated Man: The Ethics of Genetic Control* (New Haven: Yale University Press, 1970).

for its own broader reasons, is tempted to push parenting toward producing a product.

The temptation to treat a child as a product doesn't simply beset the childless couple or the advocate of positive eugenics. Ambitious parents in a meritarian culture yield to the temptation when they live out their lives vicariously through the child's performance. Parenting includes two demands always in tension with one another. On the one hand, parents need to affirm the being of the child—to accept the child as he is. As Robert Frost put it, home is where, when you go there, they have to take you in. On the other hand, parents must also encourage and foster the well-being of the child. They must promote the child's excellence.

Parents find it difficult to maintain an equilibrium between these two kinds of love. Accepting love without transforming love slides into indulgence and neglect. Transforming love without accepting love badgers and finally neglects. In a meritocratic society, where the winner takes all, we have tended one-sidedly to equate good parenting with the task of transforming. We have fiercely demanded performance, accomplishment, and results. Given the warp of our culture, parents may need to recognize that parenting resembles dirt-farming more than engineering. One turns the soil, broadcasts a little seed, and prays for a little sun and rain, and hopes for the best. Ramsey may be wrong in detail, but *Fabricated Man* arises, it seems to me, with this larger cultural theme in the background.

What of issues concerning the patient as person *beyond* the confines of Ramsey's own work? I will restrict myself simply to two later issues that have surfaced: first, the limitations of a principle-oriented ethic in exploring the full moral world of patients, and second, the bearing of structural issues, such as residency training programs and the economics of health care system on the treatment of patients as persons.

Ramsey's work, like most ethics to follow in the next two decades, dealt with disease and death within the parameters of a principle-oriented theory of ethics. Philosophers and theologians concentrated chiefly on moral dilemmas that professionals face and appealed to moral principles (or paradigmatic cases) that would help solve or resolve these moral binds. This view of ethics fit smoothly in the cur-

riculum of medical schools and teaching hospitals, since medical education already focused on case studies. Moralists like Ramsey accordingly produced impressive work on a range of quandaries.

But solving problems by appeals to principles does not suffice as
insight into the ordeals patients and their families face as they endure the siege of disease and death. Such ordeals do not wholly admit of solution: they assault and test core identity. Such problems
must be faced rather than solved. I have in mind here the comment
of a friend, Mrs. Nielson, the eighty-year-old widow of a much honored Smith College president. Twenty years after his death, she said
to me, "I could do nothing about the death of my husband. The only
question I faced was whether I could rise to the occasion." With one
stroke, his death had altered her daily life and intimacy and transformed her from a person with a clear-cut public role in the college
and town into a superfluity. Certainly there were things to do and
principles needed to guide her decisions. But how could she rise to
an occasion that redefined her?

T. S. Eliot once pointed to this second range of problems. At the
close of a lecture on a serious issue in American life, an undergraduate arose to ask him urgently, "Mr. Eliot, what are we going to do
about the problem you have discussed?" Eliot replied, in effect, "You
have asked the wrong question. You must understand that we face
two types of problems in life. One kind of problem provokes the
question, 'What are we going to do about it?' The other kind poses
the subtler question, 'How do we behave toward it?'" The first type of
problem demands relatively technical, pragmatic, and tactical responses that will eliminate the difficulty; the second poses deeper
challenges that no specific policy, strategy, or behavior can dissolve.
The problem will persist. It requires behavior that sensitively, deco-
rously, and appropriately fits the perduring challenge. In Gabriel
Marcel's language, the latter type of problem resembles a mystery
more than a puzzle; it demands a restructuring of habits and rituals
more than technique.

Most deeper moral demands in life test one's personal identity:
the conflict between the generations, the intricacy of signals between the sexes, the mystery of birth, the health crisis, and the ordeal
of fading powers and death. At one level, adolescents embody a series of complex problems for their parents to solve. But most of the

turmoil occurs at deeper levels, as parents seek to cope with changes in the child's identity—and, even worse, the child's challenge to their identity as parents. Parents find it difficult enough to take in their stride the profound changes which their children undergo in the hormonal tide of adolescence. But they discover to their dismay that the child also redefines them as old—"out of it"—just when they feel themselves to be at the peak of their powers. (Our eldest child made this redefinition clear to my wife and me when at fourteen she took to walking twenty yards ahead of us or twenty yards behind us to signal to the world that she did not emerge from anything so gross as a human family.)

Health crises confront their victims with something to do and things to decide, but, far more profoundly, such crises assault identity—they force their victims to decide who and how they will be. The successful businessman who ponders how to save his limited and valuable time carries his cell phone into his Mercedes. It lets him pursue his business even while stalled in a traffic jam. But suddenly a blood clot stalls in his coronary artery; the rescue unit pulls him out of his car and wheels him into an intensive care unit. Now he finds his time even more limited than he thought. The catastrophe confronts him with problems to solve, but these problems pale before the deeper question: Who and what is he, now that he has suffered this explosion from within? Accustomed to commanding his world, the patient suddenly finds himself helpless in the hands of the nurses down the hospital corridor; used to total obedience from his subordinates, he discovers that the very humblest of those subordinates, his own body, has rebelled against him.

Once we dig deeper into the patient's personal ordeal, we recognize that most hard cases entail two decisions. First, and most obviously, at the level of hospital policy one must resolve the original dilemma—should one shift to palliative care? Should one pull the plug? Second, the patient and family must decide and resolve to make good on the decision; they must marshal the personal resources to see it through. Most hard choices produce a coefficient of adversity; that is, they generate a rough patch afterward regardless of the decision. They require the courage that Saint Thomas Aquinas defined as firmness of soul in the face of adversity.

On the whole, ethics oriented to principles—ethics of the sort that Ramsey wrote and that dominated the field for the next two decades—emphasizes the original dilemma mentioned in the previous paragraph. Ethical reflection oriented to the virtues must focus on the second decision as well: How does one stand by and make good in the aftermath of the original choice?

While emphasizing the importance of the second decision, one should neither isolate it from the original decision nor exaggerate it. The two decisions and the resources they require often interconnect. The wise resolution of the original quandary, for example, often depends upon a choir of virtues: wisdom, courage, self-restraint, fidelity, humility. Further, the determination to make good on the decision often depends upon the soundness of the original choice and the adroit resolution of a series of secondary issues that flow from it. Clearly, an agent's resolve doesn't make a bad original choice good. But just as clearly, my resoluteness, or the lack of it, in carrying forward a decision can affect mightily, for good or ill, the result; and reflexively, my subjective irresolution can often create havoc in an otherwise unexceptionable original choice.

Medical ethics has tended to explore those moral issues that cluster around the important question "What are we going to do about it?" but at the expense of those deep, troubling issues facing patients as persons and their families. How can they manage—whatever the event or the decision—to rise to the occasion?

In such matters, patients are not merely decision makers but also, at least in some way, authors of their lives. And authors do not write in a vacuum, but in the setting of those great shaping narratives, those mythic forms, that help supply them with their perceptions of the world and themselves, and give them some cues for their behavior. Ramsey and other ethicists of his generation trafficked chiefly in quandaries and searched for principles and policies to order practices in the setting of large institutions—an important task indeed. Others, subsequently, have turned to narrative ethics in order to flesh out and shape the stories of the patient as person. Generally, caregivers attracted to this broadening of the subject of biomedical ethics beyond quandary ethics comprise those professionals with more extended contact with patients and their families—those engaged in primary and extended care, hospice care, and, of course, nurses, some social workers, and chaplains.

Respect for the patient as person also poses structural issues about the organization of residency training programs and the economics of the health care system. Medical education and residency training must be organized in such a way as to develop the young physician as a good teacher of patients. I read Ramsey's book just before spending a year as an observer at a distinguished teaching hospital. In that particular hospital, the tight scheduling of morning rounds discouraged the teaching of patients. Patients tended to be teaching *material* rather than themselves taught. On a typical morning, the attending physician on the floor accompanied a small platoon of young clerks and residents, all of them bristling with good health. Twenty patients had to be seen in an hour and fifteen minutes, a ration of but three to four minutes to a bed. The patient, meanwhile, had just awakened. He had spent the night mulling over the five or six things that he wanted to bring up with his doctors, but suddenly found himself caught like a deer in the glare of headlights. He hurriedly voiced one or two things on his list before the procession moved on to other beds and into the hallway. There the serious teaching took place as the attending physician and retinue discussed the case, sotto voce, before traveling to the next room. Young physicians-to-be, of course, surely need the hallway instruction. Patients do serve as teaching material in a teaching hospital. But if residents are to practice competently and respectfully in their own right, and if teaching is an important part of patient compliance and collaboration in preventive, rehabilitative, and long-term care, then the teaching hospital needs to structure education so as to produce professionals who, rather than opaquely performing procedures, genuinely profess what they know.

Residency training programs may have improved since my year as an observer, but economic issues and marketplace pressures today have systematically depersonalized medical care. We have entered the era of turnstile medicine. In the name of productivity (read efficiency and cost-saving), a doctor's average contact time with a patient, one gathers, has dropped from twenty-seven minutes to sixteen minutes and less. The technique of rapidly moving people through a system has become an art of which Walt Disney is the twentieth-century master. Disney's theme parks enclose an expensive piece of real estate that, much like a hospital, imposes chronic costs. One makes money as a for-profit or breaks even as a non-profit institution by moving people through the system efficiently and rapidly.

Turnstile medicine also skews the art of healing. We can define healing as an art rather than an applied science because the individual patient it serves does not merely illustrate a general scientific principle into which the patient disappears entirely. Each patient is a full-bodied person with her own history and universe. Her diabetes may, more or less, illustrate a generalization about a particular disease. And, if we are to heal rather than treat, we cannot tidily separate the host from the disease or vice versa. Diagnosing, treating, and helping the ill person face her disease require knowing the patient, her habits, and, in some measure, her world, pressures, and strains. These complex undertakings surely draw on science, but the physician must artfully marshal the generalizations of science to heal the person rather than merely treat the disease. Such doctoring takes time, and institutional pressures today move in another direction. The rapid processing of patients through hospitals, offices, and clinics neglects the patient as person as much as the jammed schoolroom of thirty-five or forty children crowds out the student as a person. In addition, there are those who do not have assured passage through the turnstile at all—44 million people with no health insurance and another 40 million under-insured.

Not that Ramsey was unaware of systemic issues. Toward the end of *The Patient as Person* he calls the "matter of ordering our medical priorities and ordering our overall social priorities, including medical needs in [a] rational way . . . the most incorrigible social and ethical question . . . concerning medical practice, and indeed concerning social policy at large." He asks: "Who shall say or how do we go about deciding what sorts of medical services should be given priority over others, and how much of a nation's resources should be spent on medical care in comparison to other claims and needs?" Ramsey opens the door to such systemic issues; he calls for reflection on our priorities in the production and distribution of the good of health care. However, he chooses not to walk through that door, and indeed, he concedes, with what Al Jonsen calls "uncharacteristic humility," "I do not know the answer to these questions, nor how to go about finding the answer."[3]

3. Ramsey, Paul, *The Patient as Person* (New Haven: Yale University Press, 1970), p. 268; Jonsen, p. 219; *Patient as Person*, p. 272.

Only slowly in the 1980s did bioethicists take on the vexing issue of justice in the health care system, which eventually led to the aborted effort to achieve comprehensive health care reform in 1993. In that year, the media and therewith the United States riveted attention on the dramatic possibility (or threat) of health care reform emanating from Washington. However, while the media reported daily on the odds of legislative change, they barely noticed the stealth revolution in health care occurring below the radar screen. Dramatic changes largely spread, not from D.C., but from Louisville, Kentucky, and Knoxville, Tennessee, with profound consequences for patients.

Why did Ramsey shy away from the systemic allocative issues in health care? Probably his commitment to developing exceptionless rules, rather than the virtue of intellectual humility, explains his reluctance. He knew that allocative issues could not be resolved by appeal to exceptionless rules. No moralist could offer a tidy hierarchical ordering of competing goods and services to guide allocations within health care (heart disease versus cancer versus arthritis versus preventative care) or allocations between health care and other human goods (the fundamental goods of food, clothing, shelter, or basic education) and the higher goods (of advanced education and the arts). Thus Ramsey, in effect, surrendered the issue of health care to the political process.

Ramsey's hesitation as an ethicist may result from his attraction to an ethics of duty and his no-holds-barred wrestling match with Joseph Fletcher, the situational ethicist, whose commitment to an ethic of love led him to suspect any and all rules except to do the most loving thing in the particular situation. Ramsey feared that situational ethics would leave everything awash in the sea of the relative and ultimately justify the expedient. In defense of an individual life as "noninterchangeable, not substitutable, and not meldable with other lives," Ramsey believed that Christian ethics (and medical research and care) called for an ethic of love that embodied itself in "exceptionless moral rules."[4] Such rules would compare with the just war proscription against direct attack on noncombatants; they would seek out the neighbor's good, and not the good overall. He

4. Ramsey, Paul, *Ethics at the Edges of Life* (New Haven: Yale University Press, 1978), p. xiv; Werpetowski, William, and Stephen D. Crocco, *The Essential Paul Ramsey* (New Haven: Yale University Press, 1994), p. xix.

was seeking rules that would "build a floor under the individual fellow man by minimum faithfulness-rules," which are "unexceptional."[5]

The image of "building a floor" is telling. To be sure, Ramsey's ethical floor is not a minimal level of duty accommodating the mediocre. Rather it imposes a strenuous (one of his favorite words) demand on researchers and clinicians that they conform scrupulously to the canons of patient loyalty as they engage in inquiries and offer services. An ethical floor provides a firm resistance to any and all rationalizations on behalf of medical progress and ingenious interventions that might distract physicians from their exceptionless responsibilities to their patients as persons.

Yet, the image of a floor inadequately describes the full range of the moral life; it requires a building above it. Indeed, the etymological root for the word *ethos* suggests as much. The word *ethics,* derived from *ethos,* traces back in the Greek language to the dwelling place of an animal. The animal needs a habitat, a sheltering arrangement of space that accommodates its varying needs and movements. Similarly, human beings, naked apes, the most extraordinary, complicated, and vulnerable of animals, need not simply a dwelling place that shelters them from the elements, but an *ethos,* a range of customs, practices, and ways of being that protect and support not only human survival but flourishing.

Of course, if one thinks not simply of a floor but of an entire dwelling, then the legislative analogy of firm, exceptionless rules does not fully describe what humans need. They require, to be sure, moral laws that do not admit of breach, lest a society lapse into anarchy or neglect some of its members, but they also need a building that anticipates the full range of activities and goods to be sustained in a human household. At this point, the language of ethics overlaps with that of aesthetics. Ethicists, and the moralist in us all, must contend with questions of relative size and proportions and multiple uses of space, and must reckon with changing needs and claims.

Answers to such allocative questions spill over into the arena of the aesthetic, but they are not merely decorative. Such decisions about allocations of space, balance, and proportion represent declarations

5. Ramsey, Paul, *Deeds and Rules in Christian Ethics* (Edinburgh: Oliver and Boyd, 1965), pp. xx, 133.

about the kind of beings we are, the overriding ends to which we aspire, and the goods and burdens that of necessity and by grace we may be called upon to share.

In his book *The Morality of the Law,* which supplied the background for the distinction between disciplinary rules and ethical considerations in the legal code, Lon Fuller of Harvard Law School recognized that a *legislative* metaphor shapes the notion of disciplinary rules whereas an *aesthetic* metaphor shapes the ethics of aspiration to ideals which are, at best, approximated, but not perfectly realized. I do not know whether Ramsey read Fuller, although he might have gotten the distinction by another route.

Ramsey's own mentor, H. Richard Niebuhr, who was given to typologies in ethics and who trafficked in metaphors, recognized that the dominant metaphor for a deontological ethics is legislative. What are the rules by which we must live and practice, all violations subject to sanction? (In theological discourse, the prominence of exceptionless duties in the moral life led to the metaphor of the Kingdom of God.) But Niebuhr also recognized a second type of moral discourse associated with a teleological ethic—ethics oriented to fundamental ends, goals, and purposes to which one aspires. Here the shaping metaphor is aesthetic rather than legislative. One focuses on humans not as legislators but as makers, sculptors, builders, and constructors—and builders not simply of products but of edifices that ultimately reflect the builders themselves and their ways of being. (In theological discourse, the prominence of teleological language about ends led to language about the vision of God.)

In the strictest sense of the term, Paul Ramsey was no moral visionary. He shied away from questions of proportion and balance in the arrangement of a health care system: in its production of services, its setting of priorities within the several goods of health care, and the competition of the good of health care with other fundamental goods. Still, he certainly led a judiciary, concerned to protect the unique, inviolable, irreplaceable, noninterchangeable, not substitutable, and not meldable individual life, especially regarding those not in a position to protect themselves.

In fact, I think ethics has more to offer regarding the contours of a health care system and the characteristics that such a system ought to display, because a society reckons with three basic features of health care: it is a fundamental good; it is not the only fundamental good; and it is a public good.

Because health care is a fundamental good, it ought to offer universal access and a comprehensive range of services, its distribution of benefits and burdens ought to be fair, and it should be of high quality, and responsive to some choice. Because it is not the only fundamental good and it competes with other fundamental and higher goods, it must be efficient and cost-effective. Finally, because it is a public good, a health care system must increase the provider's sense of responsibility for the skill he exercises as a calling and the consumer's sense of responsibility for collaborative self-care. No system, however ingeniously devised, can gratify all wants, tamp down all worries, or remove the mark of mortality from our frame.

Moralists are not authorized or endowed with the exclusive capacity to address the relative weight and balance of these several considerations, and are certainly not in a position to settle these matter for the ages. The route to moral reflection does not pass exclusively through philosophy or theology departments. As Samuel Johnson remarked, "We are all moralists perpetually, geometers only by chance." However, the political process is not fully itself if it does not reckon with the connection between ethics and politics. Ethics focuses on the pursuit of the good; politics on the common good. Oxbridge got it right when it linked the study of politics, economics, and philosophy. And I suspect Paul Ramsey might have broadened his approach, if he saw what can happen to the patient as person in the midst of turnstile medicine. He might have paid as much attention to economics now as he paid to Supreme Court decisions then.

I have hesitated to use the phrase "the structure of the revolution in bioethics." The phrase is a little too orotund for the man whose work we recall. Ramsey once said that he viewed it as his vocation simply to keep the conversation going—a modest goal, which I like. It reminds me of T. S. Eliot's complaint about American poets: rather too often, they aspire to be major poets and fall flat in overreaching themselves. America lacks the tradition of minor poets who bless us twice over. They produce something of intrinsic worth and, in doing so, also keep the great tradition alive.

At the close of one of the weekend sessions of younger ethicists who gathered with Ramsey several times a year at the Princeton Center for Theological Inquiry, he took the group to the Princeton cemetery, to the gravesite of Jonathan Edwards, a veritable monadnock among theologians whose writing on ethics Ramsey was editing for the Yale series of Edwards's collected works. As the group of us left the grave, Ramsey pointed to another site, a respectful distance away, but in the general vicinity of Edwards's grave, and said: "That's where I will be buried." I thought that decision was about right, a respectful distance but very much in the vicinity.

This new edition, some thirty years after the first publication of the Beecher Lectures, makes it clear. He has offered enduring service in keeping the conversation alive.

William F. May
2001

Preface

This volume undertakes to examine some of the problems of medical ethics that are especially urgent in the present day. These are by no means technical problems on which only the expert (in this case, the physician) can have an opinion. They are rather the problems of human beings in situations in which medical care is needed. Birth and death, illness and injury are not simply events the doctor attends. They are moments in every human life. The doctor makes decisions as an expert but also as a man among men; and his patient is a human being coming to his birth or to his death, or being rescued from illness or injury in between.

Therefore, the doctor who attends *the case* has reason to be attentive to the patient as person. Resonating throughout his professional actions, and crucial in some of them, will be a view of man, an understanding of the meaning of the life at whose first or second exodus he is present, a care for the life he attends in its afflictions. In this respect the doctor is quite like the rest of us, who must yet depend wholly on him to diagnose the options, perhaps the narrow range of options, and to conduct us through the one that is taken.

To take up for scrutiny some of the problems of medical ethics is, therefore, to bring under examination at once a number of crucial human moral problems. These are not narrowly defined issues of medical ethics alone. Thus this volume has—if I may say so—the widest possible audience. It is addressed to patients as persons, to physicians of patients who are persons—in short, to everyone who has had or will have to do with disease or death. The question, What ought the doctor to do? is only a particular form of the question, What should be done?

This, then, is a book *about ethics,* written by a Christian ethicist. I hold that medical ethics is consonant with the ethics of a wider human community. The former is (however special) only a particular case of the latter. The moral requirements governing the relations of physician to patients and researcher to subjects are only a special case of the moral requirements governing any relations be-

tween man and man. Canons of loyalty to patients or to joint adventurers in medical research are simply particular manifestations of
canons of loyalty of person to person generally. Therefore, in the
following chapters I undertake to explore a number of medical
covenants among men. These are the covenant between physician
and patient, the covenant between researcher and "subject" in experiments with human beings, the covenant between men and a
child in need of care, the covenant between the living and the dying,
the covenant between the well and the ill or with those in need of
some extraordinary therapy.

We are born within covenants of life with life. By nature, choice,
or need we live with our fellowmen in roles or relations. Therefore
we must ask, What is the meaning of the *faithfulness* of one human
being to another in every one of these relations? This is the ethical
question.

At crucial points in the analysis of medical ethics, I shall not be
embarrassed to use as an interpretative principle the Biblical norm
of *fidelity to covenant,* with the meaning it gives to *righteousness*
between man and man. This is not a very prominent feature in the
pages that follow, since it is also necessary for an ethicist to go as far
as possible into the technical and other particular aspects of the
problems he ventures to take up. Also, in the midst of any of these
urgent human problems, an ethicist finds that he has been joined—
whether in agreement or with some disagreement—by men of various persuasions, often quite different ones. There is in actuality a
community of moral discourse concerning the claims of persons. This
is the main appeal in the pages that follow.

Still we should be clear about the moral and religious premises
here at the outset. I hold with Karl Barth that covenant-fidelity is
the inner meaning and purpose of our creation as human beings,
while the whole of creation is the external basis and condition of the
possibility of covenant. This means that the conscious acceptance of
covenant responsibilities is the inner meaning of even the "natural"
or systemic relations into which we are born and of the institutional relations or roles we enter by choice, while this fabric provides
the external framework for human fulfillment in explicit covenants
among men. The practice of medicine is one such covenant. *Justice,
fairness, righteousness, faithfulness, canons of loyalty,* the *sanctity*

of life, *hesed, agapé* or *charity* are some of the names given to the moral quality of attitude and of action owed to all men by any man who steps into a covenant with another man—by any man who, so far as he is a religious man, explicitly acknowledges that we are a covenant people on a common pilgrimage.

The chief aim of the chapters to follow is, then, simply to explore the meaning of *care,* to find the actions and abstentions that come from adherence to *covenant,* to ask the meaning of the *sanctity* of life, to articulate the requirements of steadfast *faithfulness* to a fellow man. We shall ask, What are the moral claims upon us in crucial medical situations and human relations in which some decision must be made about how to show respect for, protect, preserve, and honor the life of fellow man?

Just as man is a *sacredness in the social and political order,* so he is a *sacredness in the natural, biological order.* He is a sacredness in bodily life. He is a person who within the ambience of the flesh claims our care. He is an embodied soul or ensouled body. He is therefore a sacredness in illness and in his dying. He is a sacredness in the fruits of the generative processes. (From some point he is this if he has any sanctity, since it is undeniably the case that men are never more than, from generation to generation, the products of human generation.) The sanctity of human life prevents ultimate trespass upon him even for the sake of treating his bodily life, or for the sake of others who are also only a sacredness in their bodily lives. Only a being who is a sacredness in the social order can withstand complete dominion by "society" for the sake of engineering civilizational goals—withstand, in the sense that the engineering of civilizational goals cannot be accomplished without denying the sacredness of the human being. So also in the use of medical or scientific technics.

It is of first importance that this be understood, since we live in an age in which *hesed* (steadfast love) has become *maybe* and the "sanctity" of human life has been reduced to the ever more reducible notion of the "dignity" of human life. The latter is a sliver of a shield in comparison with the awesome respect required of men in all their dealings with men if man has a touch of sanctity in this his fetal, mortal, bodily, living and dying life.

Today someone is likely to say: "Another 'semanticism' which is somewhat of an argument-stopper has to do with the sacredness or inviolability of the individual." [1] If such a principle is asserted in gatherings of physicians, it is likely to be met with another argument-stopper: It is immoral not to do research (or this experiment must be done despite its necessary deception of human beings). This is then a standoff of contrary moral judgments or intuitions or commitments.

The next step may be for someone to say that medical advancement is hampered because our "society" makes an absolute of the inviolability of the individual. This raises the spectre of a medical and scientific community freed from the shackles of that cultural norm, and proceeding upon the basis of an ethos all its own. Alternatively, the next move may be for someone to say: Our major task is to reconcile the welfare of the individual with the welfare of mankind; both must be served. This, indeed, is the principal task of medical ethics. However, there is no "unseen hand" guaranteeing that, for example, *good* experimental designs will always be morally *justifiable*. It is better not to begin with the laissez-faire assumption that the rights of men and the needs of future progress are always reconcilable. Indeed, the contrary assumption may be more salutary.

Several statements of this viewpoint may well stand as mottos over all that follows in this volume. "In the end we may have to accept the fact that some limits do exist to the search for knowledge." [2] "The end does not always justify the means, and the good things a man does can be made complete only by the things he refuses to do." [3] "There may be valuable scientific knowledge which it is morally impossible to obtain. There may be truths which would be of great and lasting benefit to mankind if they could be discovered, but which cannot be discovered without systematic and sustained violation of legitimate moral imperatives. It may be necessary to choose between knowledge and morality, in opposition to our long-standing

1. Wolf Wolfensberger, "Ethical Issues in Research with Human Subjects," *Science* 155 (January 6, 1967): 48.

2. Paul A. Freund, *Is the Law Ready for Human Experimentation?*, *Trial* 2 (October–November 1966): 49; "Ethical Problems in Human Experimentation," *New England Journal of Medicine* 273, No. 10 (September 10, 1965): 692.

3. Dunlop (1965), quoted in Douglass Hubble, "Medical Science, Society and Human Values," *British Medical Journal* 5485 (February 19, 1966): 476.

prejudice that the two must go together." [4] "To justify whatever practice we think is technically demanded by showing that we are doing it for a good end . . . is both the best defense and the last refuge of a scoundrel." [5] "A[n experimental] study is ethical or not in its inception; it does not become ethical or not because it turned up valuable data." [6] These are salutary warnings precisely because by them we are driven to make the most searching inquiry concerning more basic ethical principles governing medical practice.

Because physicians deal with life and death, health and maiming, they cannot avoid being conscious or deliberate in their ethics to some degree. However, it is important to call attention to the fact that medical ethics cannot remain at the level of surface intuitions or in an impasse of conversation-stoppers. At this point there can be no other resort than to ethical theory—as that elder statesman of medical ethics, Dr. Chauncey D. Leake, Professor of Pharmacology at the University of California Medical Center, San Francisco, so often reminds us. At this point physicians must in greater measure become moral philosophers, asking themselves some quite profound questions about the nature of proper moral reasoning, and how moral dilemmas are rightly to be resolved. If they do not, the existing medical ethics will be eroded more and more by what it is alleged *must* be done and technically *can* be done.

In the medical literature there are many articles on ethics which are greatly to be admired. Yet I know that these are not part of the daily fare of medical students, or of members of the profession when they gather together as professionals or even for purposes of conviviality. I do not believe that either the codes of medical ethics or the physicians who have undertaken to comment on them and to give fresh analysis of the physician's moral decisions will suffice to withstand the omnivorous appetite of scientific research or of a therapeutic technology that has a momentum and a life of its own.

The Nuremberg Code, The Declaration of Helsinki, various

4. James P. Scanlan, "The Morality of Deception in Experiments," *Bucknell Review* 13, No. 1 (March, 1965): 26.

5. John E. Smith, "Panel Discussion: Moral Issues in Clinical Research," *Yale Journal of Biology and Medicine* 36 (June, 1964): 463.

6. Henry K. Beecher, *Research and the Individual: Human Studies* (Boston: Little, Brown, 1970), p. 25.

"guidelines" of the American Medical Association, and other "codes" governing medical practice constitute a sort of "catechism" in the ethics of the medical profession. These codes exhibit a professional ethics which ministers and theologians and members of other professions can only profoundly respect and admire. Still, a catechism never sufficed. Unless these principles are constantly pondered and enlivened in their application they become dead letters. There is also need that these principles be deepened and sensitized and opened to further humane revision in face of all the ordinary and the newly emerging situations which a doctor confronts—as do we all—in the present day. In this task none of the sources of moral insight, no understanding of the humanity of man or for answering questions of life and death, can rightfully be neglected.

There is, in any case, no way to avoid the moral pluralism of our society. There is no avoiding the fact that today no one can do medical ethics until someone first does so. Due to the uncertainties in Roman Catholic moral theology since Vatican Council II, even the traditional medical ethics courses in schools under Catholic auspices are undergoing vast changes, abandonment, or severe crisis. The medical profession now finds itself without one of the ancient landmarks—or without one opponent. Research and therapies and actionable schemes for the self-creation of our species mount exponentially, while Nuremberg recedes.

The last state of the patient (medical ethics) may be worse than the first. Still there is evidence that this can be a moment of great opportunity. An increasing number of moralists—Catholic, Protestant, Jewish and unlabeled men—are manifesting interest, devoting their trained powers of ethical reasoning to questions of medical practice and technology. This same galloping technology gives all mankind reason to ask how much longer we can go on assuming that what can be done has to be done or should be, without uncovering the ethical principles we mean to abide by. These questions are now completely in the public forum, no longer the province of scientific experts alone.

The day is past when one could write a manual on medical ethics. Such books by Roman Catholic moralists are not to be criticized for being deductive. They were not; rather they were commendable attempts to deal with concrete cases. These manuals were written with the conviction that moral reasoning can encompass hard cases, that ethical deliberation need not remain highfalutin but can "subsume" concrete situations under the illuminating power of human moral reason. However, the manuals can be criticized for seeking finally to "resolve" innumerable cases and to give the once and for all "solution" to them. This attempt left the impression that a rule book could be written for medical practice. In a sense, this impression was the consequence of a chief virtue of the authors, i.e., that they were resolved to think through a problem, if possible, *to the end* and precisely with relevance and applicability in concrete cases. Past medical moralists can still be profitably read by anyone who wishes to face the challenge of how he would go about prolonging ethical reflection into action.

Medical ethics today must, indeed, be "casuistry"; it must deal as competently and exhaustively as possible with the concrete features of actual moral decisions of life and death and medical care. But we can no longer be so confident that "resolution" or "solution" will be forthcoming.

While no one can do ethics in the medical and technological context until someone first does so, anyone can engage in the undertaking. Anyone can do this who is trained in one field of medicine and willing to specialize for a few years in ethical reasoning about these questions. Anyone can who is trained in ethics and willing to learn enough about the technical problems to locate the decisional issues. This is not a personal plea. It is rather a plea that in order to become an ethicist or a moral theologian doctors have only to quit resisting being one. An ethicist is only an ordinary man and a moral theologian is only a religious man endeavoring to push out as far as he can the frontier meaning of the practice of a rational or a charitable justice, endeavoring to draw forth all the actions and abstentions that this justice requires of him in his vocation. I am sure that by now there are a number of physicians who have felt rather frustrated as they patiently tried to explain to me some technical medical circumstance I asked about. At the same time, I can also testify to some degree of frustration as I have at times patiently tried to explain some of the things that need to be asked of the science and methods of ethics. Physicians and moralists must go beyond these positions if we are to find the proper moral warrants and learn how to think through moral dilemmas and resolve disagreements in moral judgment concerning medical care.

To this level of inquiry we are driven today. The ordinary citizen in his daily rounds is bound to have an opinion on medical ethical questions, and physicians are bound to look after the good moral reasons for the decisions they make and lead society to agree to. This, then, is a plea for fundamental dialogue about the urgent moral issues arising in medical practice.

No one can alter the fact that not since Socrates posed the question have we learned how to teach virtue. The quandaries of medical ethics are not unlike that question. Still, we can no longer rely upon the ethical assumptions in our culture to be powerful enough or clear enough to instruct the profession in virtue; therefore the medical profession should no longer believe that the personal integrity of physicians alone is enough; neither can anyone count on values being transmitted without thought.

To take up the questions of medical ethics for probing, to try to enter into the heart of these problems with reasonable and compassionate moral reflection, is to engage in the greatest of joint ventures: the moral becoming of man. This is to see in the prism of medical cases the claims of any man to be honored and respected. So might we enter thoughtfully and actively into the moral history of mankind's fidelity to covenants. In this everyone is engaged.

The present volume is based on the 1969 Lyman Beecher Lectures at the Divinity School and the School of Medicine of Yale University. A gift of Henry W. Sage (then of Brooklyn, New York), accepted by the Yale Corporation on April 21, 1871, founded this lectureship in honor of Lyman Beecher (of the class of 1797, Yale College), who died January 10, 1863. The first lecture was given by Henry Ward Beecher on January 31, 1872. For almost a century this distinguished series of lectures has been addressed to the faculty, students, and alumni of the Yale Divinity School in annual spring convocation. Among the lecturers are the names of men whose story is that of the church in America and of religious scholarship in the modern period. To mention a few: Phillips Brooks, Washington Gladden, Henry van Dyke, George Adams Smith, Lyman Abbott, Francis G.

Peabody, Charles R. Brown, P. T. Forsyth, J. H. Jowett, Charles H.
Parkhurst, Henry Sloan Coffin, Harry Emerson Fosdick, W. R. Inge,
George A. Buttrick, Ernest Freemont Tittle, William Lyon Phelps,
Bromley Oxnam, Reinhold Niebuhr, H. H. Farmer, Leslie Weather-
head, W. H. Auden, Halford E. Luccock, Lesslie Newbigin.

I was permitted to join this lustrous succession as a result of a
decision made by the Yale Corporation in May, 1882, with the au-
thorization of the donor, that thereafter the lecturer might address
himself to any branch of pastoral theology or any other topic appropriate to the work of the Christian ministry; by the donor's authori-
zation and the Corporation's decision in December, 1893, that a
layman instead of a minister might be appointed to deliver the
course of lectures on the Lyman Beecher foundation; and—finally—
by the invitation of the faculty of Yale Divinity School, who gave me
my seminary and graduate education. The proposal was that the
1969 Lyman Beecher Lectures be an inter-faculty event, sponsored
jointly by the School of Medicine and the Divinity School of Yale
University, and that the theme of my lectures be devoted to medical
ethical questions. On each of the four nights, I would be joined by
a panel of commentators, consisting of physicians and medical school
professors and theologians—Protestant, Catholic and Jewish. During
the day visiting experts, medical and religious, were to lead seminars
at both the Divinity School and the School of Medicine. In addition,
there were to be seminars in critical response to the Beecher Lectures led by students in ethics at the Divinity School, medical students, and students in the Law School.

A grand idea—to which my initial response was that I should emi-
grate to Canada since I am conscientiously opposed to being made a
guinea pig even in the noblest of causes! I judged at once, of course,
that I needed to know how medical men themselves discuss the
questions they confront. It was my great, good fortune at this point
to receive from the Joseph P. Kennedy, Jr. Foundation the first grant
for the study of medical ethics which they have awarded. For this I
am greatly indebted to Sargent and Eunice Kennedy Shriver, to
whom I here give the meager thanks that words can indicate.

Other gratitudes follow. I was appointed the Joseph P. Kennedy,
Jr. Foundation Visiting Professor of Genetic Ethics at the Medical
School of Georgetown University. This was a research appointment

for two spring semesters in 1968 and 1969. It enabled me, a Protestant Christian ethicist, to be located in the middle of a medical school faculty—not on its periphery—and to begin some serious study of the moral issues in medical research and practice. The word *genetic* in that title was a term of art, invented to avoid calling me "Visiting Professor of Obstetrics and Gynecology," referring to the department where I was administratively located. Dr. Paul Bruns, Chairman of the Department, and Dr. André Hellegers, Professor of Obstetrics and Gynecology, arranged biweekly conferences for my instruction. On these occasions a physician who was a member of the faculty of Georgetown Medical School would present an analysis of some preappointed topic and his point of view on such issues as medical experimentation involving human subjects, researches upon fetal life, the definition of clinical death, the patient's right to be allowed to die, organ transplantation, genetic counseling, etc. Thus, I could put my questions to experts in many fields of medicine, overhear discussions among them, and begin to learn how teachers of medicine, researchers, and practitioners themselves understand the moral aspects of their practice. Participating in these meetings were also theologians from seminaries and departments of religion in the Washington area and scientists from other departments of Georgetown University and from the National Institutes of Health, Bethesda, Maryland.

From each meeting and from subsequent conferences with individual doctors I came away with a year's work to do before I, a layman, could venture to say anything about a single medical ethical question. Still I am grateful for the "cultural shock" as well as for the instruction I received. I am especially indebted to those of my colleagues at Georgetown who—in addition to Dr. Bruns and Dr. Hellegers—took the time to read one or another of the following chapters and discussed them with me: Dr. Robert C. Baumiller, S.J., genetics; Dr. Charles A. Hufnagel, heart surgeon and chief of surgery; Dr. George E. Schreiner, hemodialysis; Professor Thomas King of the Department of Biology—and Dr. Leon Kass, biochemist at N.I.H. and now Executive Secretary, Committee on the Life Sciences and Social Policy, National Academy of Science; Professor Irving Ladimer of the Department of Community Medicine at Mt. Sinai School of Medicine and now with the United Health Foundations in

New York; and Dr. Laurence R. Tancredi, formerly of the National Center for Health Services Research and Development of the Department of Health, Education and Welfare. If there is weak reasoning or bad medicine or just plain error in the following pages, it is because I got them back in faster than André Hellegers and Leon Kass could get them out: these two men gave a great deal of time to my undertakings.

It remains for me to thank Dean Robert C. Johnson of the Yale Divinity School and Dean Frederick C. Redlich of the Yale School of Medicine for the welcome they gave me on the occasion of the Lyman Beecher Lectures, April 14–17, 1969. Harry B. Adams, Associate Dean of the Yale Divinity School, served as chairman of the planning committee and during those four days seemed also to be chairman of logistics and triage. I thank also my great and good friends James Gustafson, Julian Hartt, and Paul Minear of the divinity faculty for their too lavish introductions.

Other participants in the program as respondents or as seminar leaders were Dr. Henry K. Beecher, Dorr Professor of Research in Anaesthesia, Harvard Medical School; Edward F. Dobihal, Jr., Chaplain, Yale–New Haven Hospital and Clinical Associate Professor, Yale Divinity School; Dr. Jay Katz, Professor of Law and Psychiatry, Yale Law School; Dr. Irving Ladimer, Associate Clinical Professor, Department of Community Medicine, Mt. Sinai School of Medicine, now with the United Health Foundations; James T. Laney, Professor of Christian Ethics, Vanderbilt Divinity School and now Dean, Chandler School of Theology, Emory University; Dr. Howard Levitin, Associate Professor of Medicine and Associate Dean, Yale School of Medicine; Richard A. McCormick, S.J., Professor of Moral Theology, Bellarmine School of Theology; Ralph B. Potter, Jr., Professor of Social Ethics, Harvard Divinity School; Dr. Frederick C. Redlich, Professor of Psychiatry and Dean, Yale School of Medicine; Dr. Richard A. Selzer, Clinical Associate in Surgery, General Surgeon, Department of University Health, Yale; Richard B. Sewall, Master of Ezra Stiles College and Professor of English, Yale; and Seymour Siegal, Professor at the Jewish Theological Seminary of America.

If the sponsors of the 1969 Lyman Beecher Lectures are of the opinion that the goal of interdisciplinary analysis of important moral questions was achieved, this is due in no small measure to the distinguished respondents and seminar leaders who added a wider context of discussion and a greater range of problems and perspectives than one lecturer could supply.

Last but not least, I owe appreciation to my secretaries in Washington, Miss Mabel Riollano and Mrs. Nina Blakney, who were uniformly efficient and helpful. To my colleagues at Princeton who may have been cheered by my absence but whose continuing academic duties I did not share while on leave. To Margaret (Mrs. Ernest W.) Lefever who prepared the index swiftly and well, and whose home and friends in Washington became mine. To Mrs. Jane Isay for her remarkable combination of ebullience and competence as my editor at the University Press. To my daughter, to whom I dedicate this book with deepest affection, who from the practice of her profession learned many of the same things I was belatedly learning with effort.

It is appropriate to release this book to the reader with the words I used at the first of the series of Lyman Beecher Lectures at Yale University—words I owe to a wise physician, Dr. Paul Bruns:

> A physician-friend of mine (who has read my undertakings) tells me that at the outset I should say that these lectures will ask more questions than they will answer, will pose questions that may be unanswerable, will answer questions seldom asked and particularly questions physicians never thought of asking, and won't answer the questions doctors did ask.
>
> I stipulate that to do any one of these things shall be deemed success and that I enroll in any of these undertakings only on a "Pass-Fail" basis. Stiffer competition or any more severe judgment would be too much for me.

P. R.

Princeton, New Jersey
May 1970

THE PATIENT AS PERSON

1

Consent as a Canon of Loyalty with Special Reference to Children in Medical Investigations

The voluntary consent of the human subject is absolutely essential. This means that the person involved should have legal capacity to give consent; should be so situated as to be able to exercise free power of choice, without the intervention of any element of force, fraud, deceit, duress, overreaching, or other ulterior form of constraint or coercion; and should have sufficient knowledge and comprehension of the elements of the subject matter involved as to enable him to make an understanding and enlightened decision. This latter element requires that before the acceptance of an affirmative decision by the experimental subject there should be made known to him the nature, duration, and purpose of the experiment; the methods and means by which it is to be conducted; all inconveniences and hazards reasonably to be expected; and the effects upon his health of person which may possibly come from his participation in the experiment.

Articles of the Nuremberg Tribunal

When first I had the temerity to undertake some study of ethical issues in medical practice, my resolve was to venture no comment at all—relevant or irrelevant—upon these matters until I informed myself concerning how physicians and medical investigators themselves discuss and analyze the decisions they face. One then finds himself in the midst of a remarkable professional ethics. Actual performance, of course, may often be quite different from the principles endorsed by the profession. However, whether performance falls below the stated principles cannot itself be measured except in terms of these same principles of medical ethics stated and generally agreed to. The first thing to note is, therefore, that there is no profession that comes close to medicine in its concern to inculcate, transmit, and keep in constant repair its standards governing the conduct of its members.

One need not read very far in medical ethics—and especially not in the literature concerning medical experimentation or the ethical "codes" that have been formulated since the medical cases at the Nuremberg trials—without realizing that medical ethics has not its sole basis in the overall benefits to be produced. It is not a consequence-ethics alone. It is not solely a teleological ethics, to use the language of philosophy. It is not even an ethics of the "greatest possible medical benefits for the greatest possible number" of people. That calculus too easily comes to mean the "greatest possible medical benefits regardless of the number" of patients who without their proper consent may be made the subjects of promising medical investigations. Medical ethics is not solely a benefit-producing ethics even in regard to the individual patient, since he should not always be helped without his will.

As stated in the *Ethical Guidelines for Organ Transplantation* of the American Medical Association,[1] so also of medical experimentation involving human subjects: "Man participates in these procedures: he is the patient in them; or he performs them. All mankind is the ultimate beneficiary of them." Observe that the respect in which man is the patient and man the performer of medical care or medical investigation (the relation between doctor and patient/subject) places an independent moral limit upon the fashion in which the rest of mankind can be made the ultimate beneficiary of these procedures. In the language of philosophy, a deontological dimension or test holds chief place in medical ethics, beside teleological considerations. That is to say, there must be a determination of the rightness or wrongness of the action and not only of the good to be obtained in medical care or from medical investigation.

A crucial element in answer to the question, What constitutes right action in medical practice? is the requirement of a reasonably free and adequately informed consent. In current medical ethics, this is a chief *canon of loyalty* (as I shall call it) between the man who is patient/subject and the man who performs medical investigational procedures. Physicians discuss the consent-requirement just as ethicists discuss fairness- or justice-claims: these tests must be satisfied along with the benefits (the "good") obtained.

1. Report of the Judicial Council, E. G. Shelley, M.D., Chairman, and approved by the House of Delegates of the American Medical Association, June 1968.

Ethics in the Consent Situation

A theologian or moralist, of course, is not the one to say anything about "ethics in the consent situation." He cannot tell us what the principle of an informed consent requires in actual application. This, physicians and investigators and boards of their peers must do. That is to say, the practical applications of the requirement of an informed consent is always the work of prudence, which does not mean caution but practical wisdom in the appraisal of cases and specific situations. This is rightly the matter that is under discussion in the literature of medical ethics and in consultations among physicians and investigators themselves.

It is possible to parody the consent-requirement by simply writing out all the details and the possible consequences that would have to be mentioned in order for a patient to be fully informed. If that is the meaning of informed consent, then major operations that are quite ordinary might get few takers, or be performed only upon patients who are frightened to death. Likewise, it is possible to analyze the motivations of normal volunteers so as to cast total doubt upon the freedom of their choice. But then one casts doubt as well upon most human decisions, such as the decision to become a physician or a minister.[2] But a choice may be free and responsible despite the fact that it began in emotional bias one way rather than another, and consent can be informed without being encyclopedic.

For this reason I referred a moment ago to "a reasonably free and adequately informed consent." It is the meaning of this that is chiefly under discussion when physicians and investigators talk about the consent-requirement. They are trying to compose their prudence in aptly applying the principle or developing a common aptitude for extending the principle of consent to new sorts of

2. "Studies have revealed that physicians are afraid of death in greater proportion than control groups of patients. This is a fascinating statistic, and, if true, it is likely to reflect the doctor's perturbation and confusion in a situation reputed to be natural" (Charles D. Aring, "Intimations of Mortality: An Appreciation of Death and Dying," *Annals of Internal Medicine* 69 [July 1968]: 139). See *Death and Dying: Attitudes of Patient and Doctor* (New York: Group for the Advancement of Psychiatry, 1965), vol. 5, Symposium 11, pp. 591–667. What similar studies, or Rorschach inkblot tests, would show about theologians or ministers, I do not know.

cases or for making a concrete application of it in a given case. A theologian or moralist can as such have only some opinions about that. It is not the task of moralists to give an account of ethics in the consent situation, although they may pertinently comment upon the ethics of consent itself, as I propose to do in this chapter.

I will observe concerning applications of the consent-requirement only that physicians and investigators lean on a slender reed if they suppose that "situation ethics" correctly describes how principles apply in medical practice.[3] Situation ethics proposes that our moral reasoning and practice should be based on a readiness to violate some moral requirement or to set it aside in the face of wholly unique situations that call for exceptions to be made. To the contrary, unless I have totally misunderstood the literature dealing with medical experimentation, the practical question is always about the *meaning* of the consent-requirement in concrete cases of its application. About this a moralist knows nothing unless he happens also to be a physician-investigator, or has at least acquired considerable specific knowledge of all that is at stake in the case or the sort of cases in question. However, a moralist may presume to draw attention to the fact that the discussion in medical ethics is always about the meaning of the consent-requirement in practical application. It is not about supposed reasons for violating or setting this principle aside, or about the justification of quantity-of-bene-

3. An example of this misconception is the excellent article by Delford L. Stickel, "Ethical and Moral Aspects of Transplantation," *Monographs in the Surgical Sciences* 3, no. 4 (1966): 267–301. Situation ethics is assumed as the framework or the approach to be taken to all medical ethical questions. This theory is set forth at some length. Yet in the substance of the ethics and the norms applied we find the following: (1) "In the care of a patient who is a prospective cadaveric donor, treatment which is solely for the purpose of obtaining a healthy graft ought not to be undertaken" (p. 289); (2) "The principle that consent by parent, guardian, or court on behalf of a minor is not valid except for procedures which benefit the minor" was left intact by the ruling in the identical-twin kidney transplant cases, which the author endorses (pp. 284–85); (3) A quotation—with evident approval—from Pope Pius XII: "I think an overwhelming majority of physician-experimenters, if not thoroughly aware of the nature of the original patient-physician relationship, are so deeply rooted in the democratic spirit that they agree and will continue to agree, that the use of force is not justified on a single person, even if millions of other lives could be saved by such an act. They realize that the act would not just save millions of lives but that, as an amoral act from the standpoint of democratic brotherhood, it might create millions of amoral sequels, and that the moral history of mankind is more important than the scientific" (Stickel, p. 274; *Acta Apostolicae Sedis* 44 [1952]: 779).

fit-"exceptions" to this requirement (which would *maxim*-ize the principle or reduce it to a mere guideline). Where the ethics of the medical profession no longer speaks of *codes,* it speaks instead of *principles*—whose meaning in application is under constant review. The applications are for the doctor or the investigator and their peers to determine, while the principles accord with the ethics of a wider human community.

The Ethics of Consent

Hopefully while not exceeding an ethicist's putative competence or trespassing upon the competence of medical men, I wish to undertake an analysis of the consent-requirement itself. The principle of an informed consent is a statement of the fidelity between the man who performs medical procedures and the man on whom they are performed. Other aspects of medical ethics—for example, the requirement of a good experimental design and of professional skill at least as good as is customary in ordinary medical practice— treat the man as a purely passive subject or patient. These are also the requirements that hold for an ethical experiment upon animals. But any human being is more than a patient or experimental subject; he is a *personal* subject—every bit as much a man as the physician-investigator. Fidelity is between man and man in these procedures. Consent expresses or establishes this relationship, and the requirement of consent sustains it. Fidelity is the bond between consenting man and consenting man in these procedures. The principle of an informed consent is the cardinal *canon of loyalty* joining men together in medical practice and investigation. In this requirement, faithfulness among men—the faithfulness that is normative for all the covenants or moral bonds of life with life— gains specification for the primary relations peculiar to medical practice.

Consent as a canon of loyalty can best be exhibited by a paraphrase of Reinhold Niebuhr's celebrated defense of democracy on both positive and negative grounds: "Man's capacity for justice makes democracy possible; man's propensity to injustice makes democracy necessary." [4] Man's capacity to become joint adventurers

4. *The Children of Light and the Children of Darkness* (New York: Scribner's, 1949), p. xi.

in a common cause makes the consensual relation possible; man's propensity to overreach his joint adventurer even in a good cause makes consent necessary. In medical experimentation the common cause of the consensual relation is the advancement of medicine and benefit to others. In therapy and in diagnostic or therapeutic investigations, the common cause is some benefit to the patient himself; but this is still a joint venture in which patient and physician can say and ideally should both say, "I cure."

Therefore, I suggest that men's capacity to become joint adventurers in a common cause makes possible a consent to enter the relation of patient to physician or of subject to investigator. This means that *partnership* is a better term than *contract* in conceptualizing the relation between patient and physician or between subject and investigator. The fact that these pairs of people are joint adventurers is evident from the fact that consent is a continuing and a repeatable requirement. We can legitimately appeal to permissions presumably granted by or implied in the original contract only to the extent that these are not incompatible with the demands of an ongoing partnership sustained by an actual or implied *present* consent and terminable by any present or future dissent from it. For this to be at all a human enterprise—a covenantal relation between the man who performs these procedures and the man who is patient in them—the latter must make a reasonably free and an adequately informed consent. Ideally, he must be constantly engaged in doing so. This is basic to the cooperative enterprise in which he is one partner.[5]

At the same time, just as Lincoln said concerning political cov-

5. Cf. "The conduct of the consent situation is decisive for the patient's or volunteer's sense of being respected as a person . . ." "What is permanent in the consent situation is the encounter between selves when the limits of one self touch the limits of another." "The principle of *mutuality between persons,* or 'perceived effective decision making' is the relevant ethical principle for the consent situation." In that case, there simply *are* human rights and dignity which "cut across the general social principle of least suffering" and place limits upon the ethics of medical science's mission. We must "draw the line of ethical seriousness across the activities in medical research . . . at the question of consent," even if not *only* there. (John Fletcher, "Human Experimentation: Ethics in the Consent Situation," Symposium on Medical Progress and the Law, *Law and Contemporary Problems* [Autumn 1967], pp. 632, 633, 646, 639, 632).

enants among men that "no man is good enough to govern another
without his consent," so there is also this same negative warrant for
the requirement of consent in the relation between those who perform and those who are the patients in medical procedures. No
man is good enough to experiment upon another without his consent. The same can be said of the doctor-patient relation having
treatment in view. No man is good enough to cure another without
his consent. This holds without exception for ordinary medical
practice. This is the negative premise of the contract between physician and patient, even if it serves mainly to direct us to the positive
pole, to the need for a patient's partnership in his own cure.

In medical treatments, however, there is one clearly definable
exception from the requirement of expressed consent, which does
not weaken the general rule governing medical practice by consent
alone. This is the sort or class of cases in which consent may properly
be assumed or implied when men are in extreme danger and cannot
themselves consent explicitly. When a physician stops on the high-
way to bind up the wounds of accident victims, he is not liable to
suit for malpractice (where "Good Samaritan" laws are in force)
on the grounds that an unconscious man "constructively" consented
to procedures from which he suffered harm. The law rightly protects
the doctor in such errands of mercy. Indeed we might say that if a
doctor stops on the road to Jericho, instead of passing by on his way

---

Thus, treating the experimental subject "as an end also" (Kant), perceived effective
partnership and mutuality between the persons involved in research is the essential
moral meaning of the consent-requirement. This was marvelously confirmed by
Renée C. Fox's *Experiment Perilous* (Glencoe, Ill.: Free Press, 1959), a sociological
study of the roles and stresses of doctors and patient-subjects investigating Addison's
disease, the effects of total adrenalectomy, etc. The Group "dealt with patients as if
they were professional equals"; they treated their patients as "personal associates and
professional colleagues," correcting in part the patients' "sense of having lost the
right to be active, independent and self-determining as they were in their days of
health"; most of the patients felt that "the 'concern for the welfare of others' that
characterized their ward made it morally superior in some ways to the 'world of
wellness' from which they had been removed" (ibid., pp. 85, 105, 123, 141). This was
as it should be in a joint venture among men; and then, upon this foundation, the
researchers could afford to draw the line of moral seriousness elsewhere: they were
most concerned about whether the good consequences for others that might come from
the experimental treatments and operations they performed were worth the hazards
accepted by these patients.

to read a research paper before a scientific gathering or to visit his regular, paying customers, he is self-selected as good enough to practice medicine without the needy man's expressed consent.

In general, however, I suggest that man's propensity to overreach a joint adventurer even in a good cause makes consent necessary. This has to be said even if it is also true that this requirement is no substitute for—and indeed there can be no substitute for—the wisdom and moral integrity of the medical practitioner. That integrity still needs to be sustained in its setting in a system of medical "checks and balances" anchored in the requirement of consent.

The foregoing paragraphs describe the basis of the requirement that experimentation involving human subjects should be undertaken only when an informed consent has been secured. There are enormous problems, of course, in knowing how to subsume cases under this moral regulation expressive of respect for the man who is the subject in medical investigations no less than in applying this same moral regulation expressive of the meaning of medical care. What is and what is not a mature and informed consent is a preciously subtle thing to determine. Then there are questions about how to apply this rule arising from those sorts of medical research in which the patient's knowing enough to give an informed consent may alter the findings sought; and there is debate about whether the use of prisoners or medical students in medical experimentation, or paying the participants, would not put them under too much duress for them to be said to consent freely even if fully informed. Despite these ambiguities, however, to obtain an understanding consent is a minimum obligation of a common enterprise and in a practice in which men are committed to men in definable respects. The *faithfulness*-claims which every man, simply by being a man, places upon the researcher are the morally relevant considerations.[6] This is the ground of the consent-rule in medical practice, though obviously medical practice has also its consequence-features.

Indeed, precisely because there are unknown future benefits and precisely because the results of the experimentation may be believed

6. Sir Harold Himsworth said (1953) that the spirit of the Hippocratic Oath can be given in a single sentence: *Act always so as to increase trust* (quoted by Ross G. Mitchell, "The Child and Experimental Medicine," *British Medical Journal* 4, no. 1 [March 21, 1964]: 726). This might better read: *Act always so as not to abuse trust; act always so as to exhibit faithfulness,* to deserve and inspire trust.

to be so important as to be overriding, this rule governing medical experimentation upon human beings is needed to ensure that for the sake of those consequences no man shall be degraded and treated as a thing or as an animal in order that good may come of it. In this age of research medicine it is not only that medical benefits are attained by research but also that a man rises to the top in medicine by the success and significance of his research. The likelihood that a researcher would make a mistake in departing from a generally valuable rule of medical practice because he is biased toward the research benefits of permitting an "exception" is exceedingly great. In such a seriously important moral matter, this should be enough to rebut a policy of being open to future possible exceptions to this canon of medical ethics. On grounds of the faithfulness-claims alone, we must surely say that future experience will provide no morally significant exception to the requirement of an informed consent—although doubtless we may learn a great deal more about the meaning of this particular canon of loyalty, and how to apply it in new situations with greater sensitivity and refinement —or we may learn more and more how to practice violations of it.

Doubtless medical men will always be learning more and more about the specific meaning which the requirement of an informed consent has in practice. Or they could learn more and more how to violate or avoid this requirement. But they are not likely to learn that it more and more does not govern the ethical practice of medicine. It is, of course, impossible to demonstrate that there could be *no* exceptions to this requirement. But with regard to unforeseeable future possibilities or apparently unique situations that medicine may face, there is this rule-assuring, principle-strengthening, and practice-upholding rule to be added to the requirement of an informed consent. *In the grave moral matters of life and death, of maiming or curing, of the violation of persons or their bodily integrity, a physician or experimenter is more liable to make an error in moral judgment if he adopts a policy of holding himself open to the possibility that there may be significant, future permissions to ignore the principle of consent than he is if he holds this requirement of an informed consent always relevant and applicable.* If so, he ought as a practical matter to regard the consent-principle as closed to further morally significant alteration or exception. In this way he braces himself to respect the personal subject while he treats him as patient or tries procedures on him as an experimental subject for the good of mankind.

The researcher knows that his judgment will generally be biased by the fact that he strongly desires one of the consequences (the rapid completion of his research for the good of mankind) which he could hope to attain by breaking or avoiding the requirement of an informed consent. This, too, should strengthen adherence in practice to the principle of consent. If every doer loves his deed more than it ought to be loved, so every researcher his research— and, of course, its promise of future benefits for mankind. The investigator should strive, as Aristotle suggested, to hit the mean of moral virtue or excellence by "leaning against" the excess or the defect to which he knows himself, individually or professionally, and mankind generally in a scientific age, to be especially inclined. To assume otherwise would be to assume an equally serene rationality on the part of men in all moral matters. It would be to assume that a man is as able to sustain good moral judgment and to make a proper choice with a strong interest in results obtainable by violating the requirement of an informed consent as he would be if he had no such interest.

Thus the principle of consent is a canon of loyalty expressive of the faithfulness-claims of persons in medical care and investigation. Let us grant that we cannot theoretically rule out the possibility that there can be exceptions to this requirement in the future. This, at least, is conceivable in extreme examples. It is not logically impossible. Still this is a rule of the highest human loyalty that ought not in practice to be held open to significant future revision. To say this concerning the there and then of some future moral judgment would mean here and now to weaken the protection of co-adventurers from violation and self-violation in the common cause of medical care and the advancement of medical science. The material and spiritual pressures upon investigators in this age of research medicine, the collective bias in the direction of successful research, the propensities of the scientific mind toward the consequences alone are all good reasons—even if they are not all good moral reasons—for strengthening the requirement of an informed consent. This helps to protect coadventurers in the cause of medicine from harm and from harmfulness. This is the edification to be found in the thought that man's propensity to overreach a joint adventurer even in a good cause makes consent necessary.

This negative aspect of the ethics of medical research is essential even if only because the constraints of the consent-requirement serve constantly to drive our minds back to the positive meaning or warrant for this principle in the man who is the patient and the man who performs these procedures. An informed consent aione exhibits and establishes medical practice and investigation as a voluntary association of free men in a common cause. The negative constraint of the consent-requirement serves its positive meaning. It directs our attention always upon the man who is the patient in all medical procedures and a partner in all investigations, and away from that celebrated "nonpatient," the future of medical science. Thus consent lies at the heart of medical care as a joint adventure between patient and doctor. It lies at the heart of man's continuing search for cures to all man's diseases as a great human adventure that is carried forward jointly by the investigator and his subjects. Stripped of the requirement of a reasonably free and an adequately informed consent, experimentation and medicine itself would speedily become inhumane.

No one today would propose to eliminate the consent-requirement directly, but this can be done more subtly, or by indirection. Even while retaining it, the consent-requirement can be effectively annulled, or transformed into a disappearing, powerless guideline, simply by writing into it a "quantity-of-benefits-to-come"-exception clause. Thus we could make ourselves ready to override or avoid the consent-requirement in view of future good to be achieved. To do this is to make ourselves conditionally willing to use a subject in medical investigations as a mere means.

Research Involving Children or Incompetents

From consent as a canon of loyalty in medical practice it follows that children, who cannot give a mature and informed consent, or adult incompetents, should not be made the subjects of medical experimentation unless, other remedies having failed to relieve their grave illness, it is reasonable to believe that the administration of a drug as yet untested or insufficiently tested on human beings, or the performance of an untried operation, may further *the patient's own recovery*.

Now that is not a very elaborate moral rule governing medical practice in the matter of experiments involving children or incompetents as human subjects. It is a good example of the general claims of childhood specified for application in medical care and research. It is also a qualification immediately entailed by the meaning of consent in medical investigations as a joint undertaking between men. Again, one has to be prudent (which does not mean overcautious or scrupulous) in order to know how to care for child-patients in this way. One must know the possible relation of a proposed procedure to the child's own recovery, and also its likely effectiveness compared with other methods that have been or could be tried. These considerations may provide the doctor with necessary and sufficient reason for investigations upon children, perhaps even very hazardous ones. One has to proportion the peril to the diagnostic or therapeutic needs of the child.

Practical medical judgment has undeniable and ominous room for its determinations, since a "benefit" is whatever is *believed* to be of help to the child. Still the limits this rule imposes on practice are essentially clear: where there is no possible relation to the child's recovery, a child is not to be made a mere object in medical experimentation for the sake of good to come. The likelihood of benefits that could flow from the experiment for many other children is an equally insufficient warrant for child experimentation. The individual child is to be tended in illness or in dying, since he himself is not able to donate his illness or his dying to be studied and worked upon solely for the advancement of medicine. Again, future experience may tell us more about the meaning of this particular rule expressive of loyalty to a human child, and we may learn a great deal more about how to apply it in new situations with greater sensitivity and refinement—or we may learn more and more how to practice violations of it. But we are committed to refraining from morally significant exceptions to this rule defining impermissible medical experimentation upon children.

To experiment on children in ways that are not related to them as patients is already a sanitized form of barbarism; it already removes them from view and pays no attention to the faithfulness-claims which a child, simply by being a normal or a sick or dying child, places upon us and upon medical care. We should expect no morally significant exceptions to this canon of faithfulness to the child. To expect future justifiable exceptions is, in some sense, already to have forgotten the child.

To the layman, the most startling chapters in Dr. M. H. Pappworth's rather too sensational volume *Human Guinea Pigs* [7] are those in which he catalogues case after case of catheterization, percutaneous biopsy, and other hazardous experiments performed upon children, or upon women and their unborn children, *having no relation to their treatment.* Experts have estimated that catheterization of the right heart causes about one death per one thousand cases; of the left heart, five deaths per one thousand cases; and that the death rate in liver biopsy is from one to three per one thousand.[8] Moreover, a study of 55 deaths from heart catheterization has shown that there is "a close relation between the mortality rate and the patient's age." Deaths from this procedure result with greatest frequency in the first two months of life.[9] A parent is competent to consent for his child, and morally may venture to consent for his child to be subjected to these hazards, if the child is afflicted by a malady that is equally or more dangerous to him and to which the investigational procedure is definitely related. The diagnostic procedure may in fact prove to be of no benefit in the child's own treatment. But no parent is morally competent to consent that his child shall be submitted to hazardous or other experiments having no diagnostic or therapeutic significance for the child himself.

Pappworth's book has been criticized for, among other things, drawing the worst conclusion from the fact that articles in medical journals reporting an experiment often fail to state that consent was obtained or how it was obtained.[10] This may be a valid objec-

7. 1. Boston: Beacon, 1968.

8. Henry K. Beecher, "Medical Research and the Individual," in Daniel H. Labby (ed.), *Life or Death: Ethics and Options* (Seattle: University of Washington Press, 1968), p. 148.

9. Eugene Braunwald, "Deaths Related to Cardiac Catheterization," *Circulation,* Supplement III to vols. 27 and 28 (May 1968), pp. 17–26.

10. This is also a reply that is often given to some aspects of Dr. Henry K. Beecher's writings on ethics in medical research—that he equates failure to mention consent with failure to obtain it. See Louis Lasagna, *Life, Death and the Doctor* (New York: Knopf, 1968), p. 255.

tion, especially since an indication that a piece of research was funded by the National Institutes of Health now means that a "peer" research committee in the medical center where the experimentation was conducted certified that consent would be obtained. But mention or failure to mention that consent was obtained is surely not the point. Nor is the point merely that, upon reading some of these cases of experiments, even hazardous ones, brought upon children with no relation to their own possible treatment, one has great difficulty understanding how any parent psychologically *could* consent to the procedure. The point is rather that morally no parent *should* consent—or be asked to consent to any such thing even if he is quite capable of doing so, and even if in fact his informed consent was obtained in all cases where this fact is not mentioned in the reports.

To attempt to consent for a child to be made an experimental subject is to treat a child as not a child. It is to treat him as if he were an adult person who has consented to become a joint adventurer in the common cause of medical research. If the grounds for this are alleged to be the presumptive or implied consent of the child, that must simply be characterized as a violent and a false presumption.[11] Nontherapeutic, nondiagnostic experimentation involving human subjects must be based on true consent if it is to proceed as a human enterprise. No child or adult incompetent can choose to become a participating member of medical undertakings, and no one else on earth should decide to subject these people to investigations having no relation to their own treatment. That is a canon of loyalty to them. This they claim of us simply by being a human child or incompetent. When he is grown, the child may put away childish things and become a true volunteer. This is the meaning of being a volunteer: that a man enter and establish a consensual relation in some joint venture for medical progress— where before he could not, nor could anyone else, "volunteer" him for submission to unknown possible hazards for the sake of good to come.

11. To base "Good Samaritan" medical care upon the implied consent of automobile accident victims is quite a different matter. A well child, or a child suffering from an unrelated disease not being investigated, is not to be compared to an unconscious patient needing specific treatment. To imply the latter's "constructive" consent is not a violent presumption, it is a life-saving presumption, though it is in some degree "false."

If the requirement of parents, investigators, and state authorities in regard to their wards is "Never subject children to the unknown possible hazards of medical investigations having no relation to their own treatment," we must understand that the maladies for which the individual needs treatment and protection need not already be resident within the compass of the child's own skin. He can properly be regarded as one of a population, and we can add to the foregoing words: "except in epidemic conditions." Dr. Salk tried his polio vaccine on himself and his own children first. Then it was tested on selected children within a normal population. This involved some risk for the children vaccinated, and for other children as well, that the disease *might* be contracted from the vaccine itself, or that there might be unexpected injurious results. But the normal population of children was already subjected to waves of crippling epidemic summer after summer. A parent consenting for his child to be used in this trial was balancing the risks from the trial against the hazards from polio itself for that same child.

Physician-investigators are often in a quandary in which they are torn between the warrants for giving an experimental drug, and the warrants for withholding it from anyone in order to test it. Neither act seems justified, or both acts are equally warranted, when there is no available remedy and the indications are that a new drug may succeed. This situation also justifies a parent or guardian in consenting for a child, since we are supposing the hazard of the proposed treatment to be less or no greater than the hazard of the disease itself when treated by the established procedures. That would be a medical trial having clear relation to the treatment or protection of the child himself. He is not made, without his consent, the subject of medical investigations of possible benefit only to other children, other patients, or for the future advancement of medical science.

These may have been the circumstances surrounding the field trial of the vaccine for rubella (German measles) made in Taiwan, if this was in epidemic conditions, or in expectation of epidemic conditions, early in 1968 by a medical team from the University of Washington, headed by Dr. Thomas Grayston.[12] The vaccine was given to 3,269 young grade-school boys in the cities of Taipei and Taichung, while roughly an equal number were left unvaccinated

12. *New York Times,* October 17, 1968.

for comparison purposes. The latter group were given Salk polio vaccine so that they would derive some benefit from the experience to which they were subjected. This generous "payment" does not alter the moral dilemma of withholding the rubella vaccine from a selected group. Yet there may have been an equipoise between the hazards of contracting rubella or other damage from the vaccine and the hazards of contracting it if not vaccinated. There could have been a likelihood favoring the vaccinated of the two comparison groups.

These considerations, we may suppose, produced the quandary in the conscience of the investigators that was partially relieved by giving the unrelated Salk vaccine to the control group. Such equipoise alone would warrant—and it would sufficiently warrant— a parent or guardian in consenting that his child or ward be used for these research purposes. In the face of actual or predictable epidemic conditions, this would be medical investigation having some measurable or immeasurable relation to a child's own treatment or protection, as surely as the catheterization of the heart of a child with congenital heart trouble may be needed in his own diagnosis and treatment; and to this type of treatment a parent may venture to consent in his child's behalf. If no gulf is to be fixed between maladies beneath the skin and diseases afflicting children as members of a population, then the consent-requirement means: "Never submit children to medical investigation not related to their own treatment, except in face of epidemic conditions endangering also each individual child." This is simply the meaning of the consent-requirement in application, not a "quantity-of-benefit-to-come"-exception clause or a violation of this canon of loyalty to child-patients.

Indeed, a stricter construction of the necessary connection between proxy consent and the foreseeable needs of the child would permit the use of only girl children in field trials of rubella vaccine. Rubella is not the most contagious type of measles. The benefit to the subjects used in these trials (which plus the consent of parents legitimated subjecting them to experiment) was mainly to prevent their giving birth to children with congenital malformations should they later contract rubella during pregnancy. Therefore, there was stronger argument for considering only girl children as part of a population in establishing the necessary connection between experiment and "treatment."

More questionable were the earlier trials of the rubella vaccine performed upon the inmates of a retarded children's home in Conway, Arkansas. These subjects were not specially endangered by an epidemic of rubella. Few of the girls among them will ever be able to become part of the population of child-bearing women, or be in danger of pregnancy while in institutions. Using them simply had the advantage that they were segregated from the rest of the population, and any degree of risk to them would not spread to other people, including women of child-bearing age.

If children are incapable of truly consenting to experiments having unknown hazards for the sake of good to come, and if no one else should consent for them in cases unrelated to their own treatment, then medical research and society in general must choose a perhaps more difficult course of action to gain the benefits we seek from medical investigations. Surely it was possible to secure normal adult volunteers to consent to segregate themselves from the rest of the population for the duration of a rubella trial.[13] That method was simply more costly and inconvenient. At the same time, this illustrates the general fact that if we as a society are to proceed to the conquest of diseases; indeed, if we are to teach medical skills with fairness and justice to the poor and the ward patients, and with no violation of the basic claims of childhood, then there must be far greater encouragement generally in our society of a willingness to engage as joint adventurers for medical progress than has been achieved, or believed morally required by the principle of consent, in the past.

A final illustration may be given of the meaning and entailments of the consent-requirement in the prism of the case of the child. This is a "borderline case" in the sense that in the present age the child in question is widely deemed a borderline instance of humanity. Dr. Geoffrey Chamberlain, visiting research fellow at George Washington University Hospital in Washington, D.C., conducted experiments on animal and human fetuses with a view to developing an artificial placenta to combat the respiratory distresses com-

13. *New York Times,* April 5, 1969, reported that a hundred monks and nuns, from both Anglican and Roman Catholic orders, living in enclosed communities, were the voluntary subjects in testing American, British, and Belgian vaccines against German measles. This project was organized and directed by Dr. J. A. Dudgeon of London's Great Ormond Street Hospital for Sick Children.

monly afflicting premature babies. The eight human fetuses ranged in weight from 300 to 980 grams. The last of these experiments is described as follows:

> A 14-year-old girl was admitted for termination of pregnancy. When the patient was seen, the uterus was at about 26 weeks' gestational size and hysterotomy was performed. A 980 gram male fetus was delivered in his amniotic sac. Umbilical vein and both arteries were cannulated with no difficulty, about 11 minutes after separation of the placenta. Blood flowed evenly into the umbilical vein but no return occurred from the arteries at first. However, brisk spontaneous flow occurred 22 minutes after birth and the fetus was established on the circuit; he stayed so for 5 hours, 8 minutes. The experiment stopped then because a cannula inadvertently slipped and could not be reintroduced. . . .
>
> Once the perfusion was stopped . . . the gasping respiratory efforts increased to 8 to 10 per minute. The fetus died 21 minutes after leaving the circuit.[14]

One might ask whether the 14-year-old aborted mother was adequately informed of the experiment to be performed on her child, or whether, herself a minor, she could have or did freely consent to it. The crux of the matter, however, is whether anyone could morally consent for a 980-gram fetus that he should be used in order for mankind to learn better how to save other premature babies in the future. He was simply not considered to be one of the patients; delivery in his amniotic sac is enough to show that. He was, of course, not a viable baby by means of incubator methods customary in any large medical center. Still these methods had greater chance of success than the experimental placenta. Moreover, it is not mentioned that the effort was to save him by ordinary or by the new means. Rather was he made an experimental subject, he not able to consent to or dissent from the role designed for him in man's medical progress. I introduce this case simply to show that, in an age in which the line between feticide and infanticide was long ago breached, this question of who can morally consent

14. Geoffrey Chamberlain, "An Artificial Placenta," *American Journal of Obstetrics and Gynecology* 100, no. 5 (March 1, 1968): 624.

for a child who cannot himself consent has large and growing rami-
fications in the ethics of medical practice and investigation. Once it is
conceded that anyone can consent to submit a child to experimentation unrelated to its own care, permissible research will then include
a number of death-dealing investigations wrought upon child-life
from which mankind can expect to learn a great deal.

The Guidelines

The foregoing considerations argue for an important revision
of the Declaration of Helsinki's *Recommendations Guiding Doctors
in Clinical Research* [15] and of the AMA's *Ethical Guidelines for
Clinical Investigation.*[16] The Declaration of Helsinki distinguished
between "clinical research combined with profession care" and
"non-therapeutic clinical research." Likewise, the AMA Guidelines
distinguish between "clinical investigation primarily for treatment"
and "clinical investigation primarily for the accumulation of scientific knowledge." In the case of the first sort of research in each of
those pairs, i.e., investigations related to patient care and primarily
for treatment, there can be no doubt that a parent or legal guardian
has the right to consent in behalf of a patient who lacks legal or
physical or mental capacity. The troublesome and questionable
point, however, is that the Declaration of Helsinki and the AMA
Guidelines grant the same power of proxy consent in the case of
nontherapeutic clinical research that is primarily for the accumulation of scientific knowledge, is not primarily for treatment, and
which may be wholly unrelated to professional care.

It is worth noting that the AMA Guidelines qualify or limit in
significant degree the power of proxy consent which yet it does not
remove as a means of procuring medical knowledge. The first provision states that minors or mentally incompetent persons may be
used as research subjects, even with the consent of their parents or
legally authorized representatives, only if "the nature of the investigation is such that mentally competent adults would not be
suitable subjects." The intent of this provision, of course, is to allow

15. Adopted by the World Medical Association in 1964. *W.H.O. Chronicle* 19 (January 1965): 31–32.

16. Adopted by the House of Delegates, American Medical Association, Nov. 30,
1966. The latter, as we shall see, is much to be preferred of the two codes in respect
to what is said of children under investigation.

for research on retardation and on the mentally ill (having possible, even if remote, relation to the patient-subject's care?). In
view of this limitation, however, one might ask why the trials of
the rubella vaccine were made upon children and not first upon
consenting adults—even if there would likely be or could be different reactions to the vaccine in children, and even if it seems best as
a matter of public policy ultimately to introduce the immunization into the population at some point in childhood.

The second limitation upon the power of proxy consent in the
AMA Guidelines is the provision that the "consent" given by a
legally authorized representative of the subject shall be given only
"under circumstances in which an informed and prudent adult
would reasonably be expected to volunteer himself or his child as
a subject." The introduction of the words "or his child" renders
the entire permission circular. It states that a parent or legal guardian may volunteer a child for research purposes under circumstances
in which an informed and prudent adult would reasonably be expected to volunteer his child as a subject. That presumes that volunteering a child as a subject can be in conformity with moral reason.
It begs the entire question whether anyone can properly consent on
another's behalf that this other become a subject of investigation
primarily for the accumulation of scientific knowledge.

Nevertheless this second provision states an important guideline
or rule of thumb for determining what should be done or not done
after a child is legitimately within an experiment in the first place.
To bring a child within the ambit of medical investigation requires
(1) some relation to his own treatment and (2) informed parental or
guardian consent. As to this, men must make prudent judgment
concerning the meaning and the bearing of the test of the patient's
possible treatment and concerning what constitutes a reasonably
free and adequately informed consent on the part of parents. One
need not yet weigh the hazards of the procedure that is contemplated. It is enough to know that this is a well child or one suffering
from an unrelated disease to know that no one should consent to
bring him within the ambit of medical investigations having unknown hazards, pain, or discomfort, and promising no benefit to
the child himself. When, however, a child is properly a subject
under research in diagnostic or therapeutic investigations, it then
becomes important to weigh the hazards to which he would be ex-

posed against risks from the illness itself or from using already established procedures.[17] If the child is not being used as a mere means, it then is important to determine what means to use. Then the test of what an informed and prudent adult would reasonably do to himself or allow to be done to his own child is of some help—

17. An estimation of various hazards may be of some importance in determining who, for given experimental purposes, should be regarded as a child. A minor can under some circumstances consent to an operation; or, along with his parents, to give a kidney to a needy twin. But children in their early teens are excluded from competence to consent to hazardous operations; then, only parental consent in the presence of a child's need for treatment can authorize them. But a young child might well be mature enough to consent to a controlled toothpaste test, or to a program of physical exercise whose results are to be studied.

While subscribing to the prohibition of nontherapeutic experiments on children the Medical Research Council of Great Britain introduced some degree of latitude into our understanding of who is a "child" ("Responsibility in Investigations on Human Subjects," *British Medical Journal* 2, no. 5402 [July 18, 1964]: 179):

> In the strict view of the law parents and guardians of minors cannot give consent on their behalf to any procedures which are of no particular benefit to them and which may carry some risk of harm. Whilst English law does not fix any arbitrary age in this context, it may safely be assumed that the Courts will not regard a child of 12 years or under (of 14 years or under for boys in Scotland) as having the capacity to consent to any procedure which may involve him in an injury. . . . In the case of those who are mentally subnormal or mentally disordered the reality of the consent given will fall to be judged by similar criteria to those which apply to the making of a will, contracting a marriage, or otherwise taking decisions which have legal force as well as moral and social implications. When true consent in this sense cannot be obtained, procedures which are of no direct benefit and which might carry a risk of harm to the subject should not be undertaken. . . .
>
> Investigations that are of no direct benefit to the individual require, therefore, that his true consent to them shall be explicitly obtained. After adequate explanation, the consent of an adult of sound mind and understanding can be relied upon to be true consent. In the case of children and young persons the question whether purported consent was true consent would in each case depend upon facts such as the age, intelligence, situation, and character of the subject, and the nature of the investigation. When the subject is below the age of 12 years, information requiring the performance of any procedure involving his body would need to be obtained incidentally to and without altering the nature of a procedure intended for his individual benefit.

The first sentence of the first paragraph *prohibits* proxy consent to procedures of "no particular benefit" and which "*may* carry some risk of harm," i.e. any risk, to children. It has been contended that this would *permit* proxy consent where there is "no discernable risk." That, surely, is to argue from silence, and contrary to the main purpose of the text. See William J. Curran and Henry K. Beecher, "Experimentation in Children," *Journal of the American Medical Association* 210 (October 6, 1969), pp. 77–83.

but even then only of *some* help, as in the case of the Golden Rule, Do unto others as you would have them do unto you; or the second love-commandment, You shall love your neighbor *as yourself*. In that case, everything depends on how you love yourself, or what you might want others to do to you. There are some terrible ways of fulfilling those commandments. Just so, in the test proposed, for whether to proceed with the treatment or a diagnostic or therapeutic investigation, everything depends on what a man would be willing to have done to himself or his own child. Some stories of earnest investigators in the past are not altogether reassuring in this regard.

Nevertheless, neither the law nor medical ethics can get along without the concept of the reasonable man. The test of what an informed and prudent adult would reasonably be expected to have done to himself or his child affords some limits, *provided that* the child qualifies as a subject of investigation because of his own need. Of the two internal tests in this provision, a reference to the norm of what he would reasonably allow to be done to a loved one, such as a child, is perhaps a better test than what he might reasonably want done to himself in therapy or for the accumulation of scientific knowledge.

So much is this the case that, reading some accounts of experiments involving children as subjects, one finds it incredible to believe that a parent could have been fully informed of the procedure and its hazards and still have consented. One counts on the psychological incapacity of normal parents to consent to expose their own children to experiments, especially hazardous ones. This is the reason that failure to mention consent in reports of some experiments on children seems unimportant. If mentioned, the consent would normally be unbelievable, or believed not to have been an informed consent if it was secured. In these matters we do not ordinarily have in mind the parents in battered-children cases, but rather an (ideal or average) norm of parenthood and what may reasonably be expected of informed and prudent parents.[18] Therefore,

18. Parents in these cases may not have subjectively departed from this norm. Instead, the explanation may be that "parents tend not to distinguish between research and treatment, and hence entertain an inner sentiment that the procedure, even when they are told it is nonbeneficial, holds out some hope for their improvement" (Fletcher, "Human Experimentation," pp. 635–36). Also, parents are "consent-prone" out of gratitude to the doctor and desire to cooperate with him in every way possible. Such

our supposition that parents psychologically cannot consent to expose their children to medical investigations having unknown risks and unrelated to their own treatment prevents the question whether they *morally* should do so (if they could) from arising in our minds.

It is well to remember that the meaning of the word "hazardous" is a matter for prudent judgment in actual application within an already legitimate consent situation. Still no one can draw up rules for the application of principles. If one wants to abide by the rule, "Never drive while drunk," it is necessary for him to know something of the meaning of intoxication and its degrees. So also Plato said that even a philosopher needs practical wisdom in order to find his way home at night. Likewise, with regard to "hazardous" when seeking or giving legitimate parental consent, it is possible to parody the requirement by pointing out that even the introduction of an aspirin into an organism has its perils. But perils admit of degrees; and it is to an estimation of these objective hazards that our attention is directed by the rule of thumb that tells an investigator to bring to mind his own child. But we have seen that this maxim begs the question of proxy consent in providing a practical test for it. It is better to express the principle of consent itself in terms that make plain the need for *subsequent* practical judgment in comparison of hazards, and to say in regard to children in medical research that no one ought to consent for a child to be made the subject of medical investigations primarily for scientific purposes and unrelated to his own care, treatment, and protection.

Still, the test of what a "reasonable man" would do in the case of his own child or other loved one affords a kind of test for the care that ought to be extended not only to children needing investigation for the sake of their treatment but as well to subjects in investigations that have in view only the accumulation of medical knowledge. This is a rule of thumb or guideline of some importance for ethics in the consent situation. It serves as a sort of guideline in that it limits action and severely directs our attention to the

considerations as these, however, should strengthen the requirement of an understanding consent in a doctor's or a researcher's definition of his duty when tempted to use children having serious, unrelated diseases as subjects. Even so, it remains incomprehensible how parents, *if they were informed*, could consent for their *normal* children to be entered into nonbeneficial experiments, having unknown risks in addition to those of ordinary daily life.

degree of objective hazard or likelihood of injury which the subject may suffer.

An entirely opposite verdict must be delivered upon this provision insofar as it recommends using "circumstances in which an informed and prudent adult would reasonably be expected to volunteer himself" as the standard for determining those circumstances in which a child may be volunteered by someone else. This is simply wrong and dangerous advice. An informed and still prudent adult may often be expected to engage himself, or even be commended for volunteering himself, as a joint adventurer in the common enterprise of human medical progress under circumstances in which he ought by no means ever volunteer another without that other's own actual consent. Lord Kilbrandon, in his opening remarks at the Ciba Foundation Symposium, shifted the burden of a parent's judgment to whether he could rightfully *withhold* his child from experimentation. "I doubt whether," he said, "parents are entitled to withhold, on the part of their child, consent which, when adult, the child might probably give himself." [19] This, of course, is how one would proceed in "constructively" arriving at the child's will in case he needs to undergo a hazardous diagnostic or therapeutic procedure. But to say the same in the case of nonbeneficial research would be to treat the child as not a child, to treat him as an already consenting adult. Moreover, Kilbrandon's line of reasoning would go further and allow the child to be treated as one who, when adult, might probably be willing to make himself a martyr in the cause of medical progress. That will have to wait upon the event—unless child-life is to be violated and the duties of parenthood are to be denied.

Thus, provision 4.C.ii. of the AMA Ethical Guidelines for Clinical Investigations is either (1) false, insofar as it counsels investigators, parents, or legally authorized representatives of children to do to children always as they would will be done to themselves (this ignores the important difference made by the actual wills of free and informed consenting adults in justifying entrance into experiments for the sake of benefits to come); or it is (2) circular and ques-

---

19. In G. E. W. Wolstenholme and Maeve O'Connor (eds.), *Ethics in Medical Progress: With Special Reference to Transplantation,* Ciba Foundation Symposium (Boston: Little, Brown, 1966), p. 2.

tion-begging, insofar as it counsels investigators, parents, and legally authorized representatives of persons legally, physically, or mentally incapable of consenting, to substitute their own consent for that of "incompetent" subjects, provided (so around the reasoning goes) they do this only under circumstances in which an informed and prudent parent might reasonably be expected to volunteer his own child as subject of investigations wholly unrelated to his own treatment (this takes something that was brought into moral question, and *is* quite questionable, to be part of the answer to that question).

It is better to say of the consent-requirement or of the ethics of consent that this basically means that the *power* of proxy consent is not a *right;* that if men are in some sense capable of granting consent by proxy they should not for that reason do so; and that no one ought to consent for a child to be made the subject of medical investigations primarily for the accumulation of scientific knowledge, except in the face of epidemic conditions that bring upon the individual child proportionately the same or likely greater dangers. Then a parent's or a guardian's decision is precisely not based primarily on the accumulation of medical knowledge for future benefit to others (which may properly be the main factor in their own case or in an investigator's outlook). A parent's decisive concern is for the care and protection of the child, to whom he owes the highest fiduciary loyalty, even when he also appreciates the benefits to come to others from the investigation and might submit his own person to experiment in order to obtain them.

This is simply the minimum claims of childhood upon the adult community, whose members may make themselves joint adventurers or partners in the enterprise of medical advancement at cost to themselves if they will. The exclusion of a child's putative consent from the consensual community of medical progress (except when related to his own care or treatment) is the only way to give backing to the words with which (immediately after the provisions we have been discussing) the AMA Guidelines conclude: "No person may be used as a subject against his will." That surely does not mean: against his parent's or his guardian's will. It ought rather to read: No person may be used as a subject *without* his will.

A final word on the guidelines. Dr. Leo Alexander, of Tufts Uni-

versity Medical School, drafted the first version of the Nuremberg
Code—the standards used in trying the Nazi medical cases. Point 1
of this Code is printed at the head of this chapter. Dr. Alexander's
original draft of Point 1 contained a provision covering the case of
legitimate proxy consent in behalf of one group of incompetents:
the mentally ill. The judges at Nuremberg, Alexander has since
explained, "omitted from my original point No. 1 provisions for
valid consent in the case of mentally sick subjects to be obtained
from the next of kin and from the patient whenever possible, probably because they did not apply in the specific cases under trial." [20]
The Nazis simply were not doing beneficial research.

One can speculate on what might have been the consequence for
the development of later guidelines if the Nuremberg statement of
the consent-requirement had contained a provision for valid consent of next of kin limited to the diagnosis and treatment of the
incompetent patient. The framers of the Declaration of Helsinki
and of the AMA Guidelines would have had this as a model. They
would not have started from scratch. They would have been drafting a revision. They would have been forced to give positive moral
reasons for a new stipulation justifying research upon children and
other incompetents not related to their diseases or needs. They
might not have introduced both sorts of proxy consent as if they
had equal validity.

Pro and Con

To consent in place of a child means to consent *in his behalf
medically,* i.e., for medical reasons and possible benefit to him. Not
all physicians, of course, agree with this interpretation of the consent-requirement—excluding, as it does, children who are well, and
children with unrelated diseases, from medical investigations. In
order to highlight the issue of consent and what is at stake in the
prismatic case of the child, it may be helpful if we examine some of
the debate that has gone on among the medical profession.

1. The British journal, *The Lancet,* reported in its issue of

20. Leo Alexander, "Limitations of Experimentation on Human Beings with Special
Reference to Psychiatric Patients," *Diseases of the Nervous System* 27 (July 1966): 62;
"Limitations in Experimental Research on Human Beings," *Lex et Scientia* 3, no. 1
(January–March 1966): 16.

October 17, 1953 two cases of the use of infants or children in investigations unrelated to their medical welfare. In one, two hydrocephalic infants were used in tests unrelated to hydrocephalus,[21] and in the other normal children were used as controls to compare their tolerance to doubling the phenylalanine in their diets with the tolerance of PKU-retarded children to the same intake.

There ensued a controversy over the propriety of these experiments in subsequent letters to the editor of *The Lancet*. Dr. R. E. W. Fisher stated the case against them in no uncertain terms: "No medical procedure involving the slightest risk or accompanied by the slightest physical or mental pain may be inflicted on a child for experimental purposes unless there is a reasonable chance, or at least a hope, that the child may benefit thereby."[22] Drs. H. Bickel and J. Gerrard contended that the object of the phenylalanine-intake tests was simply to learn more about metabolism; that earlier tests on adults and on normal children had shown that considerably larger amounts caused no untoward effects and they wanted to find out whether doubling it would show the same, and further to assess the pathological metabolism of children with PKU; and that the experiment was closely comparable to glucose-tolerance tests in being "harmless" to the normal but important in assessing the abnormal. Glucose-tolerance tests, of course, are now established as harmless. One might question the use of well children in the original glucose-tolerance tests if that was an experiment, i.e. if it was

21. The purpose of this experiment was to see whether ammonium chloride infused intravenously for the relief of severe alkalosis could be used on children without producing toxic reactions. Five babies 2–11 weeks old with pyloric stenosis and alkalosis who might benefit were used, and two hydrocephalic babies aged 4 months with no abnormality in acid-base balance served as controls. The five improved, and happily the experimenters were able to report that the two hydrocephalic babies "remained well throughout their infusions." Their conclusion: "The intravenous infusion of ammonium chloride is an effective and rapid method of correcting alkalosis, and is safe when adequate precautions are taken" (*The Lancet*, October 17, 1953, pp. 801–04.

This calls to mind a parody of the "controlled trial" which for all its worth can become a fetish among experimenters. Suppose we take a group of ten patients with total kidney failure, it has been suggested. To five of them we give kidney transplants, and leave the remaining five without transplants. When the first group lives, while of the second all die, that "proves" that borrowed kidneys save lives.

22. For this and the following references see Letters to the Editor, *The Lancet*, November 7, 1953, p. 993.

not already known that such tests were harmless to them or that the procedure promised benefits to them at least as great as the possible harm. To a layman, what was done in the phenylalanine-intake tests seems an apt description of an experiment still having uncertain or unknown risks to the well child—else it was not an experiment.

In regard to the use of hydrocephalic infants in investigations medically unrelated to them, Dr. K. S. Holt stated the moral rule that, in his opinion, should govern research in children's diseases: "No procedure should be carried out involving risk or discomfort without a reasonable chance of benefit to that child *or other children*" (italics added). Amazingly, Dr. Holt expressed the view that his "working policy" differed only "slightly" from that expounded by Dr. Fisher. It is in reality light-years away. A child is not a piece of "childhood." Except in the face of epidemic, he is not a "part" of the whole population of children who can, therefore, without his will or not in his behalf medically, be properly made merely menial to the service of all other children. Dr. Holt's "working policy" seems only sentimentally different from taking the child—and every adult person as well—without his consent and in the absence of his own needed medical treatment, to be the passive subject of well-designed medical experimentation that has a reasonable chance of benefiting other people. Then the fact that adult consent can be consulted is not at all crucial. Would we not be back with the Nazis—except for our better experimental designs and the very important fact that we minimize the risks—or even say, in the case of children, that there must be "no *discernible* risks"—imposed on subjects for the sake of supposable or actual good to come? This is enough to show that investigation involving children as subjects is a prismatic case in which to tell whether we mean to take seriously the consent-requirement.

This particular exchange of opinions was concluded with Dr. Duncan Leys' letter in support of Dr. Fisher.[23] Leys voiced the following general principle condemning, among other things, "all procedures, whether therapeutic in intent or not, which are not designed with the sole intention of improving the lot of the individual upon whom they are performed." To this principle govern-

23. Letters to the Editor, *The Lancet*, November 14, 1953, p. 1044.

ing medical practice only one "exception" should be allowed: "when the experimental subject is an adult whose judgment is not impaired and who freely gives his consent." From this it follows immediately that "no child must ever be subjected to such an experiment." The latter restriction, in fact, tests whether "freely given consent" was ever meant seriously.

2. The previous exchange took place not far in time from the widespread acceptance of the strict consent-requirement that was used in trying the medical cases at Nuremberg. Since then the various codes of medical ethics seem to have weakened the meaning of mature and voluntary consent to experimentation, at least by explicitly allowing proxy consent to enter a child into investigations not in his own behalf medically. It is, therefore, of some importance to examine the pro's and con's of experiment upon children in a more recent case (1964).

Dr. Robert M. Zollinger et al. reported a study of the effect of removing the thymus of children upon their immune reaction.[24] It was not unusual, they judged, to dissect and remove, wholly or partially, the thymus of children undergoing major corrective heart surgery. They took eighteen children of both sexes ranging in age from $3\frac{1}{2}$ months to 18 years for whom heart surgery was indicated. Eleven were randomly selected to have total thymectomy, while the thymus of the remaining seven was left in place to serve as controls (only biopsy of the thymus was performed in these cases). The hypothesis was that the thymus has something to do with the development of an individual's "self/not-self" immune reaction. The hope was to prove whether removal of the thymus might, along with the use of immunosuppressive drugs, assist in the retention of tissue or organ transplants in the case of persons needing them. The test was to be the rapidity with which the two comparison groups of children rejected skin grafts; and, in order to conduct this test, full-thickness skin grafts had to be sutured in place on the chest wall of these children, none of whom needed skin grafts. The results failed to show any difference in "tolerance" due to thymectomy, but the research team planned to follow these children over the years

24. Robert M. Zollinger, Jr., Martin C. Lindemen, Jr., Robert M. Filler, Joseph M. Corson, and Richard E. Wilson, "Effect of Thymectomy on Skin-Homograph Survival in Children," *New England Journal of Medicine* 270 (April 2, 1964): 707–09.

with a view to finding out whether later on they evidence any lack of "thymic" lymphocytes.

This prompted a letter of protest from Dr. Byron H. Waksman.[25] As to one of the points in dispute, a layman has to yield to expert opinion, which was in disagreement. Dr. Waksman believed, on evidence cited, that thymectomy on these children "must at the same time remove important defenses against infection," while for Zollinger et al that was a point to be demonstrated. The researchers charged [26] that Dr. Waksman "unfortunately implied the creation of thymectomized patients" for the purposes of their experimental procedure, having the known hazard of removing the children's defenses against infection. They appealed rather to the fact that "thymectomies were and are being performed during various thoracic procedures." Theirs was only a controlled *observation* of these patients. No additional thymectomized victims were created.

What then should be said of the small remaining point, namely, that to secure comparison groups the researchers intervened on a practice and deliberately removed the thymuses of eleven and left in place those of seven of these children? This is not exactly a case in which the possible benefits of one form of therapy are judged to be about the same of another, and medical decision is in equipoise —it being as wrong to withhold as to use a new and as yet an inadequately tested treatment. Still Zollinger et al. apparently believed that no harm would come from excising the thymus or from leaving it in. As it turned out, this proved true on one check of these patient's immune response, although the hypothesis was that this *might be* decreased. The hypothesis would not have been worthwhile if there were known to be no risks, or if the risks were known to be as great either way. The procedure used would have been a redundant one, not an experiment. Since, however, in the heart surgery going on at the time some thymuses were taken and others left, the researchers could argue that they only imposed a little order on a random situation so that, for the purposes of this experiment, they

25. Correspondence, *New England Journal of Medicine* 270, no. 19 (May 7, 1964): 1018–19.

26. Correspondence, *New England Journal of Medicine* 270, no. 20 (May 14, 1964): 1314.

could tell which was which and make refined observation of the two groups.

If not the total thymectomies, then certainly the skin grafts were, as Dr. Waksman charged, "carried out as a purely experimental measure in subjects not having a disease to which this procedure is relevant." He asked whether "the possible transmission of serum hepatitis from skin graft donors and the unnecessary immunization against isoantigens" in these already weakened patients "were sufficiently offset by the usefulness of the data obtained to be worth risking in these subjects." Whether these hazards were offset is, of course, one part of the medical judgment to proceed with the experiment. It is also the very thing a true volunteer would weigh in making a mature and informed consent. Dr. Waksman himself does not take into account the special moral problem of using children in this experiment when he simply asks "if the long-term hazards, unknown at present, were duly noted and called to the subjects' attention"—one of whom was 3½ months old!

In any event Zollinger et al. gave an inadequate reply to the question Waksman asked. The research team said: "We believe the homografts introduced few new isoantigens beyond those already received in the multiple transfusions required in open-heart surgery. In this setting the added hazards in this investigation were believed to be reasonable." I should say that this was a decision the investigators had *first* to make, but that the decision was finally not theirs alone. Whether the added hazards were reasonable, and whether *any* new isoantigens were acceptable beyond those already received in the multiple transfusions required in open-heart surgery, are precisely to be encompassed in the free and informed consent of a patient who thereby could legitimate his participation as a subject in an experiment that had the accumulation of knowledge and benefit to others in view. To add experimental, unknown hazards to children already weakened by open-heart surgery, or to add any new sources of infection to children already exposed by multiple blood transfusions—to do these things *without* their wills and in the absence of any relation to their own recovery—must simply be deemed unconscionable. The ritual of parental or guardian consent in place of these children's consent would not have made it less so, since the procedure consented to would clearly not have been in their behalf medically. The editorial comment on this correspondence in the *New England Journal of Medicine* [27] was therefore quite correct, if too vague, when it said: "The question is especially disturbing when it involves children who cannot speak for themselves and for whom not even the parent can honestly speak unless the particular procedure is obviously justified in each case."

3. Among the best articles to date on the child and experimental medicine is one by Dr. Ross G. Mitchell.[28] In the judgment of the present writer, Dr. Mitchell slips at the heart of his argument in taking a qualitative leap to be only a quantitative move along a spectrum of types of experiment on children. I shall point this out first. However, in a sense this is not a very important matter in an article which evidences great sensitivity to the misuse of children and hedges experimentation upon them with many limitations. The latter are of the utmost importance.

Dr. Mitchell conceptualizes the experiments that can be carried out on children in five categories: (1) an experiment in treatment with the immediate aim of curing the child's disease; (2) an experiment on an ill child in order to find out more about his condition; (3) an experiment on an ill child in order to learn more about the disease from which he is suffering; (4) an experiment on a child who is either well or suffering from another disease in order to find out more about a particular disease; and (5) an experiment, usually on a healthy child, designed to provide information about children in general. Since more than one purpose may be served by an investigation, Dr. Mitchell rightly says that "the line between categories 2 and 3 is not a distinct one." This has been assumed in all the foregoing, whenever it was said that parents may consent to experiments to learn more about the disease from which a child is suffering if there is only some slight chance that the physicians will also learn more about his condition and that the investigation of

27. Vol. 270, no. 19 (May 7, 1964), pp. 1014–15. See also "Ethics of Human Experimentation," *British Medical Journal* 2, no. 5402 (July 18, 1964): 135–36.
28. Ross G. Mitchell, "The Child and Experimental Medicine," *British Medical Journal* 4, no. 1 (March 21, 1964): 721–27.

the disease has a remote possibility of aiding them in the investigational treatment of the child's condition.

Then Dr. Mitchell argues that "if category 3 is accepted as reasonable . . . there is little fundamental difference between it and the next category." To the contrary, categories 3 and 4 seem qualitatively quite different. In the latter case, one says to the parents, "This won't benefit your child but what we find out may help children with other diseases." But possible benefit to the child seems not to be excluded from category 3. One need *not* say to the parents—as Dr. Mitchell supposes—that "this won't benefit your child directly, but what we find out may help other children with the same disease." [29] One should, of course, make it quite clear that "this *may* not be of any benefit to your child, but we are proceeding with the investigational treatment of your child's condition, while the simultaneous investigation of the disease from which he is suffering may be of help to other children with the same disease even if it is not of benefit to him."

But that seems the most that should be said. If it is true that "whether or not the information obtained will be of help to the subject of the study can only be determined after the results have been analyzed and should not be made a condition of the experiment," it remains the case that the subject of the study *might* be benefited by its results. The latter has to be properly weighed. I have already indicated that this leaves perhaps ominously large room for the judgment of the physician-investigator. Still an estimation that there is a chance that the child will benefit remains a condition of entering him into an experiment. Dr. Mitchell does not propose the investigation of the disease to the neglect or the impairment in any degree of the investigational treatment of the child's condition. For these reasons, I do not believe Dr. Mitchell has established "the undesirability of differentiating between potentially beneficial and merely informative experiments," or that parents can give consent for a child to participate in either indifferently "with the same provisos as would pertain if they were giving permission for experiments on themselves." [30]

29. Ibid., p. 723.
30. Ibid., pp. 724, 725.

Nevertheless, it is important to notice the summary limits Dr. Mitchell imposes while still opposing "any sweeping directive to the effect that no experiments are permissible on children." A pin-prick to obtain a drop of capillary blood is painless and free of risk if properly carried out. This can be done, but "I have always considered that venipuncture in infants and young children for experimental purposes is hardly justifiable." "An experiment causing pain should never be carried out on a child." "An experiment is permissible provided that the risk does not exceed the ordinary risks of daily living. . . . Experiments carrying a greater risk may, of course, be permissible if an ill child is expected to benefit directly." "At no time should the potential scientific value of the work be used as an argument for or against carrying out an experiment . . . the importance or otherwise of the work should never be allowed to influence the decision on whether it is justifiable . . . I believe it is dangerous to suggest that an experiment which might otherwise be unjustifiable [because it uses venipuncture, causes pain, prolongs distressing symptoms, slows recovery, involves risks greater than those of daily living] is justified because it is for the common good." [31] "There are no 'inferior' children who are more suitable for experiments than others. If the proposed experiment may justifiably be carried out on any child, it may be carried out on any suitable child." Charity ward children, orphans, mentally defective or malformed children ought not be placed in a separate category. By the same token, children in hospitals are not to be used in preference to other suitable children simply because they are accessible.[32]

If we in contemporary society and in experimental work in pediatric diseases or in the testing of drugs and the treatment of children in institutions were anywhere near accepting these strictures we might not so much need the bracing principle that no one should consent for a child except *in his possible behalf medically*.[33]

31. Ibid., pp. 723, 724. As for the requirement that the experimental risk not exceed "the ordinary risks of daily living," one must ask: Is this a replacement risk or an additional risk? If additional, then the sum ipso facto exceeds the ordinary risks of daily living. If not additional, what constitutes the procedure an experiment?

32. Ibid., pp. 725–26.

33. An editorial in a recent issue of *Pediatrics* (38, no. 3 [September 1966]: 373–74), signed by Dr. William A. Silverman of Babies Hospital, New York, argued altogether

It is noteworthy that Dr. Mitchell believes that this principle is *too pliant*. The principle that experiments may be carried out only if the subject is expected to benefit, he writes, is "open to abuse through rationalization of the purpose of the experiment." [34] For this reason he prefers to prohibit definite, physiologically describable actions, conditions, or consequences. Granted that the medical researcher must also make these determinations, it still seems that something more than the pain involved, etc., could forbid taking venous blood from a child for experimental purposes. That would be if no one can validly consent in behalf of the child medically, where examination of his venous blood is no part of the investigational treatment of his condition or of the disease from which he suffers. Faithfulness to a child includes the requirement that we not inflict pain or risks in addition to those of ordinary daily living. But fidelity to a human child also includes never treating him as a means only, but always also as an end.

The use of children in research by proxy consent is a prismatic case in which to see clearly the meaning of the consent-requirement. In the case of the moral claims of the child upon us we can see clearly the claims of any fellow man not to be treated as a means only. The moral issue here does not actually depend on age, but on whether anyone should be made the property of another and disposition be made of him, without his will, that is not also in his behalf medically. We would not permit an older parent to consent for his son who is a grown man. This is not only because the son's con-

---

from the "principle of the whole." "It is unthinkable," wrote this author, "that clinical research in American children may be curtailed . . . because of the difficulties involved in grappling with the issue of 'informed consent' . . . children are no different from adults; neither must be denied the advantages that result from the accumulation of certain information. . . ." ". . . to the extent that [the unplanned, observational method of treating children] delays the solution of human problems, it is also unethical." To the core of this argument, it must simply be said that the advantages of accumulating information and eagerness not to delay the solution of human problems can lead to high crimes. In fairness, it should be said that Dr. Silverman proposes to place the consent-giving responsibility in the hands of the physician in charge of the small patient's medical care, provided he as "physician-friend" is not also the "physician-investigator" (Otto E. Guttentag, "The Problem of Experimentation on Human Beings: II. The Physician's Point of View," *Science* 117 (February 27, 1953): 207–10.

34. Mitchell, "The Child and Experimental Medicine," p. 723.

sent can be consulted. It is primarily because no man is the property of another or should be made merely menial. Where the grown
son cannot consent because of physical or mental disability, his
parent or other relative can validly consent in his behalf if this is
in his behalf medically. His welfare is then also the end in view;
he is not made into an experimental means only. So also in the case
of the small child.

What is at stake here is the covenantal obligations of parents to
children—the protection with which a child should be surrounded,
and the meaning and duties of parenthood. In veterinary medicine,
"the vet.'s 'patient' is an animal; but his client is the animal's
owner." This means that "the operative decision lies with its
owner." [35] Are we allowed to believe that an analogous situation
pertains in the triadic relation of parent-child-researcher? that the
parent is the physician's client? that the operative decision is the
parent's consent, in effect directing the disposition of the child
to ends not in his behalf? To the contrary, the doctor cannot in
respect to his small patient become the agent of another person. His
is a covenant with that patient, and faithfulness to him should be
controlling. If perfunctory consents on hospital forms are often a
kind of placebo to the experimenter's conscience, parental or guardian consent is a powerful placebo disguising the fact that these in-
terlocking covenants among men—parent-child-physician/researcher
—are on their way to being reduced to client/owner-child/object-
researcher.

The issue here is the wrong of making a human being an "object" and using him in trials not in his behalf as a subject. "In some
situations," it has been said, "such as with infants or with institutionalized lower-functioning retardates, there may be very little for
which a researcher can ask in a request for consent because whatever
a subject ordinarily has to give has never been possessed, or has already been given—or taken. . . . Unpleasant as it sounds and is,
the one thing that such a person usually still has that a researcher
may want is part of his bodily functioning." [36] In situations in which

35. "Decisions about Life and Death: A Problem in Modern Medicine." Church of
England study pamphlet (Church Information Office, Church House, Westminster
WC1, London, p. 20.

36. Wolf Wolfensberger, "Ethical Issues in Research with Human Subjects," *Science*
155 (January 6, 1967): 48, 49.

a part of a body's functioning is all a researcher wants, whom is he to ask? He cannot ask the small patient who has never possessed powers of consent which subjects ordinarily have to give. He cannot ask the retardate. He cannot ask those human beings who because of life's misfortunes have had taken from them that something else which normal subjects give in giving themselves along with their bodily functioning to the joint venture of research. If the researcher asks very little, still he asks too much when his exploration of a part of bodily function taken or conveyed to him by third-party consent is not medically in behalf of the patient-subject. True, the small patient or retardate cannot enter into the covenant making for medical progress as a human enterprise. However, this does not excuse parents, guardians, or researchers. They can still keep covenant with the child and with the individual retardate.

Anglo-American law and the ethical substance in the law as an ordering of human reality seems very clear on this point. We should bring this briefly into view. There are two different, related aspects: harmful invasions of the body (which upon expert testimony and unless informed consent to the risk can be shown may legally be judged medical negligence) and unconsented "touching" (which are still assaults even if no harm is done).[37] In the first, the dignity or degradation of the fortress of the body are at issue; in the second merely freedom from coercion (or from a harmless offense) to the will of another person. In the second case, one wrongs another human being by doing something to him without his consent; in the first case, one wrongs him by doing something that was negligently harmful. It would seem that children could be removed from the human community and deprived of the protections of the law in both respects by medical investigations upon them. They could be placed at risk of physical harm; or, with no discernible risk, they could be offensively "touched" without risk of or actual harm —unless there is a consent that can validly enter them into medical experiments. They could be *harmfully* used, or they could simply be *used* with no harm. In fact, principles in our legal tradition generally protect children from both the degradation of the body's fortress and from being treated as a means only, and not also as an

37. See Marcus L. Plante, "An Analysis of 'Informed Consent,'" *Fordham Law Review* 36, no. 4 (May 1968): 639–72.

end, even when no harm is expected or can be discerned in the result.

The courts have made it clear that "a child is not the property of its parents and may not be dealt with without regard for his best interests." [38] This means specifically, as Professor Paul Freund of the Harvard Law School pointed out, that "the law here is that parents may consent for the child if the invasion of the child's body is for the child's welfare or benefit." [39] Professor Morse continues with equal specificity: "The parental responsibility may be violated . . . if a parent or guardian exposes the child to unnecessary danger. Consequently, the parent's consent to the use of a child for clinical investigation that is not medically indicated for the benefit of the child may be of doubtful validity as a defense against a liability claim. Illness or injury may justify appropriate but unproven therapy if other procedures are unsatisfactory. But clinical investigation which is not for the purpose of treating the child cannot be assumed to be for the child's benefit simply because the child might later have the "satisfaction" or "reward" of participation in medical progress." [40] And Warren E. Burger, the Chief Justice of the U.S. Supreme Court, writing when he was Judge of the Court of Appeals, District of Columbia, stated his opinion that "No *adult* has the legal power to consent to experiments on an infant unless the treatment is for the benefit of the *infant*. . . . It is the lamentable use in experiments of such subjects as infant children, incompetents in mental institutions, unconsenting soldiers subject to military discipline—as has been done—that is indefensible; and no rational social order will or should tolerate it." [41]

Of course, no one would have us revert to the eighteenth century when Caroline, Princess of Wales, "begged the lives" of six condemned criminals for experimental smallpox vaccination, and also procured for an additional trial "half a dozen of the charity children belonging to St. James' parish." Ours is the more subtle problem of the *use* of children in research, in which the risks are minimal or

38. Howard Newcomb Morse, "Legal Implications of Clinical Investigations," *Vanderbilt Law Review* 20, no. 4 (May 1967): 754.

39. Paul A. Freund, "Ethical Problems in Human Experimentation," *New England Journal of Medicine* 273, no. 13 (September 23, 1965): 691; "Is the Law Ready for Human Experimentation?" *Trial* 2 (October–November 1966): 48.

40. Morse, "Legal Implications of Clinical Investigations, p. 755.

41. Warren E. Burger, "Reflections on Law and Experimental Medicine," Reflections on the New Biology, *U.C.L.A. Law Review* 15, no. 2 (February 1968): 438.

"negligible," but still not in their behalf medically. It is hard to see how this can be an expression of parental care (or of the state's care *in loco parentis*), or anything other than a violation of the nature and meaning of the responsibilities of parenthood as a covenant among the generations of men.

Dr. Henry K. Beecher stated our ethical quandary when he wrote that "one can fairly raise the question as to whether those responsible for children or the mentally deficient have the right to consent to something they themselves will not experience." Dr. Beecher's own view is that research upon children may be justified when "no discernible risk" is involved.[42] One can fairly raise the question how there can be no risk or no discernible risk in an experiment. When no risk is discerned, one can still fairly raise the question whether we do not always know there to be unknown or undiscerned risks if the procedure is neither proved nor redundant. The care called for by the small patient would seem to be analogous to the ethical relation protected by our law on "offensive touching" mentioned above. "What is involved" here "is the right of each of us to determine for ourselves not alone the extent to which we will share ourselves with others, but the timing and the nature of any such sharing." [43] Since "offensive touching" or "unconsented touching" is ground for legal action for assault and battery even though there has been no damage, it seems clear that *no consent* rather than *no risk* or *no discernible risk* is the decisive point at law. Only the legal fiction of parental or other representative consent keeps experiment on children from being judged to be battery even where there is no harm. This surely is the morality of the matter: a subject can be wronged without being harmed.

The room left for ethical discretion to make situational decisions

42. Beecher, "Medical Research and the Individual," p. 127; "Scarce Resources and Medical Advancement," Ethical Aspects of Experimentation with Human Subjects, *Daedalus*, Spring 1969, p. 285. In addition to the test of "no discernible risk," however, Dr. Beecher also appeals to the fact that "such work [e.g., studies of inborn errors of metabolism] is *potentially*, and sometimes unexpectedly, of direct benefit to the given subject." This, I allow, is a good reason for a seriously ill child to be subjected to experimental trial. Cf. also William J. Curran and Henry K. Beecher, "Experiment in Children," pp. 77–83; and Henry K. Beecher, *Research and the Individual: Human Studies* (Boston-Little, Brown, 1970), pp. 63–64.

43. Oscar M. Ruebhausen, "Experiments with Human Subjects," a paper presented at the annual meeting of the American Association for the Advancement of Science in New York City, December 23, 1967. *Record of the New York Bar Association* 23 (February 1968): 93.

in conducting beneficial research with children comes under the determination of what is a "benefit," weighing the nearness or remoteness of possible benefits, and telling when a minor is no longer a child but is able to give an understanding consent to a particular trial for the sake of the good of others to come. These uncertainties afford, as we have seen, such latitude that no man can relieve another of his premonitions of guilt to come whatever he decides, or lessen the stress on conscience in the situation of proxy consent to diagnostic or therapeutic investigation upon a child-life.

When one fondles or plays with an infant, he "speaks" to that child as one having individual worth; still the child may be hurt. When parents make decisions concerning a child's development or values to be imparted, and when they consent for him to undergo medical care, they have no guarantee that the benefits they seek will be forthcoming, or even that these are truly beneficial. Pediatric psychological investigations, it is often said, are always also beneficial —because the researcher gives the child more attention than the child ordinarily receives. Still, one may doubt whether more attention is always beneficial, even though a normal child has a marvelous ability to control his responses and to protect himself from "offensive observations," or he may enter freely into the game. (An anencephalitic baby discloses its impotency for further human development by the fact that it has no control of its response to environmental stimuli; such a baby has not the beginnings of the human capacity within the fortress of the body to determine the time and the nature of its sharing of himself with others.) Since, however, for the foregoing argument, a benefit is whatever is *believed* to be a benefit, many eventualities are compatible with acting on the principle that we owe the individual child the highest fiduciary loyalty we know how to perform. Basically contradictory to this it would be to consent to submit a child to procedures believed not to be in the child's behalf. Parenthood was not made for this.

Children in Institutions

Even if one granted the right of parents to consent for their children to be used in medical investigations having unknown present and future risks to them and promising future possible benefits only for others, it would still be possible to argue that children in institutions and not directly and continuously under the care of parents or relatives should *never* be so used.[44] If we are not persuaded that *because they are children* children cannot consent (nor should anyone else consent in their behalf) to experiments primarily for the accumulation of knowledge, we at least should be convinced that such experiments ought not to be performed upon children in orphanages, reformatories, or homes for the retarded *because they are a captive population.*

In discussions of the consent-requirement more attention has been paid to the question of whether and under what possible circumstances adult prisoners can validly consent to research trials than to the question of whether and under what possible circumstances there can be valid consent for children who cannot consent at all. Some authors seem to find it easier to include children by proxy, reducing consent to a merely formal requirement which can be met by someone else other than the real subject, than to include prisoners who may be under undue duress (but who, to suppose the worst, do themselves conditionally consent [45]). In an otherwise excellent article, Professor John Fletcher of Virginia Theological Seminary, for example, comes closest to ever saying "never" in ethics when he is discussing the use of prisoners, while accepting as standard the substitution of the consent of an incompetent's legal representative.[46] This anomaly or contrast in the literature of medical ethics is worth pondering.

44. World Medical Associations Draft Code of Ethics as published in the *British Medical Journal* 5312 (October 27, 1962); "Judgment Difficult," Editorial, *New England Journal of Medicine* 269 (August 29, 1963): 479–80.

45. Aristotle taught that a merchant who consents to throw all his goods overboard in a storm in order to save the ship and the lives of all on board still acts voluntarily and not from necessity or coercion. His act is "imperfectly voluntary," but still voluntary under those conditions.

46. Fletcher, "Human Experimentation," pp. 620–49. The author "agrees with those who would put the sharpest restrictions upon the use of prisoner populations in medical research, since by virtue of their imprisonment they cannot be truly said to possess an active capacity to consent. . . . [Those who have suffered] the loss of public liberty through imprisonment, should not then be made to go through the charade of seeming to possess what has been temporarily removed" ibid., p. 636). I suggest that a child, by virtue of his childhood, cannot be truly said to possess an active capacity to consent; and that it is a dangerous charade for anyone to go through the motions of consenting for him when this is not truly done *in his behalf*

The usual reasons offered for not accepting prisoner volunteers are only cautionary, even if very severe, warnings. It is not impossible in local situations to overcome them so as to secure from prisoners a reasonably free as well as an adequately informed consent. It is duress that has to be avoided—the duress to give a particular consent because of too great hope of parole. This should not be an automatic "payment." Even a pattern of always weighing heavily the consent of prisoners in considering them for parole has to be avoided. Still it is not impossible to arrange things so that a man in prison may freely volunteer to become a joint adventurer in an experiment for the sake of the knowledge and good to come, and not for the sake of the reward. It is not impossible to protect his will from duress to cooperate in such medical undertakings. To do this, some would require in the case of prisoners the complete exclusion of any possibilty of reward, or of earlier parole. This seems unfairly severe on prisoners. No one who has read the noble words of Nathan Leopold concerning the purposefulness of his own and other prisoners' participation in the malaria experiments in the Illinois State Prison during World War II can deny that prisoners *may* be as free in volunteering as persons in normal life.

If the consent of prisoners to medical experimentation is not inherently or always necessarily invalid, there may still be decisive objection to the general practice of using them. This was the most persuasive argument made by Professor David Daube in the Ciba Symposium in morally forbidding the use of prisoners as donors of organs for transplantation. Daube allowed that the pressure upon familial donors may be greater than that placed upon prisoners, but "the pressure in one's family or circle belongs to the normal burden and dignity of social existence"; this is "a pressure consonant with the dignity and responsibility of free life." This we deny to prisoners. Lord Kilbrandon made something of the same point (appealing to what philosophers call *fairness*-considerations) when he said that "when we put a man in prison we deprive him of a large number

---

medically. Particularly in regard to children in institutions, to say "never" to the consents of their legal representatives when these are not even ostensibly in the children's behalf medically would not be "to remove oneself from historical possibility" (*ibid.*, p. 636, n. 46). It would rather be to place upon ourselves the moral requirement that other historical possibilities for the accumulation of knowledge be looked for or designed.

of his consents, therefore it is perhaps distasteful to confer upon him a consent which is not for his benefit but for our own." In any case, from these considerations, Professor Daube drew a strict conclusion: "No person under any restraint whatsoever should be allowed to give consent"; "a person under restraint cannot be presumed to consent." [47] These statements—as we shall see in a moment—are applicable as well to children in institutions.

But the reasons so far cited that lend support to this sweeping conclusion are not adequate, unless imprisonment means that a man has been altogether drummed out of the human community. Since it does not, one might argue for quite the opposite conclusion. It can be contended that since we have deprived a prisoner of a large number of his consents, we should yield to his consent to do good if it is an understanding, voluntary consent. It can be contended that there are dignity and responsibilities consonant with prison life, and that under proper precautions participation in medical experimentation may be among them.

Interwoven with these considerations, however, was another that was more convincing. As Professor Daube put it: "Not all prison authorities throughout the world deserve the fullest trust"; ". . . it would be fatal to lower standards in an indirect manner, however laudable the purposes"; "I have no doubt that 99 out of 100 prisoners would have done this freely, but I wouldn't take the chance on the 100th." [48]

Dr. T. E. Starzl, and the other transplant surgeons at the University of Colorado, had used prisoner donors. He remained convinced of the *voluntariness* of their action. The program was announced in a low key, by a simple notice on the bulletin board of the prison. No pay or pardon or reduction of length of servitude was offered, and none was given. The incidence of enlistment was low. Many of those who volunteered had only a few weeks or months left to serve. These facts support the view that the prisoners' actions were volitional. They also lead us to question again whether the opportunity to make this consent should be withheld from prisoners if it is an opportunity to be presented to anyone. Still, Dr. Starzl was

47. Wolstenholme and O'Connor, *Ethics in Medical Progress,* pp. 198, 204, 205, 197, 204.
48. Ibid., pp. 198, 204

persuaded by Professor Daube for the reason stated above, and the practice was discontinued. Dr. Starzl summarized the argument very well indeed: "The use of penal volunteers, however equitably handled in a local situation, would inevitably lead to abuse if accepted as a reasonable precedent and applied broadly." [49]

This asks and gives one answer to the question: Which rule of medical practice or institutional practice, if widely adopted, can be foreseen to lead on the whole to the violation of men and to their self-violation, even if this need not be the case in each instance? Where, for example, the payment of money for blood tissue is practiced, and prisoners are not excluded from this payment, one does not have to travel far even in this enlightened land to hear rumors that local or state politicians have a concession or a kickback on the prisoner blood supply! That is wrong and was predictable, even if payment, and payment to prisoners, is not wrong in each instance.

To return to the question of investigations involving children in institutions as subjects in trials having no relation to their care, we can now say that even if this would not be (as I have argued) inherently or always necessarily wrong, still the use of captive populations of children, however equitably and safely handled in a local situation, would inevitably lead to abuse if accepted as a reasonable precedent and applied broadly. A rule of practice prohibiting the use of children in institutions simply as experimental subjects in the accumulation of knowledge for the benefit of others should govern the institutions set up to care for them. Some philosophers would call this a rule-utilitarian-rule. It is rather a rule of fidelity, expressing in a specific practice mankind's minimum loyalty to children.

The Kefauver-Harris amendments to the Federal Food, Drug, and Cosmetic Act passed in 1962 do not so rule; and the use of captive populations of children in pharmacological investigations is a practice that is not only widespread but predictably abused in this country. The bill that went before Congress for vote contained no provision for patient or subject consent. Senator Jacob Javits proposed to amend the bill to require that in investigations of a new drug the patients or subjects be "appropriately advised that such drug had not been determined to be safe in use for human beings."

49. Ibid., pp. 75–77.

The outcome of debate in the House and Senate was to make subject consent mandatory while lodging the certification of this in the investigators, not in the Food and Drug Administration. The provision finally enacted introduced proxy consent and two exceptions to the procuring of consent. As finally adopted the provision requires:

> . . . that experts using such drugs for investigational purposes certify to such manufacturer or sponsor that they will inform any human beings to whom such drugs, or any controls used in connection therewith, are being administered, or their representatives, that such drugs are being used for investigational purposes and will obtain the consent of such human beings or their representatives, except [1] where they deem it not feasible or, [2] in their professional judgment, contrary to the best interests of such human beings.[50]

The first interpretative ruling by the FDA concerning this consent requirement was not issued until August 30, 1966. Meantime, a number of investigators had thought that "not feasible" allowed them to dispense with consent if this inconvenienced the research design. In short, the provision was thought to have enacted the supremacy of *another* duty of medical experimenters, namely, to ensure that the quality of the research design is such as to secure the scientific results being sought.

The 1966 interpretative ruling, however, limited the intention of this stipulation to care for the patients or subjects consenting to drug investigations. It adopted the distinction in the Helsinki Declaration between research primarily for the accumulation of knowledge and research in therapeutic situations. No exception to the requirement of consent of the subject or his representative was allowed in the first instance. The two exceptions applied only to research having patient care primarily in view. Finally, the meaning of these exceptions was determined largely by reference to the debates in the House and Senate in 1962. "Not feasible" meant patients in coma or patients otherwise incapable of consenting whose legal representative was unavailable in an emergency. "Contrary to the best interests of such human beings" was meant to permit beneficial

50. Federal Food, Drug, and Cosmetic Act, Section 505 (i).

investigations on, for example, cancer patients without upsetting such a patient's well-being when in a physician's discretion the patient does not know he has cancer.[51]

This interpretative ruling concerning the meaning of these exceptions is dangerous if it is taken to sanction unrelated experimentation on the seriously ill or the dying without the patient's prior participatory consent. But the main thing to be said is that these stipulations are largely irrelevant to drug research. The interpretation of the "exceptions" followed the debate in Congress; but that debate about seriously ill and dying patients was also largely irrelevant to the majority of drug research. Therefore, even after these interpretations were issued, it could fairly be said of the FDA "exceptions": "Better loopholes may be invented, but this seems a good start." [52] However, seriously ill or dying patients may need an insufficiently tested drug. Then medical ethics would require that the efficacy of the new drug be predictable with some confidence; it must be more likely to work than an established remedy. But we may allow that in the course of new-drug investigations there may be cases in which, all other therapies having failed or estimated to be likely to prove less beneficial than the new drug, a patient's consent can be constructively implied as the basis of Good Samaritan emergency treatment.

Ordinarily, however, drug research is more deliberate and preplanned. What is needed are human beings willing to consent to take the drugs or to serve as anonymous controls. What is needed is an easily controlled population. The legal representative of children in institutions would ordinarily be available, if he is to be vested with the power to consent for them but not in their medical behalf. The children themselves are ordinarily under no necessity to have the drug used without delay. Reference to the use of drugs in emergencies among the specifications of a law governing investigations in drugs is exceedingly likely to come to mean that anything that delays the solution of medical problems is unethical. The research consequences are likely to become overriding. This may

51. For a full analysis of the FDA legislation and rulings, see William J. Curran, "Governmental Regulation of the Use of Human Subjects in Medical Research: The Approach of Two Federal Agencies," Ethical Aspects of Experimentation with Human Subjects, *Daedalus*, Spring 1969, pp. 552–70.

52. Oscar D. Ratnoff and Marian F. Ratnoff, "Ethical Responsibilities in Clinical Investigation," *Perspectives in Biology and Medicine*, Autumn 1967, p. 89.

happen if investigators are tempted to transfer the exceptions to the consent requirement in cases of beneficial (emergency) research to the bulk of drug research, which is nonbeneficial, and which should proceed only with the understanding of the subject. The crux, therefore, is the admission that a subject's consent can be satisfied by *his representative*.[53] This opens the door to the use of children in institutions for experimental purposes and not for drug testing that is incidental to the course of their medical care.

In 1958 and 1959 the *New England Journal of Medicine* reported a series of experiments performed upon patients and new admittees to the Willowbrook State School, a home for retarded children in Staten Island, New York.[54] These experiments were described as "an attempt to control the high prevalence of infectious hepatitis in an institution for mentally defective patients." The experiments were said to be justified because, under conditions of an existing controlled outbreak of hepatitis in the institution, "knowledge obtained from a series of suitable studies could well lead to its control." In actuality, the experiments were designed to duplicate and confirm the efficacy of gamma globulin in immunization against hepatitis, to develop and improve or improve upon that inoculum, and to learn more about infectious hepatitis in general.

The experiments were justified—doubtless, after a great deal of soul searching—for the following reasons: there was a smoldering

53. By contrast, the statement on "Clinical Investigations Using Human Beings as Subject" issued by the U.S. Public Health Service severely limits the consent of such human beings' legal representatives. "No subject may participate in an investigative procedure," it says, "unless: (a) He is mentally competent and has sufficient mental and communicative capacity to understand his choice to participate; and (b) He is 21 years of age or more, except that if the individual be less than 21, he may participate in a procedure intended and designed to protect or improve his personal health or otherwise for his personal benefit or advantage if the informed written consent of his parents or legal guardian be obtained as well as the written consent of the subject himself if he be mature enough to appreciate the nature of the procedure and the risks involved" (Department of Health, Education and Welfare, Bureau of Medical Services Circular No. 38, June 23, 1966).

54. Robert Ward, Saul Krugman, Joan P. Giles, A. Milton Jacobs, and Oscar Bodansky, "Infectious Hepatitis: Studies of Its Natural History and Prevention," *New England Journal of Medicine* 258, no. 9 (February 27, 1958): 407–16; Saul Krugman, Robert Ward, Joan P. Giles, Oscar Bodansky, and A. Milton Jacobs, "Infectious Hepatitis: Detection of the Virus during the Incubation Period and in Clinically Inapparent Infection," *New England Journal of Medicine* 261, no. 15 (October 8, 1959): 729–34. The following account and unannotated quotations are taken from these articles.

epidemic throughout the institution and "it was apparent that most of the patients at Willowbrook were naturally exposed to hepatitis virus"; infectious hepatitis is a much milder disease in children; the strain at Willowbrook was especially mild; only the strain or strains of the virus already disseminated at Willowbrook were used: and only those small and incompetent patients whose parents gave consent were used.

The patient population at Willowbrook was 4478, growing at a rate of one patient a day over a three-year span, or from 10 to 15 new admissions per week. In the first trial the existing population was divided into two groups: one group served as uninoculated controls, and the other group was inoculated with 0.01 ml. of gamma globulin per pound of body weight. Then for a second trial new admittees and those left uninoculated before were again divided: one group served as uninoculated controls and the other was inoculated with 0.06 ml. of gamma globulin per pound of body weight. This proved that Stokes et al. had correctly demonstrated that the larger amount would give significant immunity for up to seven or eight months.[55]

Serious ethical questions may be raised about the trials so far described. No mention is made of any attempt to enlist the adult personnel of the institution, numbering nearly 1,000 including nearly 600 attendants on ward duty, and new additions to the staff, in these studies whose excusing reason was that almost everyone was "naturally" exposed to the Willowbrook virus. Nothing requires that major research into the natural history of hepatitis be first undertaken in children. Experiments have been carried out in the military and with prisoners as subjects. There have been fatalities from the experiments; but surely in all these cases the consent of the volunteers was as valid or better than the proxy consent of these children's "representatives." There would have been no question of

55. J. Stokes, Jr., et al., "Infectious Hepatitis: Length of Protection by Immune Serum Globulin (Gamma Globulin) during Epidemics," *Journal of the American Medical Association* 147 (1951): 714–19. Since the half-life of gamma globulin is three weeks, no one knows exactly why it immunizes for so long a period. The "highly significant protection against hepatitis obtained by the use of gamma globulin," however, had been confirmed as early as 1945 (see Edward B. Grossman, Sloan G. Stewart, and Joseph Stokes, "Post-Transfusion Hepatitis in Battle Casualties," *Journal of the American Medical Association* 129, no. 15 [December 8, 1945]: 991–94). The inoculation *withheld* in the Willowbrook experiments had, therefore, proved valuable.

the understanding consent that might have been given by the adult personnel at Willowbrook, if significant benefits were expected from studying that virus.

Second, nothing is said that would warrant withholding an inoculation of some degree of known efficacy from part of the population, or for withholding in the first trial less than the full amount of gamma globulin that had served to immunize in previous tests, except the need to test, confirm, and improve the inoculum. That, of course, was a desirable goal; but it does not seem possible to warrant withholding gamma globulin for the reason that is often said to justify controlled trials, namely, that one procedure is *as likely* to succeed as the other.

Third, nothing is said about attempts to control or defeat the low-grade epidemic at Willowbrook by more ordinary, if more costly and less experimental, procedures. Nor is anything said about admitting no more patients until this goal had been accomplished. This was not a massive urban hospital whose teeming population would have to be turned out into the streets, with resulting dangers to themselves and to public health, in order to sanitize the place. Instead, between 200 and 250 patients were housed in each of 18 buildings over approximately 400 acres in a semirural setting of fields, woods, and well-kept, spacious lawns. Clearly it would have been possible to secure other accommodation for new admissions away from the infection, while eradicating the infection at Willowbrook building by building. This might have cost money, and it would certainly have required astute detective work to discover the source of the infection. The doctors determined that the new patients likely were not carrying the infection upon admission, and that it did not arise from the procedures and routine inoculations given them at the time of admission. Why not go further in the search for the source of the epidemic? If this had been an orphanage for normal children or a floor of private patients, instead of a school for mentally defective children, one wonders whether the doctors would so readily have accepted the hepatitis as a "natural" occurrence and even as an opportunity for study.

The next step was to attempt to induce "passive-active immunity" by feeding the virus to patients already protected by gamma globulin. In this attempt to improve the inoculum, permission was obtained from the parents of children from 5 to 10 years of age newly admitted to Willowbrook, who were then isolated from contact with the rest of the institution. All were inoculated with gamma globulin and then divided into two groups: one served as controls while the other group of new patients were fed the Willowbrook virus, obtained from feces, in doses having 50 percent infectivity, i.e., in concentrations estimated to produce hepatitis with jaundice in half the subjects tested. Then twice the 50 percent infectivity was tried. This proved, among other things, that hepatitis has an "alimentary-tract phase" in which it can be transmitted from one person to another while still "inapparent" in the first person. This, doubtless, is exceedingly important information in learning how to control epidemics of infectious hepatitis. The second of the two articles mentioned above describes studies of the incubation period of the virus and of whether pooled serum remained infectious when aged and frozen. Still the small, mentally defective patients who were deliberately fed infectious hepatitis are described as having suffered mildly in most cases: "The liver became enlarged in the majority, occasionally a week or two before the onset of jaundice. Vomiting and anorexia usually lasted only a few days. Most of the children gained weight during the course of hepatitis."

That mild description of what happened to the children who were fed hepatitis (and who continued to be introduced into the unaltered environment of Willowbrook) is itself alarming, since it is now definitely known that cirrhosis of the liver results from infectious hepatitis more frequently than from excessive consumption of alcohol! Now, or in 1958 and 1959, no one knows what may be other serious consequences of contracting infectious hepatitis. Understanding human volunteers were then and are now needed in the study of this disease, although a South American monkey has now successfully been given a form of hepatitis, and can henceforth serve as our ally in its conquest. But not children who cannot consent knowingly. If Peace Corps workers are regularly given gamma globulin before going abroad as a guard against their contracting hepatitis, and are inoculated at intervals thereafter, it seems that this is the least we should do for mentally defective children before they "go abroad" to Willowbrook or other institutions set up for their care.

Discussions pro and con of the Willowbrook experiments that have come to my attention serve only to reinforce the ethical objections that can be raised against what was done simply from a careful analysis of the original articles reporting the research design and findings. In an address at the 1968 Ross Conference on Pediatric Research, Dr. Saul Krugman raised the question, Should vaccine trials be carried out in adult volunteers before subjecting children to similar tests? [56] He answered this question in the negative. The reason adduced was simply that "a vaccine virus trial may be a more hazardous procedure for adults than for children." Medical researchers, of course, are required to minimize the hazards, but not by moving from consenting to unconsenting subjects. This apology clearly shows that adults and children have become interchangeable in face of the overriding importance of obtaining the research goal. This means that the special moral claims of children for care and protection are forgotten, and especially the claims of children who are most weak and vulnerable. (Krugman's reference to the measles vaccine trials is not to the point.)

The *Medical Tribune* explains that the 16-bed isolation unit set up at Willowbrook served "to protect the study subjects from Willowbrook's other endemic diseases—such as shigellosis, measles, rubella and respiratory and parasitic infections—while exposing them to hepatitis." [57] This presumably compensated for the infection they were given. It is not convincingly shown that the children could by no means, however costly, have been protected from the epidemic of hepatitis. The statement that Willowbrook "had endemic infectious hepatitis and a sufficiently open population so that the disease could never be quieted by exhausting the supply of susceptibles" is at best enigmatic.

Oddly, physicians defending the propriety of the Willowbrook hepatitis project soon begin talking like poorly instructed "natural lawyers"! Dr. Louis Lasagna and Dr. Geoffrey Edsall, for example, find these experiments unobjectionable—both, for the reason stated

56. Saul Krugman, "Reflections on Pediatric Clinical Investigations," in *Problems of Drug Evaluation in Infants and Children,* Report of the Fifty-eighth Ross Conference on Pediatric Research, Dorado Beach, Puerto Rico, May 5–7, 1968 (Columbus: Ross Laboratories), pp. 41–42.

57. "Studies with Children Backed on Medical, Ethical Grounds," *Medical Tribune and Medical News* 8, no. 19 (February 20, 1967): 1, 23.

by Edsall: "the children would apparently incur no greater risk than they were likely to run by nature." In any case, Edsall's examples of parents consenting with a son 17 years of age for him to go to war, and society's agreement with minors that they can drive cars and hurt themselves were entirely beside the point. Dr. David D. Rutstein adheres to a stricter standard in regard to research on infectious hepatitis: "It is not ethical to use human subjects for the growth of a virus for any purpose." [58]

The latter sweeping verdict may depend on knowledge of the effects of viruses on chromasomal difficulties, mongolism, etc., that was not available to the Willowbrook group when their researches were begun thirteen years ago. If so, this is a telling point against appeal to "no discernible risks" as the sole standard applicable to the use of children in medical experimentation. That would lend support to the proposition that we always know that there are unknown and undiscerned risks in the case of an invasion of the fortress of the body—which then can be consented to by an adult in behalf of a child only if it is in the child's behalf medically.

When asked what she told the parents of the subject-children at Willowbrook, Dr. Joan Giles replied, "I explain that there is no vaccine against infectious hepatitis. . . . I also tell them that we can modify the disease with gamma globulin but we can't provide lasting immunity without letting them get the disease." [59] Obviously vaccines giving "lasting immunity" are not the only kinds of vaccine to be used in caring for patients.

Doubtless the studies at Willowbrook resulted in improvement in the vaccine, to the benefit of present and future patients. In

58. *Daedalus*, Spring 1969, pp. 471–72, 529. See also pp. 458, 470–72. Since it is the proper business of an ethicist to uphold the proposition that only retrogression in civility can result from bad moral reasoning and the use of inept examples, however innocent, it is fair to point out the startling comparison between Edsall's "argument" and the statement of Dr. Karl Brandt, plenipotentiary in charge of all medical activities in the Nazi Reich: "Do you think that one can obtain any worth-while, fundamental results without a definite toll of lives? The same goes for technological development. You cannot build a great bridge, a gigantic building—you cannot establish a speed record without deaths!" (quoted by Leo Alexander, "War Crimes: Their Social-Psychological Aspects," *American Journal of Psychiatry* 105, no. 3 [September 1948]: 172). Casualties to progress, or injuries accepted in setting speed limits, are morally quite different from death or maiming or even only risks, or unknown risks, directly and deliberately imposed upon an unconsenting human being.

59. *Medical Tribune*, February 20, 1967, p. 23.

September 1966, "a routine program of GG [gamma gobulin] administration to every new patient at Willowbrook" was begun. This cut the incidence of icteric hepatitis 80 to 85 percent. Then follows a significant statement in the *Medical Tribune* article: "A similar reduction in the icteric form of the disease has been accomplished among the employees, who began getting routine GG earlier in the study." [60] Not only did the research team (so far as these reports show) fail to consider and adopt the alternative that new admittees to the staff be asked to become volunteers for an investigation that might improve the vaccine against the strand of infectious hepatitis to which they as well as the children were exposed. Instead, the staff was routinely protected earlier than the inmates were! And, as we have seen, there was evidence from the beginning that gamma gobulin provided at least some protection. A "modification" of the disease was still an inoculum, even if this provided no lasting immunization and had to be repeated. It is axiomatic to medical ethics that a known remedy or protection—even if not perfect or even if the best exact administration of it has not been proved—should not be withheld from individual patients. It seems to a layman that from the beginning various trials at immunization of all new admittees might have been made, and controlled observation made of their different degrees of effectiveness against "nature" at Willowbrook. This would doubtless have been a longer way round, namely, the "anecdotal" method of investigative treatment that comes off second best in comparison with controlled trials. Yet this seems to be the alternative dictated by our received medical ethics, and the only one expressive of minimal care of the primary patients themselves.

Finally, except for one episode the obtaining of parental consent (on the premise that this is ethically valid) seems to have been very well handled. Wards of the state were not used, though by law the administrator at Willowbrook could have signed consent for them. Only new admittees whose parents were available were entered by proxy consent into the project. Explanation was made to groups of these parents, and they were given time to think about it and consult with their own family physicians.[61] Then late in 1964 Willow-

---

60. *Medical Tribune*, February 20, 1967, p. 23.
61. Krugman, "Reflections on Pediatric Clinical Investigations," p. 41–42.

brook was closed to all new admissions because of overcrowding. What then happened can most impartially be described in the words of an article defending the Willowbrook project on medical and ethical grounds:

> Parents who applied for their children to get in were sent a form letter over Dr. Hammond's signature saying that there was no space for new admissions and that their name was being put on a waiting list.
>
> But the hepatitis program, occupying its own space in the institution, continued to admit new patients as each new study group began. "Where do you find new admissions except by canvassing the people who have applied for admission?" Dr. Hammond asked.
>
> So a new batch of form letters went out, saying that there were a few vacancies in the hepatitis research unit if the parents cared to consider volunteering their child for that.
>
> In some instances the second form letter apparently was received as closely as a week after the first letter arrived.[62]

Granting—as I do not—the validity of parental consent to research upon children not in their behalf medically, what sort of consent was that? Surely, the duress upon these parents with children so defective as to require institutionalization was far greater than the duress on prisoners given tobacco or paid or promised parole for their cooperation! I grant that the timing of these events was inadvertent. Since, however, ethics is a matter of criticizing institutions and not only of exculpating or making culprits of individual men, the inadvertence does not matter. This is the strongest possible argument for saying that even if parents have the right to consent to submit the children who are directly and continuously in their care to nonbeneficial medical experimentation, this should not be the rule of practice governing institutions set up for their care.

Such use of captive populations of children for purely experimental purposes ought to be made legally impossible. My view is that this should be stopped by legal acknowledgment of the moral invalidity of parental or legal proxy consent for the child to procedures having no relation to a child's own diagnosis or treatment.

62. *Medical Tribune*, February 20, 1967, p. 23.

If this is not done, canons of loyalty require that the rule of practice (by law, or otherwise) be that children in institutions and not directly under the care of parents or relatives should *never* be used in medical investigations having present pain or discomfort and unknown present and future risks to them, and promising future possible benefits only for others.

In 1967, after a study of twenty-one New York City municipal hospitals, State Senator Seymour R. Thaler proposed an amendment to the New York State Civil Rights bill that would apply sweepingly to all medical research and to all research involving children as subjects. Some of the provisions of his amendment could be applied more narrowly to captive populations of children. Senator Thaler would require the "voluntary informed written consent of adult patients used in medical experiment and would prohibit research on children unless authorized by a 'court of competent jurisdiction.'" His bill stipulated that the court may authorize a medical experiment or other medical research upon a minor when such experiment or research is related to the minor's physical or mental ailment and upon a finding by the court that the best interests of the minor would thereby be served. It was the provision placing all research upon children under courts of competent jurisdiction that caused the furor. Dr. Saul Krugman, chairman of pediatrics at New York University, called the bill "a disaster—a real disaster," if passed.[63]

The version of this bill introduced by Senators Thaler and Lent in 1969 does not entirely invalidate parental consent. This, however, is set within the context of the creation of a state board on human research charged with responsibility to formulate rules and regulations and to require the establishment of institutional and regional screening committees. The bill provides that "no person shall be used in human research without his or his parent's, guardian's or legal representative's prior written informed consent, but the board may make such exceptions as it may prescribe where the proposed subject is incompetent to give such consent . . ."[64]

63. *New York Times*, January 20, 1967. Krugman was one of the physicians who conducted the Willowbrook experiments.

64. An Act To Amend the Education Law, in Relation to the Regulation of Research on Human Subjects, in Senate, 1969–70 Regular Session, Cal. No. 1865, 4652–A, February 14, 1969.

The objection to this legislation can be only the resistance of researchers to the development of public policy in this regard, by law and through regulatory agencies. There are more regulations governing animal experimentation than govern human experimentation; more laws regulating the interstate transportation of bodies than regulate the interstate transportation of dying patients (who may be eligible organ donors when they are pronounced dead); a great mass of case law having to do with medical negligence in cases of treatment but little that deals with investigations primarily for the accumulation of knowledge. This situation is not likely long to endure.

For this reason, let us look briefly at another attempt to draft appropriate legislation—this time not by a state senator but by Frank P. Grad, Adjunct Professor of Legislation and Associate Director of the Legislative Drafting Research Fund at Columbia University Law School. In a paper before a conference sponsored by the New York Academy of Sciences, Professor Grad stated the principle that runs throughout our legal and moral tradition. "The rationale," he wrote, "which allows parents or guardians to consent on behalf of their children or wards in the therapeutic situation are not clearly applicable to the non-therapeutic one. . . . There is no clear reason why a parent should be given the power to consent to expose his child to a risk, where taking the risk is not clearly in the child's interest or for his benefit. Nor is there any reason why a lawyer-guardian sitting in his downtown office ought to be free to expose his incompetent ward in a state hospital to hazards which he has neither chosen, nor which he has the competency to choose, for himself. Consent on behalf of minors and incompetents has, therefore, been rather closely circumscribed." [65]

But in the model legislation accompanying his paper, Professor Grad suggested the unqualified enactment of this principle only in

65. Frank P. Grad, "Regulation of Clinical Research by the State," Conference on New Dimensions in Legal and Ethical Concepts for Human Research, New York Academy of Sciences, New York City, May 19–21, 1969. Professor Grad resolved the alleged problem of drawing the line between therapeutic and nontherapeutic research by imagining a patient to ask: "'Doctor, are you doing this for me, or am I doing this for you?' If the physician can truthfully answer that he is doing it for the patient, then it is clearly therapeutic research. If, on the contrary, the subject is undergoing a particular procedure not for his own benefit but for that of the re-

the case of incompetents other than children as such. "Valid consent for an incompetent to become a subject may be given by his legal guardian," the draft legislation reads, "only if the human experimentation or research bears directly upon such incompetent's disability." That statement might have been repeated with regard to subjects judged incompetent for reasons of age. Instead, the draft reads: "Valid consent for a person under the age of eighteen years may be given by his parent or legal guardian only if there is no reason to believe that the human experimentation or research will result in physical or psychological injury or harm."

In other words, these legislative proposals would bring under public scrutiny both the parental consents obtained and the physiologically describable acts to be used in medical research. Neither would actually rule out the power of the consent of parents to enter their children into nontherapeutic medical trials. I suggest that— short of prohibiting the latter—our legislation would still need to go further than these proposals. Parental responsibility is necessarily weakened when children are institutionalized, when they are no longer directly, daily, and continuously under our care.

If we are going to count on parental and familial consent as sufficient protection of child-life, this should be only when parents are constantly placed on their mettle in the daily life of the home. If we then fail our children, this may be, as Professor Daube said, among the normal burdens, hazards, and dignity of a child's daily life. But surely we have the wisdom to know that even ordinary parental care must slacken when children are away in institutions; this is even more true when parents grievously need to place a child in an institution in order to provide at all for his care.

If, then, we are not going to invalidate the consents of parents and relatives except in the case of investigations proximately or remotely related to a child's own treatment, there can be no valid argument against doing exactly this in the limited case of children in orphanages, reformatories, or homes for the retarded. The legal

---

searcher in the pursuit of a scientific goal, then the procedure is non-therapeutic." The thesis of this chapter is that since the child-patient cannot ask that question, what he is doing for the researcher is simply being done to him, while what is done to him by way of treatment or investigational treatment, with legitimate parental or guardian consent or by his implied consent, has the patient as an end in view.

representatives of such children—even if parents—should be able to make decisions only in the stated medical interests of the children themselves if they are part of a captive population. To require a showing that this in fact is what is being done would be a proper additional arrangement guaranteeing that institutions for the care of children exist in fact only to care for them according to the canons of the highest loyalty, and not for the accumulation of knowledge having no stated benefit to these children themselves. Then parents and medical experimentation in general in the case of children might be moved to come up to the standards of our institutions.

2

On Updating Procedures for Stating That a Man Has Died

Death must be held compatible with heartbeat and circulation artificially maintained.

Helen Lane died of cancer more than fifteen years ago. Yet she is living, in the cellular meaning of life, and today she is still called by her proper name in laboratories all over the world. Cancer researchers use the logo "HeLa" for this line of cells, composed of the first two letters of the two names by which Helen Lane was known and addressed when otherwise alive. This woman's cells live on, each having the genotype that constituted all her generic and individual attributes; and in a sense she still has the cancer that once was said to have caused her death. It was Dr. George Gey of Johns Hopkins University who bestowed upon her this factitious "immortality" and, it may well be, the capacity for her life to be of unique service to humanity long after her "moment of death." Thus, Helen Lane today is probably the most ubiquitous human being in the world, at least since the Lutherans declared that the risen body of Christ possesses the attribute of omnipresence belonging before to God the Father!

The Challenge to Old-Fashioned Death

But cellular life is not what we mean by being alive. To pronounce someone dead never waited for cellular death finally to occur. Life means the functioning of the integrated being or physiological organism as in some sense a whole. Death means the cessation of this functioning. This in turn depends on the integrated functioning of certain great organ systems.

In the past death meant, clinically, the irreparable cessation of spontaneous cardiac activity and spontaneous respiratory activity. The abolition of the functions of heart and lungs were required be-

fore anyone was pronounced dead. The death of other great organ
systems, such as the liver or kidneys, or the destruction of the brain,
caused the death of the individual through its fatal effect upon the
functions of heart and lungs.

A physician checked by the means available to him. He did
this by observing the movement of breathing in the patient or by
using a mirror to detect slight emissions of breath; by listening for
the heartbeat or by electrocardiogram. Brain life or the life of the
central nervous system was determined crudely, by reflex actions or
by looking at the wound. It remains the case that the determination
that "clinical death" has occurred depends on what clinic you are
in.

This definition of death may be significantly changed by the end
of this decade. An increasing number of experts and committees
of medical faculties or associations are calling for an updating of
the meaning of death—or, if not for revision in the clinical concept
of the moment of or the meaning of death, for an updating of the
clinical tests for determining that a patient has died. Some have
suggested that the perfection of the electroencephalograph makes it
possible to add brain death to the cessation of spontaneous respiration and circulation in determining that death has occurred, or even
to shift decisively or altogether to a concept of brain death.

The definition of life in terms of heart and lungs and brain
reminds us of the primitive psychophysiology of the Bible. The
difference is that a few more organ systems were included in this
ancient account of what it means to be a man alive. Prophet and
psalmist pray God to "try the reins," i.e., the kidneys, the site of
conscience. Deuteronomy 12:23 declares that "the blood is the life";
and Leviticus 17:14, that "the life of all flesh is the blood thereof."
The Scriptures frequently speak of men's "bowels of compassion."
And men are commanded to love the Lord their God with all their
hearts, souls, minds, and strength. This primitive psychology dis-
tributing the capacities of man to the various organ systems was not
only figuratively but literally meant; not only literally meant but
figuratively—for everyone of the capacities of men who are flesh.
Everywhere it was *the life* that was at issue. The Scriptures know
no life that is not embodied life; no man whose life is not (in
Karl Barth's terms) the soul (the subject) of his body, and the body

of his soul. Neither does a contemporary physician know any other life in the practice of medicine and the care of his patients (whatever else he may say or think about the "soul"). In this sense no Biblical theologian should take umbrage at the suggestion that a pronouncement of death is a medical question. What personal life do we know except within the ambience of a bodily existence? What other death do we know?—whether or not the responsibility for pronouncing death should be lodged solely with physicians.

Therefore, I venture to say that Isaiah or Jeremiah would have understood the problem that came upon us dramatically in the late 60's of the twentieth century when tissue transplantation finally reached the heart. Why should this have caused such a stir? The transplantation of the heart is only the most recent achievement in the use of human tissues in medical practice with its supporting medical research for the past four or five decades.[1] It is an interesting question why the transplantation of the heart aroused so much more discussion, and indeed controversy, than was the case in regard to other vital organs.

The answer to this question is deeper than sentiment. There was sentiment enough. The site of love and the habitat of the soul—celebrated in the poetry and psalms of all ages—had now been replaced by a simple pump. What is man now that his heart has been reduced to a replaceable muscle? Lord Byron (hightailing it out of Athens) could write: "Maid of Athens, ere we part / Give, O give, me back my heart / Or, since that has left my breast, / Keep it now and take the rest." The heart seemed an appropriate part to take for the whole, for the essential Byron. It would not have sounded the same if he had said, "Maid of Athens, ere we sever / Give, O give me back my liver"! Yet the liver is physiologically no less necessary than the heart for there to be life or any human being.

1. The remarkable story of the research and development of tissue transplantation is told in Francis D. Moore, *Give and Take: The Development of Tissue Transplantation* (Philadelphia and London: Saunders, 1964), and in Harold M. Schmeck, Jr., *The Semi-Artificial Man: A Dawning Revolution in Medicine* (New York: Walker, 1965). Dr. Moore is Moseley Professor of Surgery, Harvard Medical School, and Surgeon-in-Chief at Peter Bent Brigham Hospital in Boston, Massachusetts. Mr. Schmeck, a science writer for the *New York Times,* also gives a readable and (despite the sensationalism of the title) an informative and scientifically sound account of the medical investigations, trials, and accomplishments that together have achieved in recent years an increasing success in organ repair and transplantation.

Beyond sentiment, it is life that has palpably been touched, and our understanding of life and death has been put in question. The astonishment as well as the concern that arose at once over the news of the first heart transplant is to be explained by the fact that the heart is an unpaired organ whose functioning along with that of other vital organs is our life, and by the fact that it is an unpaired organ that "ticks." Because we feel its functioning, the heart has for us a significance that, for example, the liver (another unpaired and equally indispensable organ) does not have. This is paralleled only by respiratory functioning, which gives the lungs a significance that similarly paired organs (e.g., the kidneys) do not have. Thus, in human experience the "heart" and the "breath of life" have an importance that is attested to both by ancient lore and by the heart-lung machine. We feel both our breathing and our heartbeat; and, by comparison at least, we are only vaguely aware of the functioning of other great organ systems that may also constitute our being alive. Heart and lungs are the only organs whose cessation of function is perceived to lead to immediate death. It takes a greater sophistication to learn the central importance of the brain, for example, or to be persuaded to shift our concept of the meaning of life and death to brain life and brain death. This is what I mean by saying that because the heart is an unpaired organ that "ticks" it is understandable that grave human questions arose—questions of the meaning of life and death—when the heart was transplanted.

Perhaps in principle these same questions were raised by open heart surgery, by the heart-lung machine, and by the insertion of artificial cardiac valves—in which procedures also the heart may be stopped for hours and started again. Still it required the transplantation of the heart-pump from one human being to another to heighten the imagination to apprehend what may be at issue in all these procedures. What we apprehend, however, by means of heightened imagination is the same thing, namely, the question of whether heart function can or should be eliminated from the definition of being alive and being dead. This is the reason a number of proposals for updating the meaning of death have been stimulated by, or found their occasion in, the transplantation of hearts. This seemed to strike at the foundations of not only medical definitions of life and death but as well of a more ancient wisdom concerning the life and the acceptable death of all flesh. Only a mechanical notion (if such a notion could be deeply held and felt "along the pulses") that man's embodied life consists of an ensemble of "parts" would not have been shaken. That notion is gaining on us.

What Death Is and Telling That Death Has Occurred

To enter this discussion it is essential to separate the concept of death from the problem of determining the moment of death. It is also essential to separate the concept of death from the problem of establishing the procedures for stating or pronouncing death on the basis of any one concept.[2] We should not confuse the definition of what death is with the problematics of whether there is a moment when death occurs. Neither should we confuse the definition of what death is with a discussion of the methods by which it shall be determined that death has occurred. These are not the same questions, and when we understand that they are not we shall see that the meaning of death may be radically revised or updated while the criteria or the procedures for determining whether death (on any one understanding of it) has occurred may still include some refinements of rather old-fashioned clinical tests.

No doubt there are various levels of death (clinical death, physiological death, organ death, cellular death). No doubt also life and death fall within the continuum of all life's processes. In one sense no life has begun since three billion years ago, nor has any life died. (Not even cremation—which in the ecology of life on this planet has been compared to an organic farmer burning his leaves— succeeds in transforming life without remainder into inorganic matter.) No doubt also the individual dies biologically by degrees, and the "moment" of death is only a useful fiction.

These facts are not crucial when, in a medical-ethical context, we ask the meaning of life and death. This is to ask when in the continuum of the beginning of life there is a human life among us, and when in the continuum of the dying process there is a life still among us who lays claim to the immunities, respect, and protection which in ethics and/or by law are accorded by men to a fellow man. Even if the "moment" of death is actually a span of time, pronounce-

2. Gunnar Biörck, "On the Definitions of Death," *World Medical Journal* 14 (1967): 138.

ment of death has this significance: that we need some procedure
for determining when a life is still with us, making its moral claims
upon us, and when we stand instead in the presence of an unburied
corpse. If it is a fiction,[3] the "moment" of death has this signal
usefulness: that by a declaration of death a concept of what life is
and of what death is are applied in an actual judgment to particular
cases. If dying is actually a process, our situation in regard to life and
death is simply that to which Dr. Johnson pointed when he said
that the fact of twilight does not abolish the distinction we are able
to make between daylight and darkness.

No more should the definition of what death is be confused with
the methods by which it shall be determined that death has occurred. One of these may undergo change without changing the
other; or both may be revised in the light of contemporary knowledge. One may update the definition of death to mean brain death
and also propose that brain tests (EEG) be exclusively used, or that
brain tests (EEG) be made controlling in decisions that death has
occurred even when the other spontaneous vital signs are still
present. On the other hand, one may update the concept of death to
mean brain death, while only refining the *criteria* for determining
this and adding brain tests (EEG) to the received clinical indices.
Finally, it is theoretically possible still to hold that life means the
integrated functioning of heart and lungs and brain and to conceive
that death is the permanent disintegration and final stoppage of all
these natural functions, while simply refining the procedures for
determining that death in this sense has occurred.

Even in the face of the EEG, one can define the tests of the life
of the organism as a whole as the intake (lungs), distribution (heart,
the circulation of the blood), and the utilization of oxygen (by all
organs, of which the brain is most vulnerable to anoxia). Centuries
ago this was called the "vital spirit." On this view, death means the
permanent disintegration and cessation of the spontaneous and integrated functions of intake, distribution, and utilization of oxygen.
This may happen within the system beginning with the destruction
of the brain's utilization of oxygen; or it may happen by respiratory
blockage or by cardiac arrest. The destruction of one leads finally
to the abolition of the others of these vital functions. If physiological

3. "The Moment of Death," editorial, *World Medical Journal* 14 (1967): 133.

death means the disintegration and ultimately the total absence of the natural functions of heart and lungs and brain, the clinical signs may still be refined and measured by modern instruments, in addition to other procedures for telling that death has occurred. When all signs are gone, then one knows the "vital spirit" has departed and life as a whole has ceased.

Theoretically there are these three possible ways, in differing combinations, of updating the concept of what death is and also updating our procedures for stating that death has occurred. The first position is the most radical, suggesting that the meaning of death be now understood as brain death and also that the criteria for determining this be shifted exclusively or almost exclusively to the electroencephalograph.[4] This seems to be the view of a number of individual physicians and scientists, and there is widespread public opinion that this is what is going on. However, this view has not been endorsed, so far as I know, by any responsible committees appointed to study this question. The second position would take the meaning of death philosophically to be brain death, but would hold that there are still a number of tests for this in addition to a patient's electroencephalogram taken at designated intervals of time. The third position affirms that the theoretical meaning of death is about what it always was, namely, the permanent disintegration and cessation of heart, lung, and brain activity; but that the tests for determining death in this sense ought to be extensively refined for the protection of physicians and patients alike.

There is a great deal of confusion in the discussion of this question because of a widespread popular misconception that the medical profession is rallying to the first and more radical of these views.

4. On this view that life means brain life, or on any view that assigns even a degree of primacy to the brain as the site of human consciousness, any attempt to maintain a human brain alive (as has been done in animals) in isolation from any body or means of communication and of action (as a prelude to "brain transplants") would be subject to an absolute moral prohibition. The preponderant opinion is that brain transplants are quite impossible, since science cannot implant a brain in a new body and hook it up with that body's senses and its conscious and unconscious activities. My point, however, is an ethical one: men cannot morally get to know whether this can be done or not, since no one should maintain a human being alive in such impenetrable darkness while testing to see whether he can be given new means of bodily contact and communication, and be brought again into the land of living utterances.

Moreover, there is not much difference between the second and third of the foregoing possibilities, if we remember that doctors are not theoreticians debating the meaning of death but practical men primarily concerned to establish agreed-upon procedures for stating that death has occurred. Various sets of criteria are currently being proposed by committees of physicians. The discussion focuses on the procedures for determining that a man has died. Physicians can afford to be nominalists about the meaning of death except as this is a function of the procedural question. While among them as well as the public at large there is a good deal of talk about brain death, it is safe to say that for the medical profession death operationally means what is stated by the use of sound and sufficient criteria for telling when a man has died. These are almost always manifold tests or procedures, not solely brain tests, if by the latter EEG is meant. A careful review of the literature on updating death will show, I believe, that there is widespread misunderstanding of "brain death" conveyed by a number of physicians and certainly present in the public mind.

We should therefore take the current discussions of death to be practical proposals for revising the procedures for stating that death has occurred, and not as discussions of the theoretical meaning of death. So understood, I am emboldened to suggest that the various accounts of how death might better be reckoned are not proposing anything very startling.

If I have not misunderstood the literature on updating death, it may be characterized in the following three ways. (1) Updating death means to clear up a dangerous ambiguity in what has been going on or was reported to have happened in some recent "pronouncements" of death and/or an ambiguity in the medical reports and news reports concerning what was done in actions entailing presumptions of death. (2) Updating death means to reject some legal definitions of death. (3) Updating death means in certain sorts of cases to dismiss machine-driven or artificially maintained signs of life. After showing the validity of each of these descriptions of what the discussion is about, I shall argue for further updating the updating of death—by clearing up a remaining ambiguity concerning when the heart should be said still to beat "spontaneously" or should be deemed no longer to evidence one of the integrated signs of life.

This three-point analysis of what updating death means to say and is actually saying, and my proposal for further clarification, can be exhibited at the outset by a "primitive" case. Suppose a leader of a Boy Scout troop on a three- or four-day hike with them over remote mountain passes. They pause to take a swim. One boy, ignoring the leader's commands, dives from a high cliff, hits his head on a sharp rock, and cleaves his brain in two. Ambulance or oxygen or respirators are nowhere near. The leader applies mouth-to-mouth resuscitation and chest artificial respiration to keep the boy's blood ventilated for hours. Finally he gives up, declaring the boy to be dead.

It would seem strange for him to report to the family that he made this determination solely upon a novel concept of "brain death," from observing the ghastly wound. And if he did this it would then seem strange for him further to alarm the family by saying that he made the determination that the boy was dead (because of the massive brain injury and his failure to restore the boy's ability to respirate) while his heart was still "spontaneously" beating, while he still had an "intact cardiovascular system." Most alarming of all it would be if the Scout leader told Mr. and Mrs. Plimpton that their son was dead from the moment his head struck the rock while the assistant Scout leader reckons he was dead when attempts to respirate ceased and his heart finally failed.

Of course, an observer of those life-saving efforts could say: "Don't stop yet. Keep applying artificial respiration. His heart is still going fine." But that description of the boy, that finding of fact, was wholly enclosed within and dependent upon continuing obedience to the imperative: "Keep respirating him." The observation that his heart still was beating was not an independent ground for the continuation of the effort to save him. It rather resulted from that effort. Once it was determined that respiration was wholly artificial and hopeless, it had already been also determined that the boy's cardiovascular system has no life of its own either. It is misleading to say that the leader stopped respiration while the heart still beat, as misleading as to say that he stopped respiration while the boy still breathed. Of course, in a sense he did both of these things. But the boy was dead in brain and lungs and heart when he did so. If the boy had no recoverable capacity to breathe by himself, he had no recoverable permanent capacity to circulate himself either. Thus, one has only to update the current updatings of death—scotching the rumor that people are going to be declared brain dead while having natural activity of heart and circulation—to effect a return to a rather traditionalistic understanding of the procedure for stating that a man has died.

The difference between this case and hospital cases is only that the Scout leader was exhausted by his efforts, while respirators are inexhaustible in sustaining breathing and, one step removed, the activity of the heart.

Updating Death

DISTINGUISHING THE DEAD FROM THE DYING OR THE "VIRTUALLY" DEAD

First, then, updating death means to clear up a *dangerous and confusing ambiguity*. In the face of the need for salvaging organs, some writers evidently fail to distinguish between the dead and the dying. "When death occurs," one important article says, "or in the alternative when death has been declared inevitable, the circulation and the respiration may be maintained by artificial means" to afford time for surgeons to remove the required organs.[5] These are precisely not alternatives in the justifiable taking of vital organs. To pronounce a condition hopeless is by no means the same as to declare that a patient has died. For the purpose of organ transplant,

5. Carl E. Wasmuth and Bruce H. Steward, "Medical and Legal Aspects of Human Organ Transplantation," *Cleveland-Marshall Law Review* 14 (1963): 466–67. "When death occurs, or in the alternative, when death has been declared *shortly inevitable* . . ." is the version of this statement in Carl E. Wasmuth, "Legal Aspects of Organ Transplantation," a paper read before the 40th Congress of the International Anesthesia Research Society, Bar Harbor, Florida, February 27–March 3, 1966. What or when death is these authors do not say. They vacillate between holding that "the lack of function of the mind alone is insufficient as evidence of death" and holding that "no longer is it adequate to talk about the cessation of respiration or to talk about the cessation or circulation as the moment of death." Instead of a determination of death, these authors simply *urge* that "with the advent of the era of transplantation of organs, medicine and humanity can no longer afford the luxury of condemning to the grave the vital organs which, if transplanted into another person, can preserve that person's life" (*Cleveland-Marshall Law Review*, p. 466). This leads them to say that a patient is accessible to the transplant surgeons when he is dead or *in the alternative* when his condition has been "pronounced hopeless," survival is impossible, death imminent (p. 467)—in order to allow time to take the body to the operating room!

or any other purpose, death cannot be reckoned from when it be-comes "virtually" certain.[6] This has to be made sun-clear, else the public is justly suspicious that "cannibalizing" organs may be the practice.

Let it be said at once that after it has been determined that a patient has died and doctors and the family are in the presence of an unburied corpse, the corpse itself can certainly be used as a "vital organ bank." The German Lutheran theologian who has written most on medical-ethical questions, Helmuth Thielicke, was commenting upon such a vital use of the body as a temporary "tissue bank" when he wrote:

> It seems to me that one should not speak in such cases of having maintained "life." For what is really maintained is merely cer-tain limited biological functions. To put it more pointedly, there has been a preservation of the vitality of specific organs of an unburied corpse. . . . One could say that while there may yet be these partial "relics of life," the organism as a whole has ceased to be. And I now ask myself whether this particular measure differs in any fundamental way from other forms of preservation—for instance those employed by an insti-tute of anatomy to make cadavers available for classroom use— other than this matter of the vitality of the specimen pre-served?
>
> This special method of conservation would then have to be understood as another achievement of modern medicine, which knows how to maintain an organ within an irreversible and lethal overall situation, and to make it organically pro-ductive again by means of transplantation. I see no reason why this should involve any ethical or religious problems. If we choose to speak of the "preservation of the vitality of specific organs," it is because the term suggests—as we intend—that what is involved here is not a theological question about the nature of man but a biological question not directly related to the values of the humanum.[7]

6. "The Moment of Death," *Medical-Legal Journal* 31 (1963): 195–96.

7. Helmuth Thielicke, "Ethics in Modern Medicine," three lectures delivered at a conference on medicine, morals, and technology sponsored by the Institute of Religion,

There are a number of cases which show the urgent need for agreement concerning the old or some new procedures for stating that a man has died. Because of doubts which arise from physicians' use of such terms as "virtual" or "imminent" death, and because of suspicions that are stirred when there seems to be a difference between the medical and the legal definitions of death, or when doctors disagree over the moment of death and yet a patient's organ is used for transplantation, these cases demonstrate that the question of how validly to state death needs to be resolved by the medical profession, and to be resolved in a way that is publicly understandable.

The urgent need to clarify these questions can be seen from the manner in which a kidney was saved and used in a transplant operation from one David Potter, who suffered extensive brain damage in a brawl in June 1963 at Newcastle upon Tyne.[8] About 14 hours after admission on June 16 to the Newcastle General Hospital, Mr. Potter stopped breathing. "Artificial respiration was then begun by machine so that one of his kidneys could later be taken for transplantation in another man." I suppose this means that if Mr. Potter had not been placed on a respirator, he at that point could have been pronounced dead because of the prompt cessation of spontaneous respiratory and cardiac activity as a consequence of his massive brain injury. On this supposition, there can be no decisive moral objection to the fact that "after 24 hours of artificial respiration a kidney was taken from the body on June 17. The respirator was then turned off. . . ." The difficulty was only that the situation was left obscure.

Texas Medical Center, Houston, Texas, March 25–28, 1968, and published in Kenneth Vaux (ed.), *Who Shall Live? Medicine, Technology, Ethics* (Philadelphia: Fortress, 1970), p. 176. Objection can be raised against this statement only because Thielicke (at the ellipsis above) says, "Quite apart from any physiological definition of death . . ."; and because his words "an irreversible and lethal overall situation" are ambiguous as to whether he means to say that the man was irreversibly dying but was maintained alive for a time or that the man was irretrievably dead but his organs were maintained alive for a time. It seems clear, however, that Thielicke mainly means to say that this is a case of the vital conservation of the single organs of an unburied corpse. That *entails* a determination of physiological death.

8. See *British Medical Journal* 2 (August 10, 1963): 394. This case was also discussed by M. Martin Halley and William F. Harvey in "Medical vs. Legal Definitions of Death," *Journal of the American Medical Association* 204, no. 6 (May 6, 1968): 423–25.

The difficulty in the Newcastle General Hospital case was that the coroner and the doctors were uncertain about what had happened or was done to Mr. Potter; and this, in turn, very clearly shows why the question of the meaning of death has been raised—occasioned—by organ transplants. The coroner was reported to have said that he thought Mr. Potter was alive when the kidney was removed on June 17, although there was no hope for him; but in his view, astonishingly, the doctors had committed no offense. The chief doctor, on the other hand, offered (it was reported) two views: (1) that Mr. Potter was "virtually dead" on June 16 when he ceased breathing, while he "legally" died when the heart ceased beating and the circulation ceased to flow on June 17 (when after the kidney had been taken the respirator was cut off) and (2) that he was "medically dead" on June 16 and "legally dead" on June 17. The legal correspondent of the *British Medical Journal* was principally concerned that these comments had opened up a difference between the legal and the medical definitions of death.

To the lay reader of this report it is, indeed, difficult to tell what happened or was done to Mr. Potter. Because it is best to think the best of everyone, I can only suppose that on June 16 Mr. Potter, already lethally brain damaged, either ceased to have spontaneous cardiac and respiratory functions or that his breathing had artificially to be maintained by respirator and this—one step removed—kept the heart beating also (i.e., successfully held at bay the death of every one of his vital signs). If so, then what followed may have been a case of (in Thielicke's words) the "preservation of the vitality of specific organs of an unburied corpse." The difficulty was that procedures were not used to determine whether this was so or not, and Mr. Potter was not pronounced dead on evidence that he was. In the case of Potter, it is reported that a jury, on the evidence, returned a verdict of manslaughter against the man said to have been involved with the patient in the fight; but in the Magistrates Court this man was afterwards convicted on a reduced charge of common assault.[9] Why was Potter's assailant guilty only of assault and the surgeons not guilty of manslaughter, or, if the doctors did

9. See "Decisions about Life and Death: A Problem in Modern Medicine," Church of England study pamphlet (Church Information House, Church House, Westminster SWI, London: 1965), pp. 36–37.

nothing wrong, why was the assailant not guilty of manslaughter? Recent proposals for *updating the procedures for stating death* are addressed exactly to these confused points.

There was similar confusion in at least one case in the United States that received wide publicity and is still in the courts. On May 13, 1968, the *New York Times* reported that on May 7 in Houston, Texas, John M. Stuckwish, a 62-year-old man, received the heart of Clarence Nicks, a 36-year-old man whose brain was severely damaged as a result of a beating. The donor's respiration ceased and brain waves were absent, according to the news report, but his heart was still functioning. The patient was pronounced dead by one physician, although another disagreed, whereupon the donor was placed on a respirator until the heart was removed three hours later. The county medical examiner anticipated difficulty in prosecuting the donor's assailants for homicide. The surgeons went ahead with the operation, however, when they were assured that they would not be prosecuted for "concealing evidence," i.e., Nicks' heart, in the chest of another man.

According to the *New York Times* of January 28, 1969, the attorney for the defendants in this case stated that "it is going to be our contention that Nicks wasn't dead." Unless there is clarification of the moment of death and agreed enunciation that death has occurred, court cases will arise not only in case of victims of brawls but also of automobile accidents involving a second driver. If, however, sound procedures for stating death are agreed to and carried out, then theologians and moralists and every other thoughtful person should agree with the physicians who hold that it is *then* permissible to maintain circulation of blood and supply of oxygen in the corpse of a donor to preserve an *organ* until it can be used in transplantation.[10] Whether one gives the body over for decent burial, performs an autopsy, gives the cadaver for use in medical education, or uses it as a "vital organ bank" are all alike procedures governed by decent respect for the bodies of deceased men and specific regulations that ensure this. The ventilation and circulation of organs for transplant raises no question not already raised by these standard procedures. None are life-and-death matters.

10. Jørgen Voigt, "The Criteria of Death, Particularly in Relation to Transplantation Surgery," *World Medical Journal* 14 (1967): 145, 146.

On July 24, 1968, the *Washington Post* reported concerning a subsequent transplant of the heart of a Houston housewife, Evelyn G. Krikorian, into the body of Fredi C. Everman of Arlington, Virginia, that Mrs. Krikorian had been dead for four days but that her heart was maintained alive during this period of time. In this case, it appears that the doctors knew what they were doing. Mrs. Krikorian was dead because there was no natural heartbeat, no spontaneous breathing, no reflexes, and no brain waves. The respirator they used did not make a person live; it only kept the heart beating by keeping the chest and lungs moving to supply oxygen to the blood. In short, the respirator was a means of sustaining specific organs in an unburied corpse. I shall argue in the sequel that a pronouncement of death, *or determining the criteria in terms of which such a judgment is to be made,* should in no measure have the need of organ recipients in view. Their need, however, can with proper precaution be made adjunct to what can be done with an unburied corpse.

The confusion and ambiguity in stating that a patient has died are well illustrated again by the case of Mrs. Barbara Ewan, who, having suffered "irreversible" brain damage from tumor aggravated by a fall on ice, was flown from the Lawrence, Massachusetts, General Hospital to St. Luke's Hospital in Houston during the night of April 6, 1969, there to have her heart implanted in the artificial-heart patient, Mr. Haskell Karp, who subsequently died.

The press reports of this extraordinary event say that Mrs. Ewan was alive during the airplane flight from Massachusetts, kept alive by injections of stimulating drugs. An anaesthesiologist, Dr. Robert Lennon, and one of her daughters accompanied her in flight. A team of four doctors, not connected with the transplant team, were waiting in Houston to pronounce her dead. Despite the extraordinary means used to keep her alive, she suffered cardiac arrest in the ambulance eight blocks away from St. Luke's. She was pronounced dead at about 7 A.M. on April 7, 1969, an hour and a half after arrival at the Houston hospital. The surgical team placed her heart in the chest of Mr. Karp at 8:30 A.M.

The first news dispatch alleged that Dr. Denton Cooley said the woman died at 7 A.M., a statement that accords with the procedure used. That same dispatch quotes him elaborating on this by saying that she had total absence of brain waves for 48 hours as well as total absence of reflexes and total absence of the ability to breathe. Still Dr. Cooley said that Mrs. Ewan died only an hour and a half before the transplant operation. The news report the next day, however, after Mr. Karp's death from pneumonia and kidney failure, attributed to Dr. Cooley the opinion that Mrs. Ewan had been medically dead 48 hours by the time the transplant began, because "she had complete brain damage and no reflexes whatsoever" and "had been supported by extraordinary means." [11]

It is really quite impossible to say what happened or was being done to Mrs. Ewan, with the consent of her three daughters, during the long overnight flight from Massachusetts to Texas, with an emergency landing in Shreveport, Louisiana, in which the plane nearly ran off the runway. Was she dying all this time, as the Houston doctors implied by their pronouncement of death? If so, this is something men are morally forbidden to do to the dying, whose care should not be disturbed by alien efforts to secure a fresh graft or to get it across a continent. If Mrs. Ewan was not dead before this flight, then someone was guilty of malpractice.

On the other hand, quite possibly Mrs. Ewan was already dead in Lawrence, Massachusetts, and should have been declared dead there. Then the artificial stimulants applied to her unburied body during its midnight ride only sustained the life of certain organs in the best available "tissue bank," the human body itself. This concept may take some getting used to, but there can be no possible ethical objection to it. Our moral concern would focus instead on what was done to Mr. and Mrs. Karp in this whole affair.

As late in the heart transplant era as the statement of the Board of Medicine of the National Academy of Science it was still being said that an independent group of expert, mature physicians "should agree and record their unanimous judgment as to the donor's acceptability on the basis of crucial and irreversible bodily damage and *imminent death*." [12] This clearly shows the urgent need for clarifica-

11. *New York Times,* April 8 and 9, 1969. A second patient flown from Lawrence, Mass. to Houston, Texas was said by the assistant administrator of the hospital to have suffered injuries "incompatible with life" (UP, April 10, 1969).

12. February 27 1968. This would seem to require no more of the donor's condition than was stated for a qualified recipient: "the presence of far advanced irreversible cardiac damage."

tion: a patient whose death is "imminent" or who is irreversibly dying is not yet dead. "A person dying is still a person living." [13] The need for clarification of procedures for stating death *held with assurance* by the medical profession is made strikingly evident by constant references, in the most up-to-date proposals, to the permissibility of stopping extraordinary treatments. The latter doctrine, we shall point out below, assumes that the patient is still alive.

According to a United Press dispatch,[14] a prominent neurosurgeon, Dr. James L. Poppen, of the Lahey Clinic and New England Deaconess Hospital in Boston, who at the request of the White House, Vice-President Humphrey, and Pierre Salinger, a Kennedy aide, flew to Los Angeles as a consultant concerning the late Senator Robert F. Kennedy's condition, said that it was his opinion that Senator Kennedy was legally and medically dead at 6:30 P.M. on Wednesday, June 5, 1968, eighteen hours after the shooting, but seven hours before he was officially declared dead at 1:44 A.M. on Thursday, June 6. It is true that at this news conference Dr. Poppen spoke of a number of other tragically important matters besides his reasons for this medical judgment; and his language may not at every point have made clear exactly what he meant. He said (if this news dispatch was correct) that when he first saw Senator Kennedy at 10 A.M. on Wednesday he "immediately" knew that he would not survive. On the other hand, he said that if the senator had survived his "intellectual faculties would not have survived," his bodily faculties would have been permanently impaired, and "he would have led a very grave and devastating existence." At the same time, Dr. Poppen offered it as his opinion that the senator was a "dead man" from the moment he was hit, although the "destruction was not complete from the moment of impact."

However, to say that a man is irreversibly dying from destruction that has been set in course is not the same as making a present judgment that he is now, irretrievably, dead. Our attention should focus, therefore, on what according to Dr. Poppen happened at 6:30 P.M. on Wednesday to support the judgment that from that point

---

13. G. B. Giertz in G. E. W. Wolstenholme and Maeve O'Connor (eds.), *Ethics in Medical Progress: With Special Reference to Transplantation,* Ciba Foundation Symposium (Boston: Little, Brown, 1966) p. 147.

14. Boston, Mass., June 7, 1968; *New York Times,* June 8, 1968.

on the senator was "medically dead" [15]; and we should focus attention on the senator's reported condition from this point on for
seven hours until he was officially declared to be dead. Dr. Poppen
said, as reported, that Senator Kennedy's electrical brain waves
stopped at 6:30 P.M. on Wednesday and never started again, although his heart still beat.

The senator's heartbeat, of course, may have been faint and
erratic, and measures supportive of heart function may have been
in use in the effort to save him. Still Dr. Poppen did not affirm that
he had any way of knowing that there was an entire and an irreversible cessation of spontaneous heart function at the time he said
that the senator was already dead. This, then, seems to be a neuro-
surgical redefinition both of the meaning of death and of the tests
for death. Death means brain death, and the criteria for this are
exclusively or almost exclusively brain tests. As reported, Dr. Poppen
said that Senator Kennedy was legally and medically dead when the
brain waves ceased, even though his heart still beat.

In order to put to ourselves the question whether it would be
right to update the definition of death to brain death alone and at
the same time to narrow the criteria to brain tests alone, we have
only to ask ourselves whether we would be willing to bury a man
whose heart still permanently beats spontaneously.[16] Alternatively,
we might ask whether we would be willing under similar conditions
to remove one of a man's vital organs for use as a "spare part" for
another patient.[17] The presence or absence of truly spontaneous

15. I strike the word "legally" from the words of the news dispatch, since it is
doubtful that the legal definition of death has so far been updated to support a verdict
that a man is dead who still has a heartbeat even if this be a reasonable medical proposal. A medical judgment that a man is dead is, of course, a legal judgment in the
sense that the law itself acknowledges that only physicians can so declare. The law
generally will and should support competent medical opinion in this matter; still the
law's endorsement of any revision of the meaning of death is necessary in determining
legal death. This endorsement need not be by legislation; it can be by case law, or
even by the law's silence in face of changing medical practice.

16. See David Daube, "Transplantation: Acceptability of Procedures and Their
Required Legal Sanctions," in Wolstenholme and O'Connor, Ethics in Medical Progress, p. 190.

17. Dr. G. P. J. Alexandre of the University of Louvain, Belgium, stated in the Ciba
Symposium mentioned in the previous footnote that "in nine cases we have used
patients with head injuries, whose heart had not stopped, to do kidney transplants"
(ibid., p. 69). Other participants in this discussion doubted that any physician, what-

cardiac activity, and other indices, ought not hastily to be removed from our tests of whether a man is still alive or has died, even if our definition of death should be largely shifted to brain death. It would be far more reasonable to open decisively the question under what conditions and by what means we should continue "heroic" efforts to save life than by an intellectual tour de force to pronounce a man dead whose heart still beats spontaneously from an altogether natural power. What should be taken to be the meaning of that sign of life will be brought under scrutiny below in my proposal for more radically updating these recent updatings of death, by clearing up a remaining ambiguity concerning when the heart should be said still to beat "spontaneously" or should be deemed no longer to evidence one of the integrated signs of life.

The current proposals for updating our procedures for stating that a man has died are directed first of all at clearing up this ambiguous language about "virtual" or "impending" death. The discussion is about giving meaning instead to the such concepts as "dead but in a state of artificial survival," "dead but maintained by artificial means," [18] artificially arrested death," [19] "suspended death," "technical life."

Thus, if a patient's brain is irreversibly dead but circulation and

---

ever he might do in the case of a paired organ such as the kidney, would be willing to remove an unpaired vital organ such as the liver or heart before spontaneous circulation had stopped (Dr. T. E. Starzl, Chief of Surgery, Veterans Administration Hospital, Denver, ibid. p. 70). Also Dr. R. Y. Calne: "If a patient has a heart beat he cannot be regarded as a cadaver" (ibid., p. 73). It should be noted, however, that Alexandre insisted that in his own practice or in proper medical practice "there has never been and there never will be any question of taking organs from a dying person who has 'no reasonable chance of getting better or resuming consciousness.' The question is of taking organs from a dead person, and the point is that I do not accept the cessation of heart beats as the indication of death" (ibid., p. 154). Since *one* of Alexandre's tests was "complete absence of spontaneous respiration, five minutes after mechanical respiration has been stopped" (ibid., p. 69), it is evident that the heartbeat that was for him no sign of life was heartbeat kept going also by the artificial respiration, not the heartbeat of hopelessly comatose patients who still respirate and whose hearts still beat. These patients he believes to be still alive and inaccessible to transplant surgeons, although there is no chance of their ever getting better.

18. Jean Hamburger and Jean Crosnier, "Moral and Ethical Problems in Transplantation," in Felix T. Rapaport and Jean Dausset (eds.), *Human Transplantation* (New York: Grune and Stratton, 1968), p. 42.

19. Bernard Nolan, "Ethical Problems in Renal Homo-transplant," *British Journal of Urology* (1967); "Life and Death: A Problem in Modern Medicine," p. 26.

respiration are maintained by artificial measures, Dr. Jørgen Voigt of Copenhagen refuses to call his condition even one of "suspended death," a term proposed by Professor Dalgaard. His reason for this is that "in the expression 'suspended death' there remains a suggestion that death has not yet occurred." [20] The same argument holds against the use of such terms as "virtually dead" with which much of the discussion of updating death has been befuddled. Instead of "suspended death" or "virtual death" or "imminent death," it would be better to say that the situation as described may be one of "technical life"; and, as Dr. Voigt says, "no one can be interested in being doomed to a 'technical life' which is not life at all but a soulless vegetative dependence upon one or more machines." [21] That would be to regard these hospital-based machines, in the absence of any evidence of brain life or of other spontaneous vital functions as proper prostheses for "men" to wear indefinitely. The trick is to find a way to see behind the look of life upon the face of death, and to learn to tell the difference between a patient who may have only "technical life" sustained in him and a patient whose death may as yet be only "virtual," "suspended," or still successfully held at bay even if imminent.

Dr. Voigt's concept of what death is, however, remains the traditional one. "The definition should read: 'Death has occurred when every *spontaneous vital function* has ceased permanently.' " [22] No more does his procedure for stating death shift to brain tests (EEG) alone. Reviewing the lists of criteria and the procedures for stating death discussed by the participants in the Ciba symposium,[23] Voigt writes that, while these may seem complicated, they do not involve anything new; and that among the clinical tests "the most important is actually the classical observation that death has occurred when spontaneous circulation and spontaneous respiration have ceased." He adds that "the question of 'cerebral death' is of significance in determining whether there are indications for continued artificial maintenance of respiration and circulation, but is not itself a criterion of death."

20. Voigt, "The Criteria of Death," p. 144.
21. Ibid., p. 145.
22. Ibid., p. 144.
23. Wolstenholme and O'Connor, *Ethics in Medical Progress*, pp. 69–71.

That may be to go too far, and to say something incompatible with Voigt's concept of what death is and his own procedure for stating that death has occurred. On the same page, Dr. Voigt declared that "in a particular case if brain function is abolished and spontaneous circulation and respiration have ceased, then I consider that the patient is dead according to the above-mentioned definition." I judge that, not ever having believed that an essentially isolated heart maintained in a condition of "technical life" or an essentially isolated pair of lungs kept going also only by the respirator belong among the signs of a patient's life, Voigt has no need to shift to an essentially isolated brain for his definition of life and death, or to brain tests in isolation from the other vital signs of life in stating when death has occurred. His view is "if even only one of the vital functions continues spontaneously, indications are present for maintaining the others artificially to the greatest possible extent and, under such circumstances, the patient remains inaccessible to the transplantation surgeons." [24]

Dr. Voigt's is the most traditionalistic of the procedures for stating death which we shall review. Perhaps he has not given sufficient consideration to the fact that, with brain function gone beyond recall, it is the now useless artificial respiration that also prolongs the functioning of the heart; that too is only a "technical life." The signs of life sustained by machine cannot be kept so entirely separate in determining whether there is life or death. However, there is perhaps another lesson to be drawn from Dr. Voigt's treatment of this question of life and death. This is that if transplant therapy is brought at all into view in this matter, there is a twin danger: some physicians

24. Ibid., p. 145. A paralyzed person maintained permanently by an iron lung still has brain life, and by Voigt's tests ample signs of life. Whether he should choose to live by this means is another question. Some among the medical profession have argued (from cases of paralytic poliomyelitis) that the fact that life can be maintained only by mechanical means is not by itself sufficient to establish death (Wasmuth and Stewart, "Medical and Legal Aspects of Human Organ Transplantation," p. 465). The artificial maintenance of respiration (and so also of heartbeat) indefinitely in patients with brainstem damage that abolishes also any powers of respiration is not to be compared with the iron lung cases. In the latter, the patient has unimpaired brain activity while respiration keeps all the other vital functions going. In the cases of massive brain damage, it does not. Respirators in these latter cases maintain respiration and *one* other vital sign, the activity of the heart. But see the discussion of the "pacemaker" cases, pp. 94–96 below.

might pronounce death and render a patient accessible for organ donation where otherwise they would not hesitate to wait, while others might hesitate to pronounce death and stop the respirator until the last flutter of a failing heart makes it quite clear that the patient is accessible to the transplantation surgeons. We shall return to this point.

REJECTING SOME LEGAL DEFINITIONS

Second, the current proposals for updating death are *rebuttals to some legal definitions* which hold that, as long as any heartbeat or respiration can be perceived, either with or without mechanical or electrical aids, and regardless of how the heartbeat and respiration are maintained, death has not occurred.[25] Recent medical literature has challenged this assumption that the perceived signs of heartbeat and respiration are "vital" signs regardless of how they are maintained.

Whether perceived signs of life are really vital signs depends on whether these are spontaneous or indefinitely maintained by artificial means. This conclusion of the physicians should be endorsed by an ethicist as often as he hears it—regardless of the legalities and even if an ethicist as such knows nothing about when or in what manner mechanical and other stimulators should be "refuted" in stating that a man has died. Surely the medical definition of death must be one that significantly alters the legal one stated above. This is also an apt moral understanding of life and death. A Church of England study pamphlet assigns the correct purpose to any use of artificial sustainers while still understanding life to be the integrated spontaneous power of all the principal vital functions. In the case of the irretrievably unconscious patient whose vital functions are maintained only by artificial means, this study declared, "the purpose of the apparatus . . . can be no more than to keep the vital organs functioning until it can be determined whether they are capable of ever functioning inde-

---

25. Halley and Harvey, "Medical vs. Legal Definitions of Death," pp. 423–24. Cf. Marshall Houts, *Death* 1.03 (4) (1967): "Death is the *final* and irreversible cessation of perceptible heartbeat and respiration. Conversely, as long as any heartbeat or respiration can be perceived, whether with or without mechanical or electrical aid, and regardless of how the heartbeat and respiration were maintained, death has not occurred."

pendently again, whether the patient is capable of ever becoming again an autonomous unit." [26]

It requires no "special situation" or concession, as Drs. Halley and Harvey seem still to believe, to affirm that a man may be dead with the irreversible cessation of cerebral function in the presence of artificially maintained respiration and continuing circulation. The difficulty—if there is one—is only in devising proper procedures for telling when these other spontaneous vital signs are independently present or absent.

DISMISSING ARTIFICIALLY SUSTAINED "SIGNS OF LIFE"

Third, updating death means, under stated conditions, to *dismiss machine-driven or artificially maintained signs of life*. This is the chief question at issue in every one of the carefully drawn proposals for updating procedures for stating that a man has died. The main issue at stake is whether and when it is proper to rebut a machine, and in particular a respirator, which is a devilishly efficient instrument.

It would, in truth, be an astonishing fruit of our technological civilization if *in mente* respirators and heart-lung machines became so integral a part of the "man alive" in his terminal illness that we could say that he "died" only when these machines were cut off, or (his brain by all indications damaged beyond recall) only that he was "virtually" dead when he irrevocably ceased to be capable of permanent, spontaneous cardiopulmonary functioning. These cases in any event are entirely different from the case of a man with extensive

26. "Decisions about Life and Death," p. 38. It is true that Pope Pius XII can be cited expressing a view in accord with the legal definitions given above. Addressing an international congress of anesthesiologists on November 24, 1957, he said, "Some considerations of a general nature permit us to believe that human life continues as long as its vital functions—distinguished from the simple life of the organs—manifest themselves spontaneously or even with the help of artificial procedures" (*Acta Apostolicae Sedis* 49 [1957]: 1033; *The Pope Speaks*, Vol. IV, p. 398). However, without making too much of the point, it is worth noting that the words "or even with the help" keep somewhat in view the fact that the purpose of artificial procedures is to determine whether vital functions are capable of ever functioning independently again. The hesitant word "even" contrasts in some not insignificant degree with the equilibrating words, "whether with or without mechanical or electrical aid" and "regardless of how the heartbeat and respiration were maintained" in the legal definitions above.

brain damage whose heart still beats from an entirely natural power. There would seem to be no need to resort to such an exclusive concept of brain death. Nor is there any need to begin to reckon death from when it became imminent, especially not if we are capable of recalling other, more reasonable medical-ethical categories such as only caring for the dying to deal fittingly with untreatable terminally ill patients.[27]

Before turning to the medical literature on this third description of updating death, there are two medical facts that should be mentioned which (in addition to bad newspaper reporting) have lent support to the mistaken notion that "brain death" is marching triumphantly down the field. The first is that, of the three great organ systems—brain and heart and lungs—the function of the brain is the only one that cannot directly be indefinitely sustained artificially. This lends a seeming decisiveness to EEG tests of brain life or death as these become clinically more reliable in comparison with equally or more reliable tests of perceptible cardiac or respiratory activity—as long as it is taken to be a matter of indifference whether the latter vital signs are spontaneous or are mechanically sustained, or if one is uncertain which is the source of the activity, and it may be ambiguously both. Proposed revisions of our ways of telling that a man has died are not so much shifts to brain tests as they are carefully drawn regulations for interruptions of the extrinsic maintenance of the other vital signs of life in order to tell whether these natural functions are or are not being restored or are capable of being resumed.

The second medical fact that must be kept in mind is that heart life is much less immediately dependent on brain life than is lung life—or than the brain is dependent on heart and lungs. Indeed, the heart is partially denervated in treating some sorts of heart trouble. If the heart is getting the wrong signals, it is more extensively denervated, and that possibly fatal procedure is itself corrected by a

27. I shall argue in the sequel that there is sufficient need and sufficient reason in the dying or dead patient's own care, and that of his family, for clarifying or revising our understanding of death. The needs of potential recipients of organs need not be brought into view even as an adjunct consideration. Indeed, I am in this chapter refraining from bringing the problematics of transplantation under direct scrutiny and from making any final judgment about the ethics of giving and receiving organs for transplants. We are concerned here with the problematics of defining death, and the ethical issues that as such this raises.

"pacemaker." And an implanted heart need not be connected up with its new brain!

If the life of the organism as a whole means the *integrated* functioning of brain and heart and lungs, we must correctly understand this integration in assessing a patient's condition. The heart can continue to beat naturally for some time after a massive brain destruction whose more immediate effect will be the abolition of the capacity to respire spontaneously. The abolition of brain activity disintegrates and finally abolishes respiratory capacity before the heart will cease to manifest all signs of rhythmic, pumping life (let alone cellular life or the electrical "life" registered by ECG). If, however, a respirator is promptly applied to maintain oxygenation, this not only maintains the signs of lung life; it also keeps heart death at bay. The artificial maintenance of lung life also sustains—by one step removed—the life of the heart. The destruction of heart life resulting from lung death following brain death can be impeded by a respirator. This, I believe, is the crux of every one of the recent discussions of updating our procedures for stating that a man has died. The decisive question raised is whether doctors should continue to regard signs of "spontaneous" heart life as evidence that the patient still lives when these signs are still present only because lung life is artificially being maintained by respirators that (it can be determined) have lost their aim or hope of ever restoring spontaneous breathing. Must they wait until the last flicker of a failing heart whose dying is being artificially prolonged as surely as is the breathing? To the contrary, ought we not to say that the seemingly natural heartbeat is also being maintained only with the help of artificial procedures?

Suppose that an operation upon a patient by open heart surgery fails. Then we ought not to think the continuing ventilation and circulation of his blood by a heart-lung machine, which is simply a shunt around the heart and lungs, are signs that he still lives. Suppose that a patient is suffering from massive brain damage. Then we ought not to think that the indefinite prolongation of his respiration by mechanical means is necessarily a sign of lung life. It is only one short step more to say that, if by careful tests it can be determined that this patient has no recoverable capacity to respirate, then neither has he any natural capacity for heart life—even though with entirely artificial and hopeless artificial respiration his heart still beats. His brain is dead, his lungs are dead, and except for the continued medical intervention to keep breathing going, his heart would already be dead. He has only an entirely technical life, just as surely as if ventilation and circulation were kept going by a heart-lung machine for an indefinite time after heart surgery failed. It is beyond me why medical judgment should not pronounce that death has occurred, if there are ways of telling that this is the situation. Placing a man with paralysis of respiratory musculature permanently on an iron lung, whose heart still beats and whose brain is alive, is not at all to be compared with the sort of case we are now considering.

In the following review of some of the literature I shall continue to use this "expanded" meaning of heart death where its "life" is sustained by artificial process (directly, or one step removed) both in analysis of the proposals and in the moral argument. My thesis is that the doctors have not gone far enough if they only elaborate procedures to remove the current medical uncertainty about whether a man is alive or dead while not also removing from the public's understanding the lingering uncertainty or ambiguity over whether a patient may be pronounced dead whose heart is not in principle dead already. To say that the heart is "virtually dead" would be no improvement over saying that the man is "virtually dead." To speak of the "life" of brain-dead patients on respirators is as misleading as to speak of the continuation of their hearts as "spontaneous." Both sets of quotation marks should be removed. The heartbeat should be described as a sign of life that is being artificially maintained no less than is respiration, and so neither are signs of life. Neither are the vital signs that were consulted for centuries in medical practice. It is a machine that is being dismissed (under carefully drawn conditions). Naturally sustained (or recoverable) life in the heart is not being removed from among the signs that a man is still alive.

It is possible to make a reference to brain death decisive in certain instances, within a traditional understanding of the integrated signs of life. Paradoxically, a return to these tests of life and death would result from updating the recent updatings of death to make it quite clear that where there is no permanent capacity to respirate there can be no permanent, natural circulation (though both can be indefinitely sustained by sustaining the first artificially). In clinically

defining death, a more forthright rebuttal of the machines and procedures that the medical profession has grown accustomed to use is
needed to reassure the public that "cerebral death, *per se,* would not
justify interruption of a respiration and a circulation maintained by
the unconscious patient independently"; that "inability of the patient
to sustain an independent existence is demonstrated by the failure of
his circulation or his respiration or both" (machine-driven perceptible signs set decisively aside); while "a cerebral 'death' would justify a decision to switch off a respirator if the patient were unable to
maintain his circulation without it." [28]

There seems to me to be a very significant remaining ambiguity
when Dr. George E. Schreiner can say, "We have seen people with
a virtual transection of the brain kept alive for days and days, simply
because there was an intact cardiovascular system and a respirator."
That "and" is no simple conjunction. There was an "intact cardiovascular system" only because there was a respirator in use for days
and days. Then in what sense was this an "intact cardiovascular system"? It was actually no less abolished than was that patient's respiratory system. But such is the influence of artificially sustained signs
of life upon all our minds, and the mind of the medical profession,
that instead of upholding a pronouncement of death in this instance
Dr. Schreiner called instead for the physician "to decide, from a set
of criteria, at which point he will stop employing extraordinary
means for the prolongation of life." [29]

In a 1964 article by Dr. Hannibal Hamlin of the Massachusetts
General Hospital, Boston, notably entitled "Life or Death by EEG,"
it is quite plain that other vital signs of life are not being dismissed
in the shift to a concept of brain death. Far from it. Hamlin's contention simply is that "the sanctity of life must not depend upon
cardiologic signs alone, with the brain excluded." Moreover, when
the brain is included, the other spontaneous signs are not excluded.
When brain tests are taken to be decisive in stating that death has
occurred, these are overriding only against cardiologic and other
signs of life when these are being maintained by artificial means.
Statements of death by EEG are not proposed in the face of the other

28. "The Cape Town Human Heart Transplants," editorial, *Medical Proceedings*
(Johannesburg) 14, no. 1 (January 13, 1968): 7.
29. Wolstenholme and O'Connor, *Ethics in Medical Progress,* pp. 73–74.

signs of life spontaneously present. The situation is simply that "when the brain is so compromised the EEG can signal a point of no return, although the cardiovascular system continues to respond to supportive therapy that produces a respectable ECG." That is to say—in the vernacular—although the heart still beats by artificial means. Again, it is the machine or the stimulants that mask the fact that death has occurred. As Dr. Hamlin puts it, "resuscitative devices can serve to maintain the look of life in the face of death." He might have gone further and said that they can maintain the look of life upon the face of death. These patients "were actually heart-lung preparations"; autopsies later revealed that their brains had liquified.[30] The trick is to devise procedures for determining this now, while fully protecting those patients whose hearts now are helped to beat by artificial means who have not already died, i.e., whose brains still function and where there is hope of permanently restoring heart life and lung life as well.

Hamlin wants a way to acknowledge "that St. Peter is *at* the Gate or Charon *at* the Crossing." He might have gone further and said, a way of determining that the Gate has already been entered and the Crossing made, although men can continue indefinitely to oxygenate and circulate blood in the bodies left behind. He wants to save the families of patients from awaiting "the grim and foregone verdict until the final [artificially maintained] beat of the dying heart has been recorded." His point is simply that "the sanctity of life is not generated by [artificially if remotely generated] cardiac signs of its presence or absence when the brain has already died." [31] Again, it is the mechanical "life"-sustainers that are rebutted. Under specifiable conditions, these are no "signs of life" at all. Still among the specifiable conditions Hamlin lists is "no spontaneous respiration," and not EEG findings alone. The concept of what death is has been changed to neurological death, but the procedure for deciding that this has occurred contains a number of clinical and EEG correlates.

It is worth noting, finally, that support for a "diagnosis of im-

30. Hannibal Hamlin, "Life or Death by EEG," *Journal of the American Medical Association* 190, no. 2 (October 12, 1964): 112, 113.

31. Ibid., p. 114. I insert "artificially maintained" and "artificially if remotely generated" in the quotations above, because heart death would have occurred but for artificial respiration; and "no spontaneous respiration for 90 minutes" is among Hamlin's tests.

mutable neurological death" will not be found in every case of deep and prolonged coma. To come to grips with the problem of the comatose patient who still lives, one has to invoke the dispensability of extraordinary, or under certain conditions of ordinary, means of saving life. This is an aspect of medical ethics specifically designed to weight the claims of still living men; of the suffering dying, whose death is "virtual" or "imminent," and not, like the definition of and tests for death, designed to tell us whether it is they or an unburied corpse in whose presence we stand.

"It is not easy to say," writes Dr. Gunnar Biörck of Stockholm, Sweden, "whether the concept of 'brain death' is in its essence different from the concept of 'heart death' otherwise than with regard to procedure"—the procedures used in stating that death has occurred. The signal difference he observes is not the concept of death itself. It is rather a procedural difference (and a difficulty) that has come about because of our extensive use of life-supporting techniques, with a resulting contrast between patients being sustained by these techniques and patients who are not. "Brain death in a patient on life-supporting techniques may precede heart death—whereas in most cases of 'spontaneous death' the reverse is true." In the former case the dying of the heart is protracted, though this may eventually occur despite intensive care methods. The use of artificial stimulants and machines to keep a patient and his vital signs "warm and rosy" have thus brought it about that there may be two times of death for a patient on intensive care measures. His brain may die one day and his heart finally fail the next. Thus "the time of death, which formerly depended mainly on factors *within* the patient may now depend increasingly on factors *outside* the patient." [32]

Even in Dr. Biörck's excellent analysis of the situation, it is evident that the externally "man-made" cardiovascular activity has too much become *the patient* in stating that he has died. The respirator has intervened to place a gulf between brain death and heart death, where formerly the one followed the other—in either direction—rather quickly. A good deal of "brain washing" of medical and paramedical personnel and the families of patients on intensive "life"-sustaining treatments has evidently taken place while hearts were being stimulated or blood was being oxygenated and circulated. The

32. Biörck, "On the Definitions of Death," pp. 138–39.

goal that medical care was aiming at has dropped from view. This was not to keep the heart going, or blood oxygenated and circulating.[33] It was rather the restoration of these as permanent *spontaneous* functions, and the recovery of the patient with at least a minimally functioning brain and central nervous system. Thus our marvelous artificial means to this end became an active part of the end itself. The artificial stimulation, ventilation, and circulation of a patient came to be taken to be signs of life, when they are only means which, hopefully, may restore life.

This is the way to understand the majority of the proposals for updating death. These are rather proposals for updating our procedures for determining that death has occurred, for rebutting the belief that machines or treatments are the patient, for withdrawing the notion that artificially sustained signs of life are in themselves signs of life, for telling when we should stop ventilating and circulating the blood of an unburied corpse because there are no longer any

33. The "life" of the heart-muscle can be closely compared, in any case, to cell life. If men did not "feel" its movement and had possessed our modern knowledge of physiology, the heart might never have been located among the integrated vital signs. On the other hand, it can be argued that the heart is an *independent* one of the integrated spontaneous signs of life, because it is so strange and wonderfully made.

The heart is muscle tissue composed of cells having the capacity to contract rhythmically. When the heart is unrecoverably disorganized and no longer can pump, the heart cells still may show signs of cellular life that, I suppose, may be inelegantly compared with the muscle tissue of frog legs "kicking" in a frying pan. But as a rhythmically functioning whole organ, the heart of a frog is often kept alive by medical students entirely separate from its body; they can stop it and start it again. In dogs, the following serious experiment was reported: a "heart-lung preparation was used which enabled us to maintain the heart in a fully perfused forcefully beating stage outside the body for as long as 16 hours. This was achieved without the application of a pump oxygenator or parabiotic perfusion, but by using the pumping force of the graft itself" (Francis Robicsek, Alan Lesage, Paul W. Sanger, Harry K. Daugherty, Vincent Gallucci, and Emanuuel Bagby, "Homotransplantation of 'Live' Hearts," *Cardio-Pulmonary Disease* [May 1967]: 8).

This explains why a pump respirator need not always be in use on a brain-damaged or comatose human patient. He may not be perceptibly breathing, he may only be given oxygen through a tube, and sometimes enough will perfuse his system to keep artificially "alive" a now essentially isolated "intact cardiovascular system." The foregoing experiment also suggests that for the purpose of cardiac transplantation the hearts of dead patients may soon be transported across a continent by means of a heart-lung preparation and not by "virtually" dead but still living patients. A human heart and lungs, kept alive in a special organ preservation machine, were recently flown the distance from San Antonio to Houston, Texas (*New York Times,* April 25, 1969).

vital functions really alive or recoverable in the patient. Thus, Professor Paul Freund observed that the report of the *ad hoc* committee of the Harvard Medical School seemed to be "a set of guidelines on how to use a respirator." [34] Proposals for updating death are carefully drawn directives for intervening upon our medical interventions in order to get in touch with the still living man or with corpse that is there.

The Harvard Report

On August 5, 1968, the *Journal of the American Medical Association* published a report of a committee of the Harvard Medical School, under the chairmanship of Dr. Henry K. Beecher, examining the definition of brain death. This article, entitled "A Definition of Irreversible Coma," [35] is worth considering as an example of the fact that updating death means (1) to clear up the ambiguity in some recent presumptions of death, and the confusion in the public mind; (2) to reject some of the legal definitions of death in terms of perceived signs, however maintained; and (3) to state exactly the procedures for dismissing machine-driven or artificially maintained signs of life.

The Harvard Report expresses the view that death should be understood in terms of "a permanently non-functioning brain" but that there are multiple and not only brain tests for this. A front-page story in the *New York Times* announced that this special Harvard faculty committee recommended that the definition of death be based on " 'brain death,' even though the heart may continue to beat." This newspaper, in its summary of the News of the Week the following Sunday, reported that "in effect, the panel said that 'a permanently non-functioning brain' was tantamount to death, even though the heart and other organs may continue to function by artificial means." [36] There is a world of difference between these two statements! This illustrates a remaining confusion that is widespread in the public mind. It also brings us to the heart of the matter, the crux of the question, as it seems to me. This is the question whether

34. Panel discussion, Second Congress on Medical Ethics of the American Medical Association, Chicago, October 5–6, 1968.

35. *Journal of the American Medical Association* 205, no. 6 (August 5, 1968): 85–88.

36. *New York Times*, August 5, 1968; *News of the Week*, August 11, 1968.

we should characterize a heart that still beats only because respiration is artificially maintained as a "spontaneously" beating heart (and so a sign of life) or by one step removed an "artificially" beating heart (and so not a sign of life, unless there is on this and other counts hope of restoring this and the other vital functions).[37]

Defining death to mean, theoretically, the "permanent non-functioning of the brain" or a comatose condition in which there is "no discernible central nervous system activity," the Harvard committee then set itself the task of determining the "characteristics" of this state of affairs. It came up with a number of indications of this, and carefully laid out the procedures by which death, in the sense explained, could be determined in a combination of ways. It suggested three sorts or groups of clinical signs or criteria for brain death, and these are followed only in the fourth place by the electroencephalograph, which it should be noted "provides confirmatory data." A flat or isoelectric electroencephalogram is, of course, "of great confirmatory value" if expertly monitored, but an electroencephalograph is not always available. If available, it is not enough.

This report, in introducing its tests for stating death, states that "in situations where for one reason or another electroencephalographic monitoring is not available, the absence of cerebral function

37. In the *Daedalus* volume on Ethical Aspects of Experimentation with Human Subjects, Dr. Beecher affirms that the crucial point was the Harvard committee's agreement that "brain death is death indeed even though the heart continues to beat." Then the problem was for the committee to agree upon "the characteristics of a permanently non-functioning brain." In refining the tests for this only some—perhaps a minority—of indefinitely comatose patients are rendered eligible to be declared dead. At the same time, and pertinent to these patients alone, Dr. Beecher affirms (among other characteristics) that "there are no spontaneous muscular movements or spontaneous respiration; artificial respiration supports the continued heartbeat" (Henry K. Beecher, "Scarce Resources and Medical Advancement," *Daedalus*, Spring 1969, pp. 291, 293). Such a heart would seem to be more than "virtually" dead already. Some other committee, or Dr. Beecher himself, may want later to propose in the medical and the public forum valid ways to declare dead the other comtaose patients who slip through the sieve of this committee's tests for "no discernible central nervous system activity." Until this is done and further procedures for stating death agreed to, it seems that deeply comatose patients, the tragic "vegetable" cases whose respiration and hearts continue naturally, fall under an ethics of caring for the dying, the not yet dead, perhaps even the not yet dying. Then it would seem less confusing to say of the limited sort of cases dealt with by the Harvard report that they have no longer any capacity on their own to respirate, nor is there any hope of recovering either heart life or lung life. This, of course, is *because* their brains suffered such massive destruction.

has to be determined by purely clinical signs, to be described, or by absence of circulation as judged by standstill blood in the retinal vessels, or by absence of cardiac activity." The introductory words of that statement imply that these are alternative tests, to be used, e.g., in a small-town clinic or by a physician treating a victim of a high-way accident remote from ambulance service or hospitals. Then absence of cardiac activity would still be used as a test. The words "to be described," introducing the report's own list of tests, which includes no discernible inner need to breathe, at least raises some question of the account to be given of such brain-damaged patient's continuing cardiac activity—sustained as it is by artificial respiration.

Then, in the summary, the Harvard Report states that "among the brain-stem-spinal mechanism [i.e., still "discernible central nervous system activity"] which are conserved for a time, the vasomotor reflexes are the most persistent, and they are responsible in part for the paradoxical state of retained cardiovascular function, which is to some extent independent of nervous control, in the face of wide-spread disorder of cerebrum, brain stem, and spinal cord." This obliquely, if only obliquely, refers to the persistence of heart activity in permanently comatose patients who still breathe from a wholly natural power. These cases are simply not covered or addressed by the Harvard Report. Then the question of what account should be given of the continuing cardiac activity in the cases addressed by the report remains open. These are cases of such massive brain damage that the patient has no recoverable capacity to respirate, or no inner need to breathe. Artificially respirated, his heart continues "indefinitely" to beat, i.e., it may not succeed in failing for days to come. The account or interpretation to be given of persisting heart activity in these patients, I suggest, should be significantly different from the account or description of the persistent heart activity in permanently comatose patients whose brains have not been so deeply damaged as to abolish also all respiratory power or need.

In addition to these expressed, if oblique, references to wholly natural and continuing cardiopulmonary functioning as among the criteria determining whether a comatose individual has any discernible central nervous system activity, the committee's description of four clinical signs of brain death can hardly be verified in a patient whose heart still beats without immediate or remote artificial support. These are (1) no receptivity or responsivity, complete lack of response to the most intensely painful external stimuli and complete lack of any manifestation of "inner need;" (2) no movement or breathing. Here we can see the meaning of "inner need": the total absence of spontaneous respiration in a patient on a mechanical respirator is established if, when the respirator is turned off for three minutes, there is "no effort" on the part of the patient to breathe spontaneously. Presumably the slightest effort to breathe (not success in doing so) would be taken as evidence of brain life, and *assisted* (as distinct from entirely *artificial*) respiration would be resumed; (3) no reflexes; and (4) flat electroencephalogram. These clinical signs of brain life or death, and how properly to apply them, are described in great detail.[38] Finally, it is suggested that all of the tests should be repeated at least 24 hours later with no change before a patient is declared dead.

As applied to the Newcastle General Hospital case, the Harvard Report would quite properly require more than a determination that after the kidney was taken from Mr. Potter "the respirator was then turned off and there was no spontaneous breathing or circulation." [39] It would require (1) three-minute cutoffs to determine a failure of natural cardiopulmonary function, repeated with no change at least 24 hour later; and (2) a declaration of death upon these evidences before the respirator could finally be turned off (or organs used in transplantation). The Harvard committee further suggests that "the decision to declare the person dead, and then to turn off the respirator, be made by physicians not involved in any later effort to transplant organs or tissue from the deceased individual."

I am assured by Dr. Beecher that these tests can be verified in the presence of a "spontaneously" beating heart. That seems strange language to a layman such as I am. Still I am assured that there is plenty of clinical evidence that a man could "flunk" all the fore-

---

38. A doctor would have to learn to tell the difference between symptoms of "inner need" to breathe and a reflex in the patient from turning off the machine. Also, if I rightly understand, a patient who has been overoxygenated may not need to breathe for more than three minutes, and should be given more time. Yet more than three minutes would be dangerous and too long for other patients. The report specifies in considerable medical detail how physicians can safely proceed along the narrow ridge of using three-minute cutoffs in testing for life or death.

39. *British Medical Journal* (August 10, 1963): 394.

going tests (and be declared dead) while his heart beats "naturally." This drives us to the crux of the matter, which is the question of the *term* we should use best to convey what the situation is. It is the respiration—artificial or natural—which alone prolongs the functioning of the heart. If the artificial respiration is prolonged beyond the point of no return of spontaneous respiration, how can the prolonged functioning of the heart be called spontaneous or natural or a permanent capacity of the patient?

I seriously suggest that subtly a radical change has taken place in the meaning of natural heartbeat as a test of life, and that this no longer means what it once always did, or what it still means in the case of patients not on respirators. It is the respirator that, one step away, is being rebutted by these tests, and not brain tests elevated or truly spontaneous heart life downgraded in the procedures by which we should tell that a man has died. It is true that the respirator may be finally cut off in some sense "while the heart still beats"; but it is also cut off "while the lungs still breathe." The situation seems not unlike the "primitive case" we considered at the beginning of this discussion. There the Scout master abandoned his efforts at chest respiration while the deeply brain-injured boy still had heart circulation, also while he still breathed. But there was in either case no recoverable permanent capacity for either function.

The committee's recommendation seems to the present writer to become confused only in a few passages in which artificially sustained, even if remotely sustained, heartbeat is taken to be a sign of life still in need of rebuttal. In past times, the report says, "the obvious criterion of no heartbeat as synonymous with death was sufficiently accurate"; but "this is no longer valid when modern resuscitative and supportive measures are used. These improved activities can now restore 'life' as judged by the ancient standards of persistent respiration and continuing heartbeat." These statements led to the ambiguous press interpretations of these recommendations. The "ancient standards of persistent respiration and continuing heartbeat" meant natural or spontaneous heartbeat. The committee is not proposing that these be set aside. It is rather proposing careful checks upon whether spontaneous respiration is or is not being restored by the use of modern resuscitative measures. It proposes that breathing entirely sustained by artificial means not be viewed as a sign of life, and that a way be found to declare a person dead and these measures withheld, even though as a consequence of the artificially prolonged breathing the "signs" of heart life are also artificially prolonged.

We noted that Helmuth Thielicke said that he saw no reason why the preservation of the vitality of specific organs of an unburied corpse should be thought to mean maintaining a man alive, or to involve moral issues of life and death. In the same vein, I might remark that I see no reason why an entirely artificial sustenance of breathing (and consequently of heartbeat) in an unburied corpse should be believed to be maintaining its "life" even to the extent the Harvard committee allows by using the word in quotation marks. This report is rather an eminently wise proposal for determining, in the face of these resuscitative measures, that the patient has died and one is now only in the presence of an unburied corpse. It is, as Professor Freund said, a set of guidelines on how to use a respirator, a proposal of procedures to be used in telling that a patient has died. It is a way to use a respirator so as to get behind its artificial process to discern an unburied body. It is an updating of the meaning of death only in the—medically quite proper—nominalistic sense that death means the procedures for stating that it has occurred. This is undergirded by a *concept* that death means a permanently nonfunctioning brain. But the *characteristics* of this state of affairs are what is chiefly in view, and this leads to the *procedures* proposed for stating that a man has, on the committee's view of what death is, actually died.

Before concluding this review of the literature on updating death, there is another sort of case, unlike brain-damaged patients, that calls for some comment. There are cases that will be brought up in seeming rebuttal of my proposal that machine-driven signs of life be more radically dismissed. I have suggested that an understanding discussion of our present problem will be furthered by ceasing to regard as a "sign of life" any heart activity that continues in *brain-damaged patients* simply because their irrecoverable respiratory power is being activated artificially. To this it may be replied that if heart activity that is remotely sustained by an outside mechanism applied to the lungs is not a sign of life, then there are a great many men carrying on their daily affairs and work in the world who are dead already! These are the people whose hearts function regularly only because of a "pacemaker."

These people provided with pacemakers have no natural or recoverable spontaneous rhythmical function of the heart. Without the pacemaker their hearts would fail, and as a consequence their brains would promptly die and respiration cease altogether. Then are they not in principle dead already? If we should not say that a massively brain-damaged patient who cannot respirate on his own is dead "although his heart still beats," why should we not say that a pacemaker patient is dead already although his brain is still (one step removed) "artificially" alive and (by another step) his respiration as well? If it is the respirator alone that by sustaining breathing also keeps the heart going in "brain dead" patients, it is also the pacemaker alone that by sustaining heartbeat also keeps the brain and lungs going in "heart dead" patients. One can obviously go too far in dismissing mechanically sustained signs of life from our understanding of the meaning of being a man alive! How shall the pacemaker cases be distinguished from the cases under discussion in revising the criteria for stating that a patient with a permanently nonfunctioning brain has died—particularly in the light of the foregoing argument for not declaring patients dead "while their hearts still beat" (or for not saying that this was what was done)? One or two provisional and perhaps prosaic rejoinders can be made to this objection, and then a crucial one.

It could be said that the pacemaker patients have intact natural functioning of two of the vital signs of life (brain and lungs) whose destruction is stayed by artificially sustaining one (the heart) indefinitely, just as "iron lung" patients also have two of the great organ systems still in full power (brain and heart), the destruction of which is stayed by permanently sustaining one (the lungs) by artificial means. However, this would not be an adequate answer, since it is technically not impossible to perfect some sort of "respirator" that could be borne on the body as conveniently as a pacemaker. Then we could sustain indefinitely two of the traditional vital signs (heart and lungs) by prostheses that men can conveniently wear, instead of by hospital-based respirators alone.[40] Then we would truly

40. As these words were being written, announcement was made of the successful use of a "diaphragm pacemaker" developed under the supervision of Dr. William L. Glenn at Yale University School of Medicine. The device uses radio waves to stimulate the phrenic nerve in the neck, which in turn causes the diaphragm to move. This

have isolated brain life as alone a sufficient warrant for indefinitely sustaining the life of the entire pulmonary-vascular system by one or more extrinsic appliances. Or it could be said that when respirators became proper prostheses, like pacemakers, then we will need to avail ourselves of Pope Pius XII's judgment that life continues as long as its vital functions manifest themselves spontaneously, or even with the help of artificial procedures.[41] After all, a pacemaker patient still has heart life, only the beat is assisted; whereas the brain dead patients identified by the Harvard report have no respiratory capacity at all, or even any manifest "need" to breathe.

The crucial answer, however, is to say that the earlier iron lung cases, the pacemaker cases, or future possible cases of the prosthetic maintenance of cardiopulmonary functioning such as I have imagined are simply not parallel with any of the cases involved in the current discussion of needed revision in our procedures for stating death. In the cases that have just been brought up, the question at issue is simply whether we have isolated brain life as sufficient to warrant continuation of procedures in the absence of natural or recoverable powers of respiration and/or circulation. Brain life, indeed is sufficient for that. But the question currently under discussion is whether we have isolated brain death as sufficient warrant for a declaration of death in the *presence* of natural or recoverable powers of respiration and/or circulation. It is one thing to declare a person to be obviously still alive so long as he has an indefinitely, fully functioning brain in the absence of heart or lung function. It would be quite another thing to declare a person dead (because his brain is past full recovery) in the presence of a still continuing, natural functioning of lungs and/or heart. It may be granted that an essentially isolated brain *life* may be quite enough to warrant continuing by any means procedures that alone indefinitely stay the abolition of that brain. The question raised by the current discussion is quite different: it is whether an essentially isolated brain *death* (or some tests for this) are enough to warrant ceasing to treat a patient as a man alive and stating that death has occurred in the presence of continuing natural functioning of either lungs or heart.

enabled a 53-year-old man, who for ten years had slept on a mechanical rocking bed, to be up and about or to lie flat and still breathe (*New York Times,* May 25, 1969). Suppose that this man needed also to wear a cardiac pacemaker: what functions would constitute his life?

41. See n. 26.

None of the proposals go so far, as we have seen. Actual or recoverable respiratory function is always a test for a still functioning brain. Since respiration is controlled by brainstem activity, only a comparatively few of the tragic comatose cases are covéred by presently proposed redefinitions of death. Within this narrow range of cases, I have urged that it is misleading and false to say that death is to be stated in the presence of a still spontaneously functioning heart.

I cannot imagine why this suggestion should meet with any resistance; it is rather a clarification of the judgments made in the cases presently under discussion. A heart that still beats in an artificially and hopelessly respirated brainstem-damaged patient is an artificially and hopelessly beating heart, and is in no way a sign of life. Nevertheless, I can too readily imagine why the suggestion may meet with resistance from some quarters. This may be because of a hope that a larger number of indefinitely comatose patients, many of whom breathe and circulate themselves, may be brought within future possible improvements or refinements of this medical determination of death. It is at least remotely possible that some proponents of the current, limited redefinitions of death may want to keep saying that death can legitimately be pronounced in the presence of a still "spontaneously" beating heart (although this is backed up by a respirator) in order by this use of language to prepare the ground for saying that brain damage not so deep as to abolish respiration (and consequently not heart function either) can be counted as death.[42]

42. It is not certain where we should locate Dr. Henry K. Beecher's position in regard to this whole range of hopelessly comatose patients. Shall they be deemed alive or dead? On the one hand, Beecher writes that "although some have attempted to make a case for the concept of a corpse as one who is unconscious and suffering from incurable brain damage, one can nevertheless orient the situation swiftly by a single wry question: 'Would you bury such a man whose heart was still beating—'" (Compare this with David Daube's insistence on the same test, n. 16 above.) On the other hand, he rightly tells us that "One can submit that life is the ability to communicate with others. . . . One can make a considerable case that if a physician judges his patient's ability to communicate as lost beyond retrieval through permanent unconsciousness, he not only may, but *must*, declare the man dead" ("Ethical Problems Created by the Hopelessly Unconscious Patient," *New England Journal of Medicine* 278 [June 27, 1968]: 4). If the latter are corpses, they will be buried or cremated while still breathing and heartbeating from a wholly natural power.

My present point is simply this: some people may want in the future to resolve the problem of "vegetable" cases by pronouncing them dead upon some humanistic defi-

This possibility may not be wrongly held open. Dr. David D. Rutstein of Harvard Medical School believes that the question has already been settled in that direction in the public mind. "Those who would replace 'irreversible brain damage' for 'total absence of the function of all organs' as satisfactory for the diagnosis of death in man," he writes, are in principle already willing to disregard the the two subcortical centers of the essentially automatic functions of respiration and circulation. Rutstein states as his opinion that "this new definition of heart donor eligibility [sic!] that substitutes 'irreversible brain damage' for 'total death' raises more questions than it answers." [43] The current proposals, however, have not included patients whose cortical brain activity alone has been destroyed. When such carefully wrought medical proposals further extending the definition of death are put forth in the public forum, they can be discussed and agreed to or rejected. Until this is done, however, one must simply say that patients who still breathe and/or circulate themselves are *not* dead. These cases are rather to be addressed by an ethics of the proper care of the still living, the dying, the not yet dying.

This brings us to the first of two final critical, or at least warning, comments upon the current discussions of the meaning of life and death which it may be proper for a moralist to contribute.

On Not Confusing Death with Stopping Extraordinary Means

After reviewing this entire discussion there are two points that one should ponder. The first question is: What may be the meaning in the peculiar fact that so often in the literature on updating procedures for stating death, appeal is made to the moral authority of Pope Pius XII speaking on the entirely different topic of the dispensability of extraordinary means *to save life?* So the Harvard Report states (quite correctly, of course) that "it is the church's view that a time comes when resuscitative efforts should stop and death be

---

nition of life. Such persons will, not unnaturally, want to hold the door open for movement in this direction, by describing the comatose patients presently under discussion and addressed by the current proposals for updating death as "dead while their hearts still beat." Obviously, however, these are radically different sorts of cases, and radically different respiratory and cardiovascular activities.

43. David R. Rutstein, "The Ethical Design of Human Experiments," *Daedalus,* Spring 1969, pp. 526–27.

unopposed." The Ciba Foundation Symposium devoted entirely to the consideration of a most extraordinary therapy quotes at length from Pius XII's November 24, 1947 statement on the dispensability of extraordinary efforts at "reanimation." [44] So also Dr. Voigt, having decisively rejected the use of the term "suspended death" because in this there remains a suggestion that death has not occurred, still felt it necessary to paraphrase these religious teachings about the dispensability of extraordinary measures when there is no hope of reviving a patient who is "virtually dead." [45]

The writ of these statements runs in an entirely different direction. Rightly declaring a patient to be dead is not the same as no longer to oppose his death. These are two different subjects for medical judgment and in medical ethics. There are good reasons under both heads for stopping so-called "life"-sustaining measures. In the case of stating that death has occurred, the reason is that there is no point in ventilating and circulating the blood of a corpse (unless the body can and should be used for a time as a vital "organ bank"). In this case, there is no death or dying any longer to be opposed (unless it be the death of transplantable organs). One then could not commit euthanasia, only attempt it. One could succeed only in mutilating a corpse if one tried. In the matter of ceasing to use extraordinary means (or useless ordinary means) and no longer opposing death, the issue is the proper care of the dying when they can no longer be cured.

As Professor David Daube has written, "The question of at what moment it is in order to discontinue extraordinary—or even ordinary —measures to keep a person alive should not be confused with the question at what moment a man is dead" or with the question of the procedures by which the presence of life or death is to be determined. "Discontinuation of such measures is often justifiable even while the patient is conscious." [46] A decision to continue or to discontinue life-sustaining treatment of a person who has suffered massive brain injury, or longer to sustain a comatose patient, or a conscious dying patient, is precisely a judgment made in the face of a life still present.

44. Wolstenholme and O'Connor, *Ethics in Medical Progress,* pp. 223–30.

45. "The Criteria of Death," pp. 144–45. There is also a reference to this body of teachings tucked away in a parenthetical remark in the editorial introducing these articles in the *World Medical Journal* 14: 133.

46. In Wolstenholme and O'Connor, *Ethics in Medical Progress,* pp. 190–91.

No matter how fine the tests for telling death, some stroke or brain-damaged patients are going to get through the net and must be declared to be still living.

Because physicians seem to pass back and forth between these two problems—defining death and only caring for the dying—may be the reason that Professor Ralph B. Potter, Jr., who was a member of the Harvard committee, is troubled.[47] To avoid premature declarations of death, he writes, the medical profession needs "a simple, chaste principle." (Stating that death has occurred needs to be based on "chaste" criteria, we can agree, but these can no longer be "simple.") On the other hand, when physicians are faced with a decision whether death should still be opposed and life prolonged, they *must* use what Potter calls a "balancing logic." Potter seems to feel that the former—declaring a patient dead—is rather a subterfuge for avoiding a balancing judgment that dying should no longer be prolonged (withholding heroic measures to save life), and that the latter is a questionable practice. Instead, these are two aspects of necessary and proper medical practice, two different responsibilities of the physician. Professor Potter may have been misled by the degree of vacillation between these two issues that is present in the literature on updating death.

When I reflect on this peculiarity that in the literature on updating procedures for stating death so often there is citation of papal and other teachings on the dispensability of extraordinary means to *save life,* I can only conclude that the physicians and committees may not be quite sure that they are using the right criteria for verifying the presence of death and the absence of life. They may not be quite sure that a heart that still beats "naturally" (when backed up by the now useless maintenance of breathing by a respirator) is no sign of life. They may not be as willing as the present writer to dismiss that sign of life as only "technical."

There is a second, and more disturbing, point to ponder as a possible explanation of this unsteadiness over whether death can be correctly stated by the proposed criteria. Now that organ transplantation has reached the heart, is there possibly a remaining fear and shadow of guilt on the part of doctors that they may be killing

47. Ralph B. Potter, Jr., "The Paradoxical Preservation of a Principle," *Villanova Law Review* 13, no. 4 (Summer 1968): 784–92.

the recipients of borrowed hearts in the course of these surgical trials, and also that this will be the case when in the future heart transplantation can properly be described as a form of therapy? In the case of patients in the last stages of heart failure, are surgeons killing in order to make alive for a time? And when hearts can be implanted earlier in the deterioration of a patient's heart, will the surgeons be killing in implanting hearts as a form of *preventive* medicine? This would seem to be so, unless an indefinitely spontaneous heartbeat is altogether excluded by a set of chaste, however complex, procedures for stating that death has occurred. None of the serious proposals go that far. Can it be that the remaining references in the literature on death to the dispensability of extraordinary means to prolong life manifest a continuing belief that heart activity still indicates the presence of life? If so—as regards recipients of hearts—the "paradoxical preservation of a principle" can be restated to read: the justification of no longer opposing by extraordinary means the death of slowly deteriorating heart patients must be retained in the argument about whether they are dead or not in order paradoxically to make room for still more spectacular measures for making them alive.

On Not Confusing Death with "Organ Donor Eligibility"

In conclusion, I shall raise one simple ethical warning concerning these discussions of the meaning of death. We have seen that the Harvard committee strongly recommends that "the decision to declare the person dead, and then to turn off the respirator, be made by physicians not involved in any later effort to transplant organs or tissue from the deceased individual." This seems to be the unanimous opinion of all who have written or spoke on this subject. Will a dying man be any less assiduously treated or cared for because he is a prospective donor? This possibility, however remote, needs to be excluded altogether. The procedure to ensure that a prospective donor's death be not *for this purpose* hastened is to establish a complete separation of authority and responsibility between the physician or group of physicians who are responsible for the care of the recipient, and the physician or group of physicians who are responsible for the care of the patient who is a prospective donor. This is generally the procedure at medical centers where the organs of unburied corpses are used in transplantation. This safeguard was the principle point adopted at a meeting of the World Medical Assembly in Sydney, Australia, where there seemed from the press report to be lively discussion but little agreement on the meaning of death.[48] This procedure for ensuring the protection of prospective donors is commonly recognized and is being adopted by the medical profession itself. It is likely also to be required by law. The National Conference of Commissioners on Uniform State Laws has drafted a Uniform Anatomical Gift Act which includes this principle of the "separation of powers" among its provisions.[49] It is to be hoped that this model bill will be adopted by the various state jurisdictions.

A comment from the point of view of religious ethics can only welcome this development. This restriction is needed among the "checks and balances" in medical institutions in order to "restrain and remedy" wrongdoing. The fact that this was first widely recog-

48. *New York Times,* August 10, 1968.

49. Section 7 (b). See also Alfred M. Sadler, Jr., and Blair L. Sadler, "Transplantation and the Law: The Need for Organized Sensitivity," *Georgetown Law Journal* 57, no. 1 (October 1968): 26–27 and 34; Delford L. Stickel, "Organ Transplantation in Medical and Legal Perspectives," *Law and Contemporary Problems* 32, no. 4 (Autumn 1967): 611. I am convinced that this proposal for the separation of responsibilities for donor and recipient is not disingenuous "window dressing" to quell the doubts of patients "unjustly suspicious" of their doctors. However, one hears expressed among physicians some cynicism about whether this constraining procedure will actually work, because of doubt that one physician will "stand up" to another when they may be colleagues in the same hospital and who in any case are professional colleagues. Realistically, Dr. M. F. A. Woodruff writes, "those looking after the injured patient can scarcely fail to know that their unseen colleagues are waiting poised for action, or that their colleague's patient is also waiting hoping desperately for a graft that will give him a chance of survival" ("Ethical Problems in Organ Transplantation," *British Medical Journal* 1 [June 1964]: 1460.

The confidence which I still retain in the worthwhileness of this proposed practice was, however, further shaken by the report that, in drafting the Uniform Anatomical Gift Act, the committee—having first determined that the physician who states the death of the donor "shall not be a member of the team of surgeons which transplants the part"—changed that in their final draft to read: "shall not participate in the procedures for removing or transplanting a part." Presumably, in the Gift statutes to be enacted the donor's physician may be *a member of the transplant team;* he only in this case may not participate in the surgery! See Sadler and Sadler, "Transplantation and the Law" p. 27. This is surely a minimum attempt to achieve the stringent requirement: ". . . it is of the greatest importance that the transplant team have the least possible contact with the physicians treating this patient before he has been pronounced dead" (Hamburger and Crosnier, "Moral and Ethical Problems in Transplantation," p. 43).

nized among the self-restraints that physicians propose to impose upon themselves, and which they affirm should in one way or another be imposed upon medical practice, shows that physicians are not on the whole believers in "participatory democracy" or in the aptness of human beings always to do the right without constraints that wisely and humanely impel them to do so.

But if this is so, what are we to say concerning updating the meaning of death, or the tests for determining when a man has died, precisely at a time when great advancement is being made in organ transplantation? The revision of procedures for stating death is a development in the intellectual order, having important practical consequences for pronouncements of death. If in the practical order we need to separate between the physician who is responsible for the care of a prospective donor, and the physician who is responsible for a prospective recipient, do we not need in the intellectual order to keep the question of the definition of death equally discrete from the use of organs in transplantation? If only the physician responsible for a dying man should make the determination that he has died, with no "help" from the medical team that has in its care a man who needs a borrowed organ, should not also the definition of death and the tests for it that he uses be ones that he thinks are sound or were agreed to by the profession without having transplantation in view? There would be too little protection of life attained in the practical order by entirely separating the authority and responsibility of the teams of physicians if the definition of death and the tests for it have already been significantly invaded by the requirements of transplant therapy. If no person's death should *for this purpose* be hastened, then the definition of death should not *for this purpose* be updated, or the procedures for stating that a man has died be revised as a means of affording easier access to organs.

This is an ethical consideration of considerable importance. There is something not a little sinister when the press can state in explaining the Harvard Report that the issue of the meaning of death has been "simmering" for some time but has presumably been brought to a boil by transplant therapy; that "many medical men fear that controversy will bedevil heart transplant efforts until the definition of death is clarified"; and quote Dr. Campbell Moses, medical director of the American Heart Association, to the effect that "until recently this was not critical, but we've got a whole new ball game now because two hours can make the difference in whether an organ is viable for transplant." [50] If a person's particular moment of dying ought not to be run into that "ball game" but ought rather to be separated from it by his own physician's independence of judgment, neither should the definition of death and of the tests for saying that a person has died. This ought to be a judgment and an agreement in medical science and practice that is also independent of whether organ transplantation is bedeviled, impeded, or assisted thereby.

The present writer was once invited by a state medical association to submit in writing a theologian's definition of "the moment of death" to a symposium on that subject to be held in 1968. My reply, of course, was to say that a theologian or moralist as such knows nothing about such questions; that the determination of death is a medical matter; and that a theologian or moralist can offer only his reflections upon the meaning of respect for life and of care of the dying, and issue some warnings of the moral complexities such as are here set down. The wording of this request seemed to me to be exceedingly significant. It said: "The purpose of this symposium is to more clearly define 'The Moment of Death' *so that* those sick people who need transplanted tissues will not be sacrificed because of a lack of a clear definition as to when the donor has died." (italics added.) This comes perilously close to unsavory talk about whether "*society* can afford to discard the organs of comatose patients if they can be used to restore health to salvageable patients" (italics added).

This is not to say that the meaning of death need not be updated, or that the medical criteria for death do not need to be clarified.

---

50. *New York Times*, News of the Week, Sunday, August 11, 1968. The news account of an interview with Dr. Henry K. Beecher on the day this report was published in the *Journal of the American Medical Association* stressed the connection of the proposed updating of death with the use of organs in transplants far more than does the report itself (*New York Times*, August 5, 1968). I would argue that there is sufficient need and sufficient reason for (1) rethinking our understanding of death and/or (2) no longer opposing death, to be found in proper attention to the patient himself. There is no need—and in fact it is a little unsavory and may finally prove dangerous—to put behind these questions an urgency to answer them anew drawn in any measure from the question: "Can society afford to discard the organs of such patients if they can be used to restore health to salvageable patients?" (Robert Reinhold's dispatch in the *Times*, ibid.).

It is only to say that death should not be updated for that purpose. I should have thought that the purpose of an symposium to define more clearly the moment of death would be so that persons who have not died shall continue to be cared for and so that persons who have died need not have "life"-sustaining measures inflicted upon their unburied corpses, needlessly and at great expense to their families. The reasons for this must be sufficient in themselves as proper medical practice. Any benefit that may accrue to other patients in this age of organ transplantation must be a wholly independent by-product of an updating of death that is already per se right and wise and a proper judgment to be made concerning the primary patient.[51] The issues that have been "simmering" for a long time must be resolved as if transplantation did not exist as a method of surgical therapy. There is sufficient need and sufficient reason for updating death so that the primary patient and his family may be treated properly. There is also sufficient need and sufficient reason, as we shall see in the next chapter, for withholding (in the face of life and without a pronouncement of death) extraordinary measures in caring for the irreversibly dying.

Unless in the current discussion of the meaning of death the medical profession keeps these considerations clear of one another, it is likely to be convicted of an overweening desire to pass from one spectacular to another—from spectacular treatment of the dying, and indeed of the dead, to spectacular use of borrowed organs. It is likely to be convicted of failure to face the urgent problem of updating the meaning of death so long as that might have placed limits upon the use of extraordinary "life"-sustaining measures, and then of radically revising the meaning of death and the tests for it when this would open the way to the use of other extraordinary life-sustaining procedures for the sake of recipients, medical progress,

51. This point is often better understood by physicians than by the public generally, or by pragmatists whose sole criterion is that the greatest good should be done. Among the participants in the Ciba Symposium, Dr. R. Y. Calne warned that "any modification of the means of diagnosing death to facilitate transplantation will cause the whole procedure to fall into disrepute with the rest of the profession"; David Daube cautioned that "a redefinition with an avowed purpose might well create doubts in the mind of the layman"; while Dr. Jean Hamburger hit the target on dead center: "Transplantation is a secondary problem which must not interfere with the search for a more accurate definition of death" (In Wolstenholme and O'Connor, *Ethics in Medical Progress*, pp. 73, 190, 206).

and "society." If good must not only be done but also seem to be done, it can seriously be suggested that every prospect of organ donation be removed from the discussion of any proposed needed revision in our understanding of death. That question can and should be allowed to rest on its own merits.

My final point is this additional one, well stated by Dr. J. Russell Elkinton: "We do not want to apply [or seem to apply] a double ethical standard: one for the unconscious patient with a head injury who is not being considered as a possible donor and another for the same kind of patient who is." [52] There would be a double ethical standard—and perhaps two moments of death—if in discussing the nature of the procedures for stating death or in applying these procedures in individual cases, the need for borrowed organs led to agreement upon procedures for stating death that for this purpose hasten pronouncements of death.

Dr. Henry K. Beecher would use the definition of death in terms of a permanently nonfunctioning brain as a heuristic device for securing organs for transplant. Updating death, he writes, is an available, "powerful means of overcoming the grave shortages" in the supply of organs. From data based on "neurological" deaths when the tissues to be transplanted would be satisfactory, and assuming no legal or logistic barriers, Beecher calculates that there could be made available in the United States each year over 10,600 cadaver kidneys for approximately 7,600 needy kidney recipients, and 6,000 livers for 4,000 potential liver recipients. In this situation, he believes that "to do nothing . . . is far more radical than to accept the tissues and organs of the hopelessly comatose." [53] This seems to be a redefinition of death with an avowed purpose. It is also a quite questionable purpose, if this purpose is permitted to become the decisive reason or any part of the reason for adopting a new understanding of when patients have died. Instead we must say of revisions of the meaning of death, if proposed for this reason, exactly the same thing as was Beecher's verdict upon human experimentation "for the good of society": to be "viewed with distaste, even alarm.

52. J. Russell Elkinton, "The Dying Patient, the Doctor and the Law," *Villanova Law Review* 13, no. 4 (Summer 1968): 746–47.

53. Beecher, "Scarce Resources and Medical Advancement," pp. 295, 296, 294.

Undoubtedly all sound work has this as its ultimate aim, but such high-flown expressions are not necessary and have been used within recent memory as cover for outrageous ends." [54]

We must appeal from the late Beecher drunk to the early Beecher sober; and, with Professor Hans Jonas, appeal from Beecher's recent words to his personal humanity and moral sensibility, for which there can be nothing but admiration. The words are, nevertheless, alarming; and Professor Jonas submitted them to irrefutable moral criticism. Where Beecher had asked, "Can society afford to discard the tissues and organs of the hopelessly unconscious patient when they could be used to restore the otherwise hopelessly ill, but still salvageable individual?" Jonas comments: " 'Discarding' implies proprietary rights—nobody can discard what does not belong to him in the first place." Then he asks: "Does society then own my body?" Moreover, if it is a question of what society can "afford" and not what should be done, Jonas calls our attention to the fact that "society can go on flourishing in every way" even if cancer, heart disease, and

54. Henry K. Beecher, "Experimentation in Man," *Journal of the American Medical Association* 169, no. 5 (January 31, 1959): 468. This was Beecher's judgment (see ibid., pp. 463, 474) not upon the Nazi medical cases but upon point 2 of the Nuremberg Code used as the standard in the trial of these cases, which reads: "The experiment should be such as to yield fruitful results for the good of society, unprocurable by any other methods or means of study, and not random and unnecessary in nature." Beecher now comes close to saying that in the concept of "neurological" death we have a powerful means of securing organs for the good of society, unprocurable by means other than by this redefinition! We can agree with the redefinition while insisting that this is warranted solely by the condition of the primary patient. There need be no decisive reference to the good of society (which, in experimentation or in transplantation, means the needs of *other* patients, present or future). Recently, Dr. Beecher repeated his earlier, sounder view: "In Rule 2, the phrase 'for the good of society' is unsavory"; ". . . the *bonum communum* was precisely the rationalization claimed by the Nazis" (*Research and the Individual*, pp. 232, 77; see also pp. 14, 47–49, 51–52, 70).

Deploring the use of terms like *hopelessly incurable* to warrant the use of terminal patients in experimentation for the good of others, Beecher inserts an exception for the "irreversibly comatose individual" needed for organ "donation" (p. 85). Because there is no precise moment of death, the Harvard committee "chose to give a definition of irreversible coma rather than to attempt a definition of death" (p. 153). That suggests the definition of a more limited class of patients who are *hopelessly incurable,* and would again make virtual or imminent death the test of organ donor eligibility. Yet in the case of the "hopelessly unconscious individual" Beecher still says, "the question is whether the *body* must be left untouched" (p. 163)!

other noncontagious diseases "continue to exact their toll at the normal rate of incidence." [55] In fact, it may be said that "society" needs these deaths, even as genetically the human race needs death.[56]

Ordinarily in discussions of such topics as medical research and organ transplantation, it is assumed that the moral claims of a patient and the claims of "society" are in parity, and that a responsible moral decision will strike some balance between these claims, bartering one against the other. Hans Jonas' chapter is an extraordinary exception to this approach. For him "the individual is the primary concrete" (his good is more or less known, while the common or public good is the unknown in such "decision-making"). This means that we must always "justify the infringement of a primary inviolability" of the individual patient or subject, while this inviolability "needs no justification itself." [57]

But, of course, the public good or the good of "society" breaks down into the good of other "primary concrete" individuals— present or future patients who need medical care. Therefore, the basic question concerns how the moral claims of others are to be factored in with an individual's interest in his own inviolability and his claim to "invasion-proof selfhood." Jonas' answer to this question is as follows. These are not claims having parity; both are not moral claims, or in the same sense moral claims. Instead, the primary inviolability is a moral claim or right needing no justification, while the "salvaging" of others is a moral call needing an answering response. The call to sacrifice from highest devotion cannot and should not be reduced to a right or a legitimate claim. "No one," neither "society" nor other men, "has the shred of a right to expect and ask these things. They come to the rest of us as a gratia gratis data." [58]

This sets in proper perspective the ethics of medicine's scientific mission. Doubtless we are committed to the promotion of medical progress. Doubtless we owe to medical practice and to "society" our

55. Hans Jonas, "Philosophical Reflections on Human Experiment," Ethical Aspects of Experimentation with Human Subjects, *Daedalus*, Spring 1969, pp. 227, 228. He might as well have asked: Do other, still salvageable patients own my body? Are my organs then "discarded" if not given to their rightful new owners?

56. Bentley Glass, *Science and Ethical Values* (Chapel Hill: University of North Carolina Press, 1965), pp. 10, 32.

57. Jonas, "Philosophical Reflections on Human Experiment," pp. 220–21.

58. Ibid., pp. 220, 222.

individual contribution to the *continued promotion* of medical progress. But this debt is owed to past "martyrs," to the doers of works of supererogatory devotion. Such a debt gives no one a right to choose martyrs for the sake of medical advance, or to allow forthcoming benefit to become a decisive reason for now revising our understanding of when a man has died. Our descendants, as Hans Jonas says, "do not have a right [a moral claim] to new miracle cures . . . we have not sinned against them if by the time they come around arthritis has not yet been conquered (unless by sheer neglect)"—neglect of the mandate continually to pursue medical advancement. "We can expect ever again the upwelling of a will to give what nobody—neither society, nor fellow man, nor posterity—is entitled to"; but this gives us no cause to base a debt of gratitude upon a moral *claim* imperatively or forcibly supplanting an individual patient's primary inviolability, and no justification for advancing the moment of declaring a patient to be dead for the avowed purpose of getting access to his organs. Progress is an optional goal. There is nothing sacred about it. In any case, "it cannot be the aim of progress to abolish the lot of mortality." Jonas rightly insists upon "the essentially 'gratuitous' nature of the whole enterprise of progress, as against the mandatory respect for invasion-proof selfhood." [59] These are not commensurables to be weighed in the same balance.

Thus, there are two pairs of ponderables that ought not to be blended or pondered together: (1) the meaning of death (or when it occurs) and the morality of sometimes ceasing to oppose death's coming; and (2) the meaning of death (or when it occurs) and other patients' need for organ transplants. Given the morality of ceasing to use extraordinary or useless ordinary means to prolong dying (as Professor Jonas said of a "defined negative condition of the brain," and could have said of a defined negative condition of the heart or the liver!), the physician is "allowed to allow the patient to die his own death by *any* definition, which of itself will lead through the gamut of all possible definitions." [60] His discussion at this point, however, shows again that to mix in any degree the definition of death with the morality of allowing to die, to condition the latter by the

59. Ibid., pp. 230, 231, 245, 234.
60. Ibid., p. 241.

former determination, or to bring the shortage of organs at all into view, can lead conscientious men to adopt only the most extremely cautious and limiting criteria for stating that a man has died.

If it is a question of breaking off a sustaining medical intervention, all we need to know is that "only permanent coma can be gained." Then we should let the patient die; but if this is *patient*-centered medical care we would "let him die all the way" and by *any* definition. For this purpose we do not need to know the borderline between life and death. If, however, a possible recipient of his organs is brought into view and if we are thinking of perpetrating an operation upon the dying man, then only the most generous location of the borderline will do.

> To use any definition short of the maximal for perpetrating on a *possibly* penultimate state what only the ultimate state can permit is to arrogate a knowledge which, I think, we cannot have. *Since we do not know the borderline between life and death,* nothing less than the maximum definition of death will do—brain death plus heart death plus any other indication that may be pertinent—before final violence is allowed to be done.

This is the only way to ensure that we do not inflict a final trauma upon the sensitivity—however diffuse and elusive—which we ourselves have been maintaining in the dying man. But Jonas' chief reason is not the patient's possible suffering, but simply "the indeterminancy of the boundaries between *life and death*" and "the inflexible principle that utter helplessness demands utter protection." This adds up to the simple and unqualified impermissibility of giving transplant surgeons access to the organs of an unconscious patient until we are *quite certain* he is dead. If it is rightful to allow to die, Jonas concludes, the patient should be let die all the way, through the gamut of all definitions.[61]

61. Ibid., pp. 244, 240, 244. Jonas' rhetoric may be misleading. Surely he cannot mean to include cellular death within the gamut of all definitions, or the beginning of decomposition of the "form" of the body. A similar viewpoint, but one less agnostic about statements of death, was expressed by Dr. John J. McCutchen in "Letters," *Journal of the American Medical Association* 204, no. 13 (June 24, 1968): 107: "Discussion of the brain's role in 'death' needs to be reopened to assure that not merely

Jonas sees quite clearly the point which is obscured by all the references to the morality of ceasing extraordinary efforts to save life in the literature on updating death. He sees that "it is one thing when to cease delaying death, but another when to start doing violence to the body; one thing when to desist from protracting the process of dying, but another when to regard that process as complete and thereby the body as a cadaver free for inflicting on it what would be torture and death to any living body." [62]

Still Professor Jonas' discussion provides the strongest demonstration of the confusion that has resulted from in any degree making research or transplant purposes adjunct to the definition or redefinition of death. Those purposes, he rightly sees, easily overstep anything definition can warrant. However, his proper concern for the invasion-proof selfhood of the primary patient, whose only death should be under discussion, leads him to the strange conclusion that "the proposed new definition of death" can authorize us "only to break off a sustaining intervention." [63] Herein Jonas leans over too far backward and falls into the same error as that of the revisionists. He connects these two opposing things: the determination of procedures for stating that a man has died, and the determination of when to break off sustaining medical interventions—a decision which supposes that the patient is still alive. It is enough to say that old or new definitions of death should have the primary patient's only death solely in mind.

To restore the balance, we must say that there are twin perils that can be avoided only by never blending or pondering together these two quite different considerations: the meaning of death (or when it occurs) and other patients' need for organ transplants. If no recipient is available, a patient's doctor often *would not hesitate to wait* before pronouncing him dead and stopping "life"-sustaining treatments. The peril is that this may no longer be so, if the question of the life or death of the primary patient is mixed, either theoretically or practi-

---

reasonable but extraordinary standards be set to protect the rights of prospective donors." That was a rather new note among physicians actively engaged in the discussion of the meaning of death. To be not only sure a prospective donor is dead but to be extraordinarily sure (among the reasonable alternative tests) is the only purpose we should have in questioning the criteria to be used in stating death.

62. Ibid., p. 244.
63. Ibid., p. 245.

cally, with the need of other patients for transplanted organs. We would not have wanted Senator Robert Kennedy's physicians to hesitate to wait before pronouncing him dead, to cease trying to save his life if they could, because someone else needed a healthy organ.

But there is another peril that is of equal importance. If no recipient is available, a patient's doctor *might not hesitate to stop*. Where recipients are in prospect a doctor may wait longer than he should in stating that life had departed, or alternatively he might hesitate to acknowledge that a still living patient requires only care and no longer any attempt to cure him. If Senator Kennedy's intellectual and bodily faculties would have been permanently impaired had he survived, and he would have led a very grave and devastating existence, we would not have wanted his physicians to hesitate to stop trying to save him lest they be suspected of making him accessible to transplantation surgeons in time for a recipient's welfare.

All things considered, the canons of the highest loyalty to the primary patient can best be secured if neither the procedures for stating death nor a decision that death has occurred are distorted by any reference to someone else's need for organs. This loyalty to the primary patient may call for waiting longer or stopping earlier than may be the case if one patient's dying (or the meaning of his death) is made adjunct to another's life.

3

On (Only) Caring for the Dying

> The wish to have a death of one's own is growing ever rarer. Only
> a while yet, and it will be just as rare to have a death of one's own
> as it is already to have a life of one's own.
> Rainer Maria Rilke.

In 1964 Dr. Belding H. Scribner, pioneer in the use of the kidney
machine at the University of Washington School of Medicine and the
Swedish Hospital, Seattle, Washington, delivered the presidential
address at the annual meeting of the American Society for Artificial
Internal Organs.[1] In his remarks on that occasion there is a striking
passage in which Dr. Scribner addressed himself to the problem of a
patient on chronic hemodialysis himself overtly terminating treatment (which Dr. Scribner, mistakenly I believe, describes as "a form
of suicide"). We should expect, Dr. Scribner said, that as chronic
kidney dialysis becomes a normal exigency of life for an increasing
number of people there will be a proportionate increase in the number of those persons who will stop or simply omit this means of their
survival. This led to speculation concerning the "death with dignity"
which medical practice might extend to such patients. Death from
chronic uremia is one of the most horrible known, involving intense
suffering, vomiting, prolongation of the dying process and great costs.
"How much more humane and less expensive it would be to offer
such a dying patient a weekly hemodialysis for a limited period"—
instead of the bi-weekly or tri-weekly blood washings needed to keep
a chronic uremia patient alive. "Then he could live a normal life
right up to the end and die quickly and without prolonged suffering."
Such a "maneuver to provide hemodialysis for a limited period"
would avoid all the suffering, but Dr. Scribner described this as
"utterly impossible under existing moral, ethical and religious guide-

1. Belding H. Scribner, "Ethical Problems of Using Artificial Organs to Sustain
Human Life," in Harold M. Schmeck, Jr., *The Semi-Artificial Man: A Dawning Revolution in Medicine* (New York: Walker, 1965).

lines." That judgment was, I believe, a completely mistaken and un-instructed verdict. Nothing in our moral tradition or religious teachings sustains the conclusion that such care cannot be extended to the dying. The proposed maneuver may or may not be illegal; it is certainly not immoral. Attending and companying with the patient in his dying is, in fact, the oldest medical ethics there is.[2]

The Problem

Shall a patient suffering from terminal illness be given life-sustaining procedures? Should he be placed on a respirator, and is there reason for ever turning off the respirator if such treatment was hopefully begun? Is there any moral difference between not starting the respirator, compared to turning it off once started? Are we bound to begin and continue the use of the intravenous drip because it is so standard a procedure? The "essentially isolated heart" can be kept beating for weeks; should this be begun or continued? Alternatively, the heart can be stopped for surgery or transplantation, while circulation of the blood is shunted around the heart and maintained, along with artificial respiration, by a heart-lung machine: are we

2. Ibid., p. 211. This, apparently, was the ethics invoked at the Renal and Electrolyte Division of the Georgetown University Hospital. There the policy in regard to patients on chronic hemodialysis is one of refusal "to exhort or importune these patients in the belief that they should have complete freedom from coercion in moving either in or out of the program." "Since brain washing can take place subconsciously during blood washing," it was necessary to hold open the category of cessation of treatment by speaking lightly, if at all, of "any obligation toward continuation under extra-ordinary measures for the prolongation of life"—which the patient may regard as "merely a prolongation of ill-health" (of which there is ample enough evidence here detailed). Of 11 patients on kidney dialysis through 1964, two voluntarily withdrew from the program: "one thought that he was dying slowly, without dignity, and leaving an unpleasant memory for his teen-age children as well as making intemperate demands on their sympathy, attention, and devotion" (George E. Schreiner and John F. Maher, "Hemodialysis for Chronic Renal Failure: III. Medical, Moral and Ethical, and Socio-Economic Problems," *Annals of Internal Medicine* 62 [March 1965]: 553–54). At about the same time two kidney-machine patients expressed the desire to discontinue. Dr. Schreiner's procedure was to give them both a good dialysis and ask them the question again when they were in excellent chemical shape. One said, "Don't listen to me, that's my uremia talking, not me. I want to stay on the program." The other, however, still had the resolve to discontinue. Schreiner was convinced that it was he and not uremia talking, that his was an "intellectually free decision," and allowed him to withdraw (as reported in G. E. W. Wolstenholme and Maeve O'Connor (eds.), *Ethics in Medical Progress: With Special Reference to Transplantation,* Ciba Foundation Symposium [Boston: Little, Brown, 1966], p. 129).

obliged to use these means, and, if sometimes not, when not? Should a hopelessly paralyzed person be placed in an iron lung for the rest of his life? Must a terminal cancer patient be urged to undergo major surgery for the sake of a few months' palliation? What of fragmented creatures in deep and prolonged coma from severe brain damage, whose spontaneous cerebral activities have been reduced to those arising from the brainstem (diencephalon, mesencephalon, pons, and medulla) but who can be maintained "alive" for years by a combination of artificial activators and by nourishment? How much blood are we going to give a terminal patient, or how many successive organ transplants? Should transfusions for the treatment of hemorrhage from a gastrointestinal cancer be discontinued, when an operation to relieve this condition is not contemplated or feasible? Is there no end to the doctor's vocation to maintain life until the matter is taken out of his hands?

Alternatively expressed, ought there to be any relief for the dying from a physician's search for exquisite triumphs over death in a sort of salvation by works? Is a quadruple amputee absolutely obliged to choose existence on such terms? If not, what right has a doctor to save his life forcibly (apart from the general benefit of pushing back the frontiers of medical science); and then by what right should medical practice advance through achieving this success by means of him? Should cardiac surgery be performed to remove the lesions that are part of the picture in cases of mongolism, from which many mercifully died before the brilliant developments of recent years?

The same sort of question can be raised about many quite standard or routine procedures. Suppose that a diabetic patient long accustomed to self-administration of insulin falls victim to terminal cancer, or suppose that a terminal cancer patient suddenly develops diabetes. Is he in the first case obliged to continue, and in the second case obliged to begin, insulin treatment and die painfully of cancer, or in either or both cases may the patient choose rather to pass into diabetic coma and a earlier death? The same question can be raised in case of the onset of diabetes in a patient who has lived to old age in an institution for the severely retarded. What of the conscious patient suffering from painful incurable disease who suddenly gets pneumonia? Or an old man slowly deteriorating who from simply being inactive and recumbent gets pneumonia: are we to use antibiotics in a likely successful attack upon this disease which from time immemorial has been called "the old man's friend"? If this is the judgment to be made in regard to the aged, what shall we say of an infant who has hydrocephalus and develops pneumonia which could cause death in a short time? Should a baby born with serious congenital defect be respirated and saved from normal dying by advanced incubator procedures, or protected from the compensating abnormality which nature has somehow provided in the form of lower resistance to ordinary infections? Shall the child who is gravely impaired by mongolism be saved by a simple treatment from an infection that could cause his death?

The question whether it is right to withhold routine procedures in these cases may remain to haunt us even if we agree with Dr. Edward Rynearson that a combination of the heroic measures that are now possible may deprive many a patient of a fulfillment of the wish to have a death of one's own. The scene Dr. Rynearson describes is one of patients with an "untreatable" disease being "kept alive indefinitely by means of tubes inserted into their stomachs, or into their veins, or into their bladders, or into their rectums—and the whole sad scene thus created is encompassed within a cocoon of oxygen which is the next thing to a shroud" [3]—separated from family, from friends, and from themselves—the victims, this physician believes, of massive and unwarranted medical interventions upon their own particular death that has seized them.

One cannot hope to resolve the legitimate disagreement of conscientious men over every one of these questions. These cases suffice to show the importance of the problem raised by asking whether, beyond many present-day efforts to rescue the perishing, there does not arise a medical duty to (only) care for the dying. But this much can be said at the outset. These questions should be resolved one way or the other as *patient* policy questions and not as public policy questions because of the scarcity of beds and other hospital resources. Unless we give an ethically valid, patient-centered answer to them, medically advanced societies will move more and more to decisions based on the numbers and needs that can be accommodated.

The public policy or hospital policy question is already enormous.

3. E. H. Rynearson, "You Are Standing at Bedside of Patient Dying of Untreatable Cancer," CA 9 (May-June 1959): 85–87.

Are we not in modern medicine, a doctor asks, "piling up one Pyrrhic victory after the other, while gradually losing the war?"[4] The public policy question in regard to relentlessly prolonging life is a serious one. "Inevitably," writes Dr. Henry K. Beecher, "with increasingly bold, venturesome, and commendable attempts to rescue the dying, there will be an accumulation of individuals in hospitals who can be kept 'alive' only by extraordinary means despite the fact that there is no hope of recovery of consciousness, let alone recovery to a functioning, pleasurable existence—all this at a cost of $25,000 to $30,000 per year." Another way to state the cost that others are paying for these "heroic" procedures is that a single irretrievably unconscious patient, or incurable patient in great pain and indignity, occupies space that could have been used by 26 other patients staying on the average of two weeks in the hospital.[5] This suggests that not only in the "disaster medicine" practiced in case of natural disasters, such as the typhoons on the Texas coast a few years ago, or designed to be used in case of nuclear attack upon cities (probably administered from the "dog and cat" hospitals left standing in the outskirts), may some form of triage become necessary. Triage sets aside the more serious casualties (as "expectants"),

4. Perrin H. Long, "On the Quantity and Quality of Life," editorial, *Medical Times* 88 (May 1960): 613. See also pp. 613–14: "All have had the experience of walking down the hospital ward and witnessing a team composed of a resident, interns, nurses, and aides laboring with a patient who has cirrhosis, and who is in 'hepatic' coma. We know that many hours and thousands of dollars may be expended in the care of this patient during the episode of coma, and that if the labors are 'successful' the patient will emerge again into a painful, hopeless existence, which will eventually be climaxed by a fatal hemorrhage, or by coma and death. Next to the cirrhotic, there is a patient suffering the tortures of the damned because of the pain of tumor metastases, who has pneumonia. He is being vigorously and successfully treated with penicillin. His suffering will be prolonged. A couple of beds away sits a thirty-five-year-old Mongolian idiot playing in a pool of his own urine and feces, saved from an early death from infection by the 'miracle' drugs. In the next ward a senile old crone gibbers at us, abandoned and totally rejected by her family, who already committed to a modern, overcrowded and understaffed modern Bedlam is waiting to recover completely from a staphylococcal bacteremia originating from a bed sore which had exposed her sacrum to the view of anyone who desired to look. At the end of the ward 'Grandma' sits by her bed staring vacantly into space, and who as Glanville Williams has pointed out so well has reached 'an age of second childhood and mere oblivion' with the loss of almost all adult faculties except that of digestion. . . ."

5. Henry K. Beecher: *Research and the Individual: Human Studies* (Boston: Little, Brown, 1970), p. 159. See also "Prolongation of Dying," *The Lancet,* December 8, 1962, p. 1205.

on whom great and lengthy effort by teams of doctors and nurses would have to be expended to save their lives, for the sake of the greater healing of a greater number.[6] Are we coming into a time when, because of the unlimited application of more and more extraordinary means of saving life, we will be tempted to apply the principles of triage under normal medical circumstances? There would be something unsavory about doing this in regard to the treatment of the dying (because his bed is needed), just as it is an unsavory fact that we recently began to think seriously about updating the definition of clinical death, not for the sake of the patient, but when potential recipients of his organs came into view.

We need rather to discover the moral limits properly surrounding efforts to save life. We need to recover the meaning of only caring for the dying, and the justification—indeed the obligation—of intervening against many a medical intervention that is possible today. This is what I mean by a *patient*-centered answer to the foregoing questions. I also suggest that a culture that defines death as always a disaster will be one that is tempted to resolve these questions in terms of triage—disaster medicine. If we do not deliberately set aside the worst cases as a matter of public or hospital policy, the terminal cases will increasingly be neglected, because, paradoxically, of other demands upon sparse medical resources in a society that knows no other ethics in regard to dying patients than always by every means to keep them "alive."

Ordinary and Extraordinary Means

In any proper discussion of the physician's duty to heal and to save life, there are three interrelated distinctions that must be taken into account. These are the distinctions (1) between "ordinary" and "extraordinary" means of saving life; (2) between saving life by prolonging the living of it and only prolonging a patient's dying; and (3) between the direct killing under certain conditions of specifiable sorts of "hopeless cases" (called *euthanasia*) and merely allowing a patient to die by stopping or not starting life-sustaining procedures deemed not morally mandatory. By making use of all these concepts, the med-

6. See Thomas J. O'Donnell, S.J.: "The Morality of Triage," *Georgetown Medical Bulletin* 14 (August 1960): 68–71.

ical ethics developed in western Christendom set its face resolutely against the direct killing of terminal patients which it judged to be murder, whatever warrants may be alleged in favor of the practice. At the same time, medical ethics in the centuries before the recent achievements in scientific medicine and technology afforded reasonable grounds for refusing to "war without retreat and without quarter" against almighty God for the last shred of sentient life, worldly value, or physiological existence in the dying man.

It is necessary for us to enter this thicket if we are to gain an adequate comprehension of what is morally required in caring for the dying. This we must do if we are concerned to explore the possible bearing of religious ethics on medical practice.[7]

It is necessary for us to enter the thicket of the several meanings the moralists had in mind for yet another reason. Physicians themselves ponder this question of the care of the dying, and they repeatedly draw a distinction between "ordinary" and "heroic" measures. The generic duty to "save life" which governs medical practice is readied for application in the moral-species terms distinguishing ordinary from extraordinary means. This tells physicians the difference between a mandatory and an elective effort to save life. Therefore, the relativity in the meanings of ordinary and extraordinary procedures is precisely a chief virtue of using this distinction in the practice of medicine. It is not—as often is said—a reason for dismissing

7. No one can deny the truth of Dr. Henry K. Beecher's observation. "It will be evident," he writes, "that Roman Catholic leaders have examined these questions with great care and have arrived at firm conclusions. It is interesting to observe that their attitudes on most such questions are remarkably similar to the Jewish. Modern Protestant theological considerations are not very helpful in the present quest." (Henry K. Beecher, *Research and the Individual*, p. 187). Cf. E. Fuller Torrey's words in the preface to the volume of essays he edited, *Ethical Issues in Medicine: The Role of the Physician in Today's Society* (Boston: Little, Brown, 1968), p. viii: "If the Catholic Church seems to be unduly criticized in some chapters, let it be remembered that the Church has often taken the lead in discussing these issues."

However, to enter the thicket of these distinctions need not mean getting stuck in the brambles. It is necessary to qualify, reform, and extend the analysis of past moralists. At the same time there can be no ethics of medical practice without discourse with all those who have examined these questions of life and death with great care in the past. It is equally certain that theological moralists can make no contribution to medical ethics or shed any light upon its lasting themes by de novo starts and stops.

the distinction as worthless.[8] This would be the conclusion only from the premise that ethics must deal in absolutes unrelated to practice, or in principles that are inapplicable. Or else dismissal of this distinction is simply a vain effort to eliminate the role of prudence (practical wisdom) in applying moral rules by demanding the certitude of secondary rules for the application of them.

First, we need in preliminary fashion to notice some important differences between the moralist's meaning and the physician's meaning when each uses the terms *ordinary* and *extraordinary*. It is, of course, difficult to generalize, and no doubt there are some doctors who are closer than others to the moralists on the point in question. Still as a general rule—if I have not mistaken the general tenor or emphasis in the medical literature—a doctor's understanding and a moralist's understanding of ordinary and extraordinary means are likely to be different in three important and related respects.

First, the doctor is apt to use the distinction to mean customary as opposed to unusual procedures. Physicians use these terms relative to the state of medical science and the healing art, by reference to whether or not a remedy has become a part of customary medical practice. In contrast, the moralists are somewhat more likely than doctors to use these terms relative to a patient's particular medical condition. While an unusual practice may become customary and the medical imperative change as medicine advances, it is also the case that the medical imperative ought to change according to the patient's condition and its "advances," no matter how usual the remedy may be for other patients or for this patient at other times. The first relativity is to the disease and to what is ordinarily done to remedy it. The second relativity is to the condition of the man who has the disease; these relative meanings lead to a definition of optional remedies in terms of what would be "extraordinary" for this individual.

Apart from what doctors may sometimes or often do in withholding or stopping treatments in particular cases, one observes in medi-

8. If it is said (Joseph Fletcher, "Elective Death," in E. Fuller Torrey [ed.], *Ethical Issues in Medicine* [Boston: Little, Brown, 1968], p. 149) that "there is no way to establish a consensus (even if desirable) as to the defining features of an extraordinary treatment," the answer is, of course not! There may be meaningful *specifications* of moral rules without *certainty* in the applications of them.

cal writings a tendency to define *extraordinary* in terms of "heroic" or unusual efforts. This is not only because doctors may be in danger of malpractice suits if they depart too far from customary medical practice in what they do or omit to do. In general, the doctor's conscience is formed in these terms; his imperative is likely to be to do everything medical science affords as established practice in the saving of life. He will justify refraining from trying some unusual remedy more readily than he can justify stopping or not using a customary procedure. He is likely to feel that the moralist's understanding of "extraordinary" grants him more liberty than either law or a proper medical conscience allow.

Second, for the moralist, a decision to stop "extraordinary" life-sustaining treatments requires no greater and in fact the same moral warrant as a decision not to begin to use them. Again if I have understood the medical literature, a physician can make the decision not to institute such treatments with an easier conscience than he can make the decision to stop them once begun. "I believe that it is of primary importance," writes Dr. Jørgen Voigt, "not to get unawares into a situation in which it may be necessary to make a decision regarding the continuation of respirator treatment. Before institution of such treatment, as with every form of therapy [such as palliative interventions in inoperatable cancer patients], a decision must be taken as to whether it is *indicated*." [9] That, of course, is true. But there should be no greater reluctance to judge that continuation of treatments is no longer indicated than to judge that they should not be begun. The moralists would support physicians in this conclusion. Since a trial treatment is often a part of diagnosis of a patient's condition, one might expect there to be greater reluctance on the part of physicians in not starting than in stopping extraordinary efforts to save life. As I understand them, physicians often have the contrary difficulty.

Putting these first two points together in summary, a doctor "is more likely to refrain from giving an antibiotic than he is to direct the withholding of nourishment. He is likely to hesitate longest over switching off the machine for artificial respiration. The reasons for

9. Jørgen Voigt, "The Criteria of Death, Particularly in Relation to Transplantation Surgery," *World Medical Journal* 14 (1967): 145.

these variations in reactions are probably psychological rather than rational." [10]

Of course, there may be no difference between the moralist and the physician on the matter of the weight given to customary medical practice and to individual medical circumstance in defining ordinary (imperative) and elective medical care of the fatally ill, or in the matter of stopping or not starting heroic efforts to save life. If no disagreement is to be found on these two points, one is likely to arise on the third.

Third, moralists almost always understand the distinction between ordinary and extraordinary procedures to refer decisively to morally relevant, nonmedical features of a particular patient's care: his "domestic economy," his familial obligations, the neighborhood that has become a part of his human existence, the person and the common good, and whether a man's fiduciary relations with God and with his fellow man have been settled. The difference between an imperative and an elective effort to save life will vary according to evaluations of these features of a human life, and a moralist's terms for expressing this final verdict are *ordinary* and *extraordinary*.

Thus, the standard definition reads as follows: "*Ordinary* means of preserving life are all medicines, treatments, and operations, which offer a reasonable hope of benefit for the patient and which can be obtained and used without excessive expense, pain, or other inconvenience. . . . *Extraordinary* means of preserving life . . . mean all medicines, treatments, and operations, which cannot be obtained without excessive expense, pain or other inconvenience, or which, if used, would not offer a reasonable hope of benefit." [11] In explanation of the moral judgment that "one may, but need not, use extraordinary means to preserve life," another writer sums up the morally relevant factors that go into determining the meaning of this by say-

10. "Decisions about Life and Death: A Problem in Modern Medicine," Church of England study pamphlet, Church Information Office, Church House, Westminster SW1, London, 1965, pp. 47. Yet many moralists would press the question," "To what medical lengths is there any obligation to go in order to administer nourishment?" (ibid., p. 27). "There would seem to be no valid distinction in principle between these different means, whether they be nourishment, antibiotics or the electric current which operates the apparatus for breathing" (ibid., p. 47).

11. Gerald Kelly, S.J., *Medico-Moral Problems* (St. Louis, Mo.: The Catholic Hospital Association, 1958), p. 129.

ing, "We may define as an extraordinary means whatever here and now is very *costly* or very *unusual* or very *painful* or very *difficult* or very *dangerous,* or if the good effects that can be expected from its use are not proportionate to the difficulty and inconvenience that are entailed." [12] It is evident that theologians mean to counsel first the patient and his family and then the physician that, in deciding concerning an elective effort to save life or elective death, it is quite proper to make a balancing judgment involving decisive reference to a number of human (nonmedical) factors that constituted the worth for which that life was lived and that may discharge it from imperative continuation. Speaking as men who are doctors and in their practice, physicians may also say the same; but it is not strictly a medical judgment to say this. This is certainly not what a physician usually means when he distinguishes between ordinary and extraordinary procedures for saving life.

It may be that medical ethics will approach the position staked out by the theological moralists if it takes seriously the banner unfurled by the World Health Organization's positive definition of *health* as general human *well-being.* An erratic application of this extensive and liberal construction of a medical judgment, however, would not suffice. It would not suffice for the medical profession to invoke the psychosocial well-being of the woman as a justification for abortion while limiting professional judgment to strictly bodily considerations in caring for the hopelessly dying. That broad definition of health will either have to be withdrawn or else consistently applied. The latter would mean that professional medical judgments assumes responsibility for the full range of human moral considerations. This would be to locate medical considerations in direct lineage with all of man's moral reflection upon the meaning of *eudaimonia* (well-being, happiness) since Aristotle!

This, I rather think, is an alarming suggestion from which the medical profession should draw back in the direction of a stricter construction of medical judgments as such. The oddity is that the medical profession seems to have adopted a comprehensive definition of health precisely in a period in which we are undertaking to conceive that inconceivable thing: a society that itself has no moral philosophy

12. Edwin F. Healy, S.J., *Medical Ethics* (Chicago: Loyola University Press, 1956), p. 67.

and no common assumptions as to the good or well-being of man which medicine sporadically invokes. Increasingly, the medical profession—if it moves from a strictly medical to a more extensive definition of health—would have to find the sources of its medical ethics not in the culture generally but by developing within its own community a moral ethos representative of mankind's general well-being. In this respect, medical ethics would be not unlike the ethics of church and synagogue. The ethics of no group today floats upon a sea of social ethics or upon a received moral philosophy or an understanding of man's well-being or that of society generally.

This being so, it would seem wise for the medical profession to hesitate before assuming, along with social scientific judgments, also the tasks of an entire moral philosophy under a definition of health as general human well-being. For this reason, in the sequel I shall sometimes speak of *the medical imperative,* at other times of *the moral imperative* in dealing with the dying. These, of course, cannot be entirely separated, because the doctor is both a physician and a man. But this does suggest a distinction between the physician *qua* physician and whatever authority or role he may have as a man in relation to the well-being of the man who is his patient. It suggests a continuing distinction between the medical meaning and the theological-moral or humanistic meaning of imperative and elective procedures for saving life. This would require that the doctor lean against his understanding of the medical imperative in order to keep it optional for his patients; and that, as a man who happens also to be a doctor, he should make room for the primacy of human moral judgment on the part of the men who are his patients, the relatives of his patients, and their spiritual counselors to elect life-sustaining remedies or to elect them not. His may be the task of only caring for the dying for reasons that are not within his special competence to determine.

The Morality of (Only) Caring for the Dying

In discussions of ordinary and extraordinary means it is commonly assumed by physicians and moralists alike that the use of all "ordinary" remedies is morally required of everyone, and that the failure to provide or use ordinary means of preserving life is the equivalent of euthanasia. The crucial question to be asked of traditional medical ethics is whether ordinary, imperative procedures can, in a proper moral judgment, become "extraordinary" and elective only. Can a patient morally refuse ordinary remedies? Can a physician morally fail to supply them or fail to continue ordinary remedies in use?

This is an unavoidable question, and one that goes to the heart of the morality of *caring*, but *only* caring, for the dying. Whoever raises this question lightly, or with a concern to disprove or dismiss past moral reflection, can only deny himself one possible source of helpful insights. Our inquiry shall concern whether and in what sense traditional medical ethical concepts and distinctions should be ethically regulative of present-day medical practice in regard to the fatally ill and the dying. During this brief journey into the meanings of the moralists, our "method" of doing medical ethics will not be to propose *replacing* definitions. Instead, our search will be for an understanding of past moral wisdom, and in this to locate places at which a *reforming* definition of one or another relevant moral concept suggests itself. In this section two such important qualifications or creative lines of development will be brought into focus which are needed to complete an ethics of caring for the dying. Then in the following section, we shall ask whether, understood in terms of these reforming definitions, the ancient distinctions between ordinary and extraordinary (as a way of telling the difference between mandatory and elective efforts to save life) do not in sum reduce to the obligation to determine when a person has begun to undergo irreversibly the process of his own particular dying; and whether with *the process of dying* (all other terms aside) there does not arise the duty only to care for the dying, simply to comfort and company with them, to be present to them. This is the positive object of our search.

Then, in subsequent sections, we shall have to ask whether, over and above only caring for the dying, there is significant meaning still remaining in the distinction between ordinary and extraordinary means as specifications of our human obligation to continue or to discontinue life-sustaining procedures in the case of persons seriously or perhaps fatally ill, but not yet irreversibly dying. In addition to positing or enforcing the duty to respect with simple acceptance the dying process of a fellow man, the question then will be: Do these terms have any relevance for the medical care of persons not yet seized by their own dying?

A good place to cut into the moralists' analysis of the question whether "ordinary" medical procedures are always imperative is with the publication of two articles by Gerald Kelly, S.J., in *Theological Studies* in 1950 and 1951.[13] Here we can plainly see how far traditional medical morality was willing to go in limiting the active use even of so-called ordinary means of sustaining life. The title of Kelly's 1950 article suggests that he answered the question just raised by distinguishing between "natural" and "artificial" among the ordinary means of preserving life. Closer examination will show that there is more to it than that; and that in fact Kelly has himself already elaborated good reasons for dispensing from ordinary natural no less than from ordinary artificial means of preserving life.

Kelly makes it quite clear that he is willing to remove "ordinary" means under certain circumstances from the class of morally or medically imperative means. Agreeing with those moralists who regard intravenous feeding as in itself an ordinary means (and who *therefore* judged it to be imperative), Kelly says instead that "even granted that it is ordinary one may not immediately conclude that it is obligatory." An ordinary means may be out of place because of the condition of a patient—as out of place as unusual or heroic procedures. In regard to the usual use of a stimulant to prolong life for only a short time, Kelly calls that also an ordinary means. In this instance he gives two reasons for dispensing with the stimulant: "since it is artificial and since it has practically no remedial value in the circumstances, the patient is not obliged to use it." [14] It is evident, however, that in Kelly's argument the latter reason is far more important than the former. His argument is quite sufficient to make it unnecessary to distinguish between natural and artificial remedies in morally evaluating whether they should be used or not.

The argument revolves around whether the means used are really *remedies* or not. One is excused from using a proposed "remedy" if it does not offer a reasonable hope of success; it is then not a remedy. Kelly is simply intent on establishing that ordinary means may be omitted. His warrant for this is "the fine distinction between omit-

13. Gerald Kelly, S.J., "The Duty of Using Artificial Means of Preserving Life," *Theological Studies* 11 (June 1950): 203–20; "The Duty to Preserve Life," *Theological Studies* 12 (December 1951): 550–56.

14. Kelly, "The Duty of Using Artificial Means of Preserving Life," p. 218.

ting an ordinary means and omitting a useless ordinary means." The uselessness of it is decisive; and it is hard to see why this does not afford us another "fine distinction," namely, that between omitting a natural means and omitting a *useless* natural means—if there is ever any need to invoke this principle in actual practice. In any case, the artificiality of the ordinary means which may be omitted Kelly puts decisively aside. Simply the fact that they are no longer *remedies* or are no longer useful in saving the life of a patient alone warrants the omission of efforts to save life. The means would have to be means-full—of use to a human life. There is no obligation to do anything that is useless.[15]

I suppose that the point in drawing attention to the fact that this argument encompasses "natural" no less than "artificial" means is simply to demonstrate how far traditionally minded moralists were in principle willing to go in ordering means to the human life they are supposed to serve. Physicians should observe this, if they are inclined in conscience to continue beyond genuine usefulness the use of means that in the course of medical progress have become "usual" or "customary," and if they are any more ready for reasons relative

15. Ibid., p. 219. Fr. Kelly's argument accepts the conclusions of Joseph V. Sullivan, and seems to go further in clarifying their grounds. Sullivan had written: "A natural means of prolonging life is, per se, an ordinary means of prolonging life, yet per accidens it may be extraordinary. . . . An artificial means of prolonging life may be an ordinary means or an extraordinary means relative to the physical condition of the patient" (*Catholic Teaching on the Morality of Euthanasia*, [Washington, D.C.: Catholic University of America Press, 1949] p. 65, original in italics). "There is an absolute norm [*sic*] beyond which means are *per se* extraordinary," Sullivan writes; and it is not entirely clear whether he intends to say this of both "natural" and "artificial" means. The latter certainly are the chief practical issues, since almost all means of preserving life are "artificial." However, when Sullivan speaks of an "absolute norm" beyond which natural or artificial means become extraordinary and elective only, it is clear that the warrant for this is *relativity* to the age and physical condition of the patient. "An aged woman sick unto death with cancer would not have to use the same means toward prolonging life as a young girl ill for the first time in her life with a hopeful future ahead. For this aged woman an operation which might prolong her life a few months or a year would be an extraordinary means" (ibid., pp. 64–65). One of this author's case illustrations justifies a physician in cutting off intravenous feeding because, however "usual" as a practice, for *a terminal patient in great pain* it is an extraordinary means and therefore need not be used (ibid., p. 72, case [R]). Here again the meaning of the medical imperative to care for the dying is relative to the physical condition of the individual patient, not alone to usual or established procedures. Then, is there any point in holding on to a distinction between "natural" and "artificial" *ordinary* means?

to the patient to omit only their spectacular or "heroic" efforts.

The present writer has removed Kelly's delaying reference to the "artificiality" of the *useless* means that may be dispensed. He, not I, embraces also "natural" means—not alone in the logic of his argument but in specific cases as well. This happened in his apparent approval of the solution of two cases by Cardinal De Lugo. If a man, about to be burned to death by his enemies, has only a few buckets of water he is obliged to use the available water if he can prevent his death; but if the use of the water would only delay the inevitable he is not bound to use it. Water would seem to be a "natural" means of putting out fire, if anything is. If anyone doubts this, the second case settles the matter. Is a starving man bound to eat food brought to him by his friends? Yes, if he can get food regularly enough to ward off death. No, if by eating he only postpones his death by starvation. In sum, a prolongation of life that "may be morally considered as nothing" is *never* imperative whether the means are "natural" or "artificial," "ordinary" or "extraordinary." [16]

Several times in the foregoing paragraphs I have suggested that in an era of scientific and technical medicine, and since few people are likely to try suicide by ceasing to eat, to talk about the moral dispensability of "natural" means of saving life may be a moot question. This is not so, since so-called "natural" means (and also artificial means) have other uses than as *remedies* or (as "means" to any future). These are things done for no purpose except to care. To give a cup of cold water to a man who has entered upon the course of his own particular dying is to slack the thirst of a man who will soon thirst again, and thirst unto death. When a man is irreversibly in the process of dying, to feed him and to give him drink, to ease him and keep him comfortable—these are no longer given as means of preserving life. The use of glucose drip should often be understood in this way. This keeps a patient who cannot swallow from feeling dehydrated, and is often the only remaining "means" by which we

16. Ibid., p. 208. For Kelly the test of human benefit is finally overriding in telling whether the use of any sort of means is imperative. The prime importance of humane considerations was thereafter made quite evident by the fact that, in his 1951 Note and following the suggestion of a number of other moralists, Kelly wrote the test of benefit or usefulness into the *definition* of ordinary and extraordinary means. This produced the "standard" definitions given on p. 122 above, which include the words "offer a reasonable hope of benefit." See Kelly, "The Duty to Preserve Life," p. 550.

can express our present faithfulness to him during his dying (since to give him water intravenously would destroy his red blood cells and directly weaken and kill him). If a glucose drip prolongs this patient's dying because of the calories that are also introduced into his system, it is not done for that purpose or as a means in a continuing useless effort to save his life.

The administration of increased dosages of pain-killing drugs in the care of the dying is, as it were, the "mirror image" of the glucose drip: these drugs are judged to be life-shortening (to an immeasurable degree, because to suffer extreme pain would also be debilitating), but they are properly to be given in order to keep the patient as comfortable as possible, to show that we understand his need for succor, and not as a "useful" means to push him beyond our love and care. All these procedures, some "natural," others "artificial," are appropriate means—if "means" they should be called—of only caring for the dying, of physically companying with the dying. They are the embodied and effective gestures of soul to soul. As such, these acknowledgments of solidarity in mortality are due to the dying man from any of us who also bear flesh. Thus do men give answer by their presence and comfort to the faithfulness-claims of persons who are passing through the acceptable death of all flesh. If death should be accepted and treatment can no longer affect it, one might even raise the question whether *glucose* water should be used to keep the dying patient comfortable. I understand that there are certain sugars which it might be possible to use to give water for hydration without metabolizing calories and prolonging the dying process.

A second place at which a liberalizing definition of our obligation to care for the dying begins to suggest itself is in Kelly's answer to the question, "Is a person who suffers from two lethal diseases obliged to take ordinary means of checking one of them when there is no hope of checking the other?" The question at issue is whether a person suffering from incurable cancer who develops diabetes is obliged to begin insulin treatment, or a diabetic who develops an incurable cancer obliged to continue on insulin, and die slowly of the cancer instead of sooner in coma. Other moralists had answered that the patient must use the insulin since that is an "ordinary" means of checking the *disease* diabetes. Kelly doubts whether a patient is bound to "prescind from the cancer in determining her obligation of using the insulin." The latter depends on two factors: that it is an ordinary means and that it offers a reasonable hope of success. The simultaneous presence of cancer throws doubt on the second stipulation. But then Kelly observes: "I think the doubt would be even stronger were there some connection between the two diseases." [17] An illustration of this would be the need for intravenous feeding *connected with* the fatal disease from which a patient is dying. Presumably Kelly would be more certain about the judgment that it is permissible to withdraw intravenous feeding in this case, although nowadays a drip is surely per se an ordinary procedure for sustaining life. Thus, in assessing mandatory and only elective remedies, Kelly moves away from judging this in terms of *single* diseases only, to connected diseases, and only hesitantly beyond that. His reasoning should be faulted only for this hesitation.

The patient is not exhaustively characterized by one disease, two separate diseases, or the interconnected diseases from which he may be suffering, both incurable, one involving prolonged dying. Ideally, Kelly wanted the description of the human act of caring for this patient to terminate in a texture of related diseases. But a proper description of the human acts of caring for mortal man terminates in that man. He is the unity of the diseases he suffers when one his quietus makes. Doctors do not treat diseases, though often they conquer them. They treat patients, and here finally all fail. If a diabetic patient need not prescind from the cancer in determining her obligation to start or to continue to use insulin, the reason is that she is the one flesh in which both diseases inhere. If to use insulin is for her quite useless, it is surely contraindicated. To move beyond the interrelation of the ills to which all flesh is heir requires that we move to *the flesh* that is heir to all its ills, indifferent to whether these ills are themselves connected or physiologically unrelated. It is this flesh, and not diseases one by one, that is the subject of medical treatment. This truth is enough to undercut the bondage of conscience to the imperativeness of "customary" or "usual" procedures for treating single diseases.

17. Kelly, "The Duty of Using Artificial Means of Preserving Life," pp. 215–16. I presume that the above debate is about the dying cancer patient or a quite advanced incurable cancer. There are, of course, stages of cancer for which treatment holds out the hope of, say, ten years of relatively normal life. The diabetes of such a patient should certainly be treated. While it may be that the disease has seized him from which he one day will die, he is not yet dying of it.

We need to ponder one further possible entailment of the reforming definition of only caring for the dying at which we have arrived. If the unity of the person in whom the diseases inhere is the important point, and not a texture of interrelated diseases, this concept has important bearing on the treatment of infants with serious congenital defects. The argument cannot always be, as Kelly seems still to contend, that "the determination of ordinary and extraordinary means begin with the mentally normal" and this be then applied without qualification to the congenitally abnormal. That requirement may hold true for the chronically defective, like infants afflicted with mongolism, who often have a satisfactory degree of human existence that is only a burden, sometimes rewarding, to others.

The theologian who recently judged that "a Downs is not a person" uttered a scandalous untruth; and the fact that our advanced societies are now launching out upon the practice of allowing to be killed in utero all who are likely to be born mentally or physically defective shows, in the prismatic case of the most vulnerable, what we are coming to think of mankind's needy and helpless life in general. Nevertheless, the "abnormal" have, at the first of life, often been seized by their particular process of dying unless medical science relentlessly intervenes. Here there are even related defects any one of which will be mortal unless we intervene to stop them in course. Since we ought not to absolutize the distinction between "usual" and "heroic" treatment of newborn babies, not to place "a monstrosity in a heating bassinet" or to stop opposing the infection to which it is prone cannot be declared morally wrong while an operation is said to be optional to provide a child who was born with congenital atresia with an artificial or implanted esophagus.[18]

"Ordinary" or imperative, and "extraordinary" or only elective treatments are, as we have seen, not fixed categories. The feeling that infants should be given the greatest protection does not alone settle what we ought to do. Life in the first of it and life in the last of it are both prismatic cases of human helplessness. The question is, What does loyalty to the newborn and to the dying require of us? Consistently, we could say that both should unqualifiedly be given every effort that might save or prolong their existence. But if a balancing judgment is permitted—even morally mandatory—concerning whether proposed remedies will be beneficial to the adult dying,

18. Kelly, "The Duty of Using Artificial Means of Preserving Life," pp. 211–12.

the same reasoning cannot be preemptorially excluded from our care
of the newborn.

If in the case of terminal patients the quality of life they can expect enters into the determination of whether even ordinary or customary measures would be beneficial and should or should not be
used, cannot the same be said of infants? It is not obvious that an
anencephaletic baby should be respirated while a grown man in prolonged coma should no longer be helped to breathe. In the first of
life, a human being may be seized by his own unique dying. Indeed,
far from taking the death of the aged and the enormous death rate
of zygotes and miscarriages to be a part of the problem of evil, a religious man is likely to take this as a sign that the Lord of life has
beset us behind and before in this dying life we are called to live and
celebrate. There is an acceptable death of the life of all flesh no less
in the first than in the last of it. An ethical man may always gird
himself to oppose this enemy, but not the religious ethical man.

The Process of Dying

In the foregoing analysis we have drawn two pivotal conclusions:
(1) that there is no duty to use useless means, however natural or
ordinary or customary in practice; and (2) that the description of
human acts of caring for the dying (or caring for the not yet dying)
terminates in the man who is the patient of these ministrations and
not in the disease or diseases he has. These are related points: in judging whether to try a given treatment one has to estimate whether
there is a reasonable hope of success in saving the man's life.

A recent essay reviewing the distinction of extraordinary from ordinary means, and the different ways in which particular cases have
been judged by traditional moralists, concludes that in the final analysis "the one general positive guideline from the past that will remain" may prove to be the directive that "the use of any means
should be based on what is commonly termed a 'reasonable hope of
success.' " [19] The residue of the distinctions we have reviewed, this
author seems to suggest, is the test of usefulness. If so, the moral
meaning of dispensable means would seem to reduce without remainder to a determination of an irreversible "process of dying."

19. Kieran Nolan, "The Problem of Care for the Dying," in Charles E. Curran
(ed.) *Absolutes in Moral Theology?* (Washington, D.C. and Cleveland: Corpus Books,
1968), p. 253.

This is certainly a principal component of the medical-moral imperative. It can certainly be said that our duties to the dying differ radically from our duties to the living or to the potentially still living. Just as it would be negligence to the sick to treat them as if they were about to die, so it is another sort of "negligence" to treat the dying as if they are going to get well or might get well.[20] The right medical practice will provide those who may get well with the assistance they need, and it will provide those who are dying with the care and assistance they need in their final passage. To fail to distinguish between these two sorts of medical practice would be to fail to act in accord with the facts. It would be to act in accord with some rulebook medicine. It would be to act without responsivity to those who have no longer any responsivity or recuperative powers.

Thus would we fail to care for them as the dying men they are, just as surely as if we failed to take account of the responsivity that the living sick or the not yet dying still have. Only a physician can determine the onset of the process of dying. For all the uncertainty, he must surely make this determination. He is bound to distinguish so far as he can between that time span in which his treatment of a patient is still a part of diagnosis and treatment—diagnosis and treatment not of the disease but of a patient's particular responsivity —and a subsequent time in which the patient is irreversibly doing his own dying. The "treatment" for that is care, not struggle. The claims of the "suffering-*dying*" [21] upon the human community are quite different from the claims of those who, through suffering, still may live, or who are incurably ill but not yet dying.

In connection with all that has just been said we should not have in mind only those patients who are in deep and prolonged coma. A conscious patient as well may have begun irreversibly the process of his particular dying; and, precisely because conscious, his claims are strong upon the human community that only care and comfort and company be given him and that pretended remedies or investigative trials or palliative operations be not visited upon him as if these were hopeful therapy. Therefore, to all of the foregoing the words of David Daube, Professor of Law at Oxford University, are pertinent. "The question of at what moment it is in order to discontinue extraordinary—or even ordinary—measures to keep a person alive,"

20. Ibid., p. 256.
21. Ibid., p. 260.

Professor Daube writes, "should not be confused with the question at what moment a man is dead" or with the question whether he is conscious or unconscious. "Discontinuation of such measures is often justifiable even while the patient is conscious." [22]

This risk-filled decision concerning the onset of a man's own process of dying can be and is made by physicians. The problem is to find the courage (and perhaps legal protection) to act upon it. Dr. John R. Cavanagh defines the "dying process" as "the time in the course of an irreversible illness when treatment will no longer influence it." [23] The patient has entered a covenant with the physician for his complete *care,* not for continuing useless efforts to *cure.* Therefore, Dr. H. P. Wasserman calls for "a program of 'pre-mortem care,' " and for the training of doctors in this, and in the diverse ways in which they may fulfill their vocation to cure sometimes, to relieve often, and to comfort always.[24]

If the sting of death is sin, the sting of dying is solitude. What doctors should do in the presence of the process of dying is only a special case of what should be done to make a human presence felt to the dying. Desertion is more choking than death, and more feared. The chief problem of the dying is how not to die alone. To care, if only to care, for the dying is, therefore, a medical-moral imperative; it is a requirement of us all in exhibiting faithfulness to all who bear a human countenance. In an extraordinary article, Dr. Charles D. Aring says flatly that "it is not to be surmised that under the most adverse circumstances the patient is not aware." [25] That may be to say too much, but it strongly suggests that the sound of human voices and the clasp of the hand may be as important in keeping company with the dying as the glucose-drip "drink of cool water" or relieving their pain.

Dr. Aring tells of the case of a man who, under continuing exotic

22. David Daube, "Transplantation: Acceptability of Procedures and Their Required Legal Sanctions," in Wolstenholme and O'Connor, *Ethics in Medical Progress,* pp. 190–91.

23. John R. Cavanagh, "Bene Mori: The Right of a Patient to Die with Dignity," *Linacre Quarterly,* May 1963 (unpaginated reprint).

24. H. P. Wasserman, "Problematic Aspects of the Phenomenon of Death," *World Medical Journal* 14 (1967): 148–49.

25. Charles D. Aring, "Intimations of Mortality: An Appreciation of Death and Dying," *Annals of Internal Medicine* 69, no. 1 (July 1968): 149.

treatments, kept asking to be returned to his ward and to within the presence of his three ward companions. Instead, "he died alone, denied what he most wanted, the unspoken comfort of people—any people—around him." This physician's judgment is that this man's "want of his friends and familiar surroundings, new though they were, should have been an imperative and taken precedence over any and all technical matters." That would have been proper "pre-mortem care" of the dying. To do this, the physician needs to become aware of his own feelings about death, and to lean against his possible proneness to visit cursorily or to pass hurriedly by the room in which lies one of his "failures." And all of us in the "age of the enlightenment" need to recognize "death's growing remoteness and unfamiliarity," the masks by which it is suppressed, the fantastic rituals by which we keep the presence of death at bay and our own presence from the dying, the inferiority assigned to the dying because it would be a human accomplishment not to do so, the ubiquity of the fear of dying that is one sure product of a secular age.[26]

There is a final entailment of caring for the dying that is required of priests, ministers, rabbis, and every one of us, and not only or not even mainly of the medical profession. "The process of dying" needs to be got out of the hospitals and back into the home and in the midst of family, neighborhood, and friends. This would be a "systemic change" in our present institutions for caring for the dying as difficult to bring about as some fundamental change in foreign policy or the nation-state system. Still, any doctor will tell you that by no means does everyone need to die in a hospital who today does so. They are there because families want them there, or because neighbors might think not everything was done in efforts to save them. They are there because hospitals are well equipped to "manage death," and families are ill equipped to do so.

If the "systemic change" here proposed in caring for the dying were actually brought about, ministers, priests, and rabbis would have on their hands a great many shattered families and relatives. But for once they would be shattered by confrontation with reality, by the claims of the dying not to be deserted, not to be pushed from the circle that specially owes them love and care, not to be denied human presence with them. Then God might not be as dead as lately

26. Ibid., pp. 141, 137, 138, 144–45, 151.

He is supposed to be. The "sealing up of metaphysical concerns," Peter Berger recently pointed out, is one of the baneful results of a "happy" childhood—a childhood unhappily sheltered from the dying in all our advanced societies.[27]

Caring for the Seriously Ill and the Irreversibly Ill

Nevertheless, it would not be correct to suggest that the distinction of extraordinary from ordinary treatments—of elective from imperative remedies—and the subtle ethical judgments falling under these heads can be reduced without significant remainder to the twin concepts of "reasonable hope of success" (usefulness) and "the process of dying." That, as we have seen, is an important component. It is, in fact, the component encompassing the duty of only caring for the dying. In this respect, the moral imperative and the medical imperative are the same. For medicine to do more or otherwise would be blameworthy. But this is not all the meaning of ordinary-extraordinary—of imperative and only elective efforts to save life.

In the remaining meaning of these concepts, the moral imperative may be more extensive than the medical imperative. The "process of dying" is not the only condition for stopping the use of medical means, although when present it is a sufficient and a morally obliging condition. Other conditions can make it morally right to stop the use of medical means, although the decision to do so may not be a strictly medical judgment. "No reasonable hope of success" (uselessness) is not the only warrant for stopping the use of medical means, although where present it is a sufficient and a morally obliging condition. Other grounds than hopelessness can make it morally right to stop the use of medical means, although the decision to cease using them is not a strictly medical judgment. Fr. Kelly speaks of "the recognized principle that an extraordinary means is not per se obligatory even when success would be certain." [28] The true humanity of

27. Symposium on "The Culture of Unbelief," held in Rome under the sponsorship of the Vatican Secretariat for Nonbelievers and the University of California at Berkeley. A second baneful effect of a happy childhood, Berger said, is "a new utopianism—a radical demand for the humanization of existing social structures," measured by "the benign character of the institutions in charge of primary socialization," family, school, playground (*New York Times*, March 26, 1969).

28. Kelly, "The Duty of Using Artificial Means of Preserving Life," p. 214.

moralists of the past led them unanimously to say that there are conditions that could make efforts to save life only elective even if they are certain to be successful. When a physician yields or—better still—himself makes room for these more extensive moral and human judgments, he likely does so as a man who is a doctor, by an exercise of the moral authority he has acquired in relation to the man who is his patient and to his family, and not by virtue of his medical expertise.

Even when he could succeed, a doctor may and sometimes should allow his medical judgment to defer to a patient's estimate of the higher importance of the worth and the relations for which his life was lived. In doing so the doctor acts the more as a man than as a medical expert, acknowledging the preeminence of the human relations in which he stands with these and all other men, rather than solely in his capacity as a scientist or as a healer.

In this age of scientific medicine and of the authority figure in a white coat, it is salutary to remind ourselves of some of the measures which, until not so long ago, no one needed to use to save his life. Fr. Kelly lists the following examples: "Leaving one's home to go to a more healthful climate; the maiden's repugnance to being treated by a (male) physician or surgeon; the amputation of a limb; other major operations, especially those involving the opening of the abdomen; and all very costly treatments." Thomas J. O'Donnell, S.J., has roundly criticized these out-of-date cases and his fellow moralists for not keeping up with advancements in medical practice.[29] Still we should notice the humane wisdom contained in some of these illustrations, a sensitivity to human factors that is too likely to be evacuated in this age of technology. We should notice the good moral reasons that could be adduced for formerly deeming only elective certain of the medical practices that have become established practices with the advancement of the science and art of medicine. Thus to accent the morally relevant features of practices and patients that made it right to elect death will be to indicate precisely those morally relevant features that had to be overridden by medical

29. Kelly, "The Duty of Using Artificial Means of Preserving Life," pp. 204–05; Thomas J. O'Donnell, S.J., *Morals in Medicine* (Westminister, Md.: Newman, 1960), pp. 63–67.

progress, and that have always to be removed or otherwise cared for if saving life under certain conditions is to be pronounced always imperative.

Leaving home. This may no longer be a test in the age of the jet airplane and the mobility of populations. Still, to say this is in a sense to call attention to the human and familial and neighborly values which have in part been destroyed by the very same achievements of a technical civilization that now make imperative many a lifesaving procedure that formerly was likely not choiceworthy. It is at least still arguable that the New York state legislator who went from Queens to Houston to wait for and receive a heart transplant, and there to die, need not have done so. Houston may be a far more beautiful city than Queens, but Queens was his own home town! There were the people and relationships that made up the fabric of his human existence, and among them he might well have chosen to die.

Repugnance. Slight support can now be given for a "maiden's" repugnance to be treated by a male physician. But repugnance in general cannot be so easily set aside as one of the right-making or wrong-making features important in deciding to submit to or not to use medical procedures. The personal repugnance of a member of the religious sect of Jehovah's Witnesses to having his life saved by a transfusion of the blood (the "life") of another human being is surely grounds for his right to be allowed to die—even if we do not, and the medical profession does not, believe that this can be "reasonably requested." This "makes the transfusion for him an extraordinary means of preserving life." [30] Moreover, a more well-founded repugnance is still a factor in assessing what the moralists used to call "notable operations." If plastic and other corrective surgery not actually needed for life or health can be justified because of the human difficulty of living with grotesque deformities or facial disfigurement, then such like consequences of surgery that alone can save life may be grounds for not choosing life under those conditions. The medical-moral imperative is not first to save the life, and then to seek over the course of future progress to provide the ancillary remedies for those human consequences. It works the other way

30. John C. Ford, S.J., "The Refusal of Blood Transfusions by Jehovah's Witnesses," *Linacre Quarterly* 22, no. 1 (February 1955): 3–10.

round: as medical progress removes or lessens the consequences that are repugnant, its elective extraordinary procedures that succeed in saving life only at the cost of "notable" and repugnant consequences may become imperative.

Very costly treatments. One moralist declared only a few years ago that in normal times $2,000 or more would constitute too great a sum for the average man; and that, if the treatment would cost that amount or more, one would not be obliged to seek treatment! To say that this statement attempts to turn ethics into an exact, monetary science would—while true—not be a proper response.[31] That statement rests rather upon a regard for the average man; and, in estimating the human burden of costly treatment, it rightly takes account of the fabric of personal relationships and values which constituted the worth for which the terminal patient has lived. Here again, the medical-moral imperative is not first to save life at these costs, and then seek by some future course of action to remedy the human costs of warding off death. It works the other way round: the social distribution of medical care, removing or lessening these human costs, can alone transform presently elective (because costly) procedures into imperative ones.

31. Healy, *Medical Ethics,* p. 68. There are other unavoidable quantitative considerations in estimating merely elective surgery or other procedures which need to be highlighted at the present moment in medical progress. "In general," John Marshall writes, "a procedure carrying a mortality of ten per cent or less may be taken as an ordinary means, and one with a mortality of twenty per cent or more is extraordinary" and therefore dispensable. Among procedures having 10 percent mortality or less, those that seriously disable are elective only, never mandatory (John Marshall, *Medicine and Morals* [New York: Hawthorn Books, 1960], pp. 12 ff; "Decisions about Life and Death: A Problem in Modern Medicine," p. 57.) At that rate, the motto over a great deal of surgery performed today as if it were imperative should read: *Choose* all you who enter here! You *must* choose before entering here! and You *may* choose not to enter here!

Another sort of unavoidable quantitative estimation encompasses the probable length of days or months or years that may be gained. Here, often, choice is placed under duress rather than held open not only by the desperation of patients but also because the medical profession means one thing by "indefinitely" while people hear another. When a physician says that a procedure will extend a patient's life "indefinitely" he means anything from somewhat more than that patient's present prognosis to n-time. An "indefinite" extension of life means in ordinary usage much more than extension beyond prognosis. A physician has to lean against his meaning in order to keep it clear that many a promised "indefinite" extension of life is *not* humanly and morally choiceworthy, or may be judged not to be.

Amputations. This, of course, is the classic example of how an operation may become "ordinary" through the advancement of medical science. Not too many decades ago every Christian moralist characterized the amputation of an arm or a leg as an extraordinary operation which no man had the affirmative obligation to endure. That was before there were anaesthetics to remove the terrible pain, or disinfectants to ward off the high probability of infection. Today, the amputation of an arm or a leg is clearly an ordinary and morally imperative means of saving life.[32] Nevertheless, it is noteworthy that the physical pain or the physical danger of infection were not the only reasons adduced for this judgment upon amputations. Even in regard to removing pain, one moralist declared at the beginning of this century that a general anaesthetic is itself an extraordinary means because it takes away reason for a time. A man might choose to do his own dying with reason and self-consciousness in exercise. Whatever we may think of that suggestion, the moralists who judged amputations to be morally dispensable were chiefly concerned to hold open the possibility that a man might not judge life to be worth living without an arm or leg. In regard to this more human and enduring disadvantage in the balancing judgment about amputations, it is the development and provisioning of subtle artificial limbs that has done most to render these operations morally choiceworthy or imperative as a means of saving life.

We should also observe that, while the advancement of the science

---

32. Amputation is now a rare hospital procedure. Still, in 1966 two brothers petitioned the New York State Supreme Court to appoint them temporary legal guardians of their 80-year-old mother "for the specific and limited purpose of executing a consent in her behalf" to amputate her right ankle and foot that were infected with extensive gangrene. The aged woman was not capable of understanding the nature of the proposed operation, and the Jewish Home and Hospital for the Aged refused to proceed without the consent of all three of her sons. One son—a physician—refused, saying, "Assaultative surgery in a terminal case in the name of an emergency is cruelty beyond description." In the case of a diabetic patient dying slowly of cancer, we asked whether she needed to prescind from her cancer in judging whether to continue insulin treatment, or choose to die in coma by stopping that treatment. In the present case, need the woman or her sons prescind from her other ailments in judging whether to approve the amputation or to allow her to die more quickly from the spreading infection? This case was complicated by the fact that a psychologist reported to the court that the patient "wants both to live and to retain her limb and is not clearly aware of the conflict implicit in these alternatives" (*New York Times,* September 21, 1966).

and art of medicine may suffice to shift a means from the elective to the imperative category, this shift does not automatically take place. Not every means for prolonging life, once it is successful and made available—even "customary" medical practice—becomes thereby ordinary and mandatory upon both patient and doctor. There are always broader human factors to be taken into account, and these always in Christian medical ethics kept the saving of life from being made an absolute and inflexible norm, a hardship inhumanly applied. Medical progress may be described as a process of constantly creating ordinary means out of extraordinary ones, but also as a process of constantly creating more and more extraordinary means that need not be used and perhaps ought not to be chosen.

As amputation of an arm or leg became ordinary, the saving of men who suffered quadruple amputation by accident or in war came into view. This as well as a number of other ways of saving life, such as organ transplantation, may be such that they can never become proper specifications of the requirement that we always should save life, or desire to live by all ordinary means. After all, the moralists' main reason for holding amputations to be only elective surgery was the "serious inconvenience of living with a mutilated body," not the pain or the risk of infection endured for only a short time. Looked at in this light, terminal wards and the present-day practice of geriatrics increasingly testify to the fact that "progress" in the science and art of medicine can also be described as the mounting use of means that are irremediably extraordinary. This also can be the result of the mistaken notion that men and medicine are required to save life by every physically effective means.[33]

Not only morally relevant features of practices but also morally

33. "Respect for life has played its part in directing scientific research towards the discovery of many new and ingenious means of keeping people alive and, paradoxically, these very discoveries have demonstrated that life may not always be good" ("Decisions about Life and Death: A Problem in Modern Medicine," p. 46.) Dr. Kenneth O. A. Vickery is reported to have said at a congress of the Royal Society of Health in London that while "serious consideration of euthanasia should be unthinkable" we cannot much longer "avoid the issue of medicated survival." His mistake was to choose an arbitrary age (80) after which such patients should not be kept alive, and to cite the case of the late President Dwight D. Eisenhower (who was 78) as an instance of the practice he deplored of maintaining "medicated survival" (*New York Times,* April 30, 1969).

relevant features of patients themselves can render merely elective remedies morally required. For example, if a person need not save his life by using exquisite or painful procedures so far as he alone is concerned, perhaps he ought to do so if he bears some special relation to the common good. It may be that the next peace congress greatly depends on him. Then extraordinary means of extending his life for yet a while longer are, for that patient, "ordinary." To gain time to put in order one's fiduciary relations with God and man—to give and receive forgiveness—may also warrant extraordinary efforts to prolong life. Thus also, it is arguable that the one hundred heart transplants performed in 1968 were warranted because these were investigative operations having in view the common good to come. As therapy they were .dispensable. The transplants were elective, however, through the consent of patients and surgeons to become coadventurers in the cause of medical progress. The experimental nature of these operations should, then, have been made very clear to recipients and donors alike.[34]

Before concluding this section on the broader, nonmedical grounds for the possible rightness of electing not to oppose death, there are two final points that need to be mentioned. A physician may, we have said, either (1) on medical grounds only care for patients who have been seized by their particular process of dying, or (2) make room for the dispensability of extraordinary life-sustaining treatments because he as a man acknowledges that there may be sufficient moral and human reasons for this decision. If he does either of these things, he has a special problem in relation to the family of a patient who is unconscious or otherwise incompetent to consent or ask that either course of action be taken. He cannot and would not proceed without the agreement of the close relatives of such a patient. His problem, however, is that the family of seriously or irreversibly ill patients and of the dying have, in this situation, an enormous load of guilt. The guilt need not be for anything overtly done in the past. It is only that every one of us has the guilt of failing to enrich the life of an ill or dying loved one as much as we might have done.

Such is the human condition, that all are responsible for all—and

34. See Chapter 6 for a longer and more careful discussion of the issue raised by heart transplants.

in face of the death of a loved one, we are guilty of many a sin of omission. Out of their guilt, members of the family are likely—at long last—to require that everything possible be done for the hopelessly ill and the dying loved one. This may mean the prolongation of dying or the continuation of extraordinary life-sustaining measures beyond reasonable moral justification. At the same time, guilt-ridden people in their grief may be unable to bear the additional burden of a decision to discontinue useless treatment, and they are often relieved if this decision is not wholly placed on them. This means that the physician must exercise the authority he has acquired as a physician and as a man in relation to the relatives and take the lead in suggesting what should be done. In doing this, the doctor acts more as a man than as a medical expert, acknowledging the preeminence of the human relations in which he with these and all other men stand. For this reason, the medical imperative and the moral imperative or permission are, while distinguishable, not separable in the person or in the vocation of the man who is a physician.

Second, while in caring for patients a moral judgment concerning mandatory and elective treatment may be based on broader grounds than a strictly medical judgment, still a physician has in relation to disease a strictly medical imperative that is more encompassing than the patient-doctor relation itself. His is the ethics of a scientific mission in regard to disease itself. He is bound by a medical imperative that is more extensive than the human and moral considerations that may warrant elective death on the part of the man who is the patient of his care. It is not contrary to the common good or to the care now needed for a doctor to admit that a patient is incurable, or that he is now dying, and to cease trying to effect his cure or prolong his dying. But, while as a doctor he should act in accord with the incurability of the patient and as a human being should act in accord with the humanity of the patient, "it would be contrary to the common good [for him] to cease trying to find a remedy for the disease itself." [35] Here the medical imperative governing a doctor's profession and specifying the requirement that he never cease trying to find the cure or relief which future patients need proves more extensive in its turn and preeminent over the humane moral judgment that can clearly warrant the choiceworthiness of death for

35. Kelly, "The Duty of Preserving Life," p. 555.

other than medical reasons in many a particular instance. The question of questions is whether both judgments (with appropriate actions) can dwell together in the same person and calling. Or must one be bartered against the other, and in practice the one weaken the other resolve?

The medical imperative to continue to try to find a remedy for incurable diseases, while admitting that a patient is incurable and while ceasing to try to effect his cure, may involve the creation of a consensual community between doctors and incurable patients in which they both become joint adventurers in the common cause of curing these diseases. No advantage should be taken of the desperation of dying men, of course; but they also should be accorded the nobility and opportunity of personally nontherapeutic service of mankind, if this is the true account of trials made upon them to save life from that disease. An understanding partnership between a physician-investigator and the dying or the incurably ill would be one way, and perhaps a satisfying way, of not dying alone.[36]

The Same Objection from Two Opposite Extremes

There are physicians, of course, who entirely agree with the moralists' distinction ethically between direct killing (euthanasia) and allowing to die, and who also affirm the importance of this distinction for medical ethics. Dr. J. Russell Elkinton of the University of Pennsylvania School of Medicine, for example, calls upon his fellow physicians to attend, in addition to their obligation to save life, to their "other obligation" to allow the patient, if he is to die, to die with

36. Professor Hans Jonas discusses medical experimentation with the dying with a profound sense that this bodily life of ours provides the basis for a dying patient's identification with a physician's research. His illness is his; in some sense it is his own dying. Therefore, in research aimed at learning more about that illness, a "residue of identification is left him that it is his own affliction by which he can contribute to the conquest of that affliction"; "the patient's own disease is enlisted in the cause of fighting that disease, even if only in others"; if sufferers from disease consent to be drawn into the investigative process, "they do so *because,* and only because, of *their* disease." They should be spared "the gratuitousness of service to an unrelated cause." In no case should the dying be told: "Since you are here—in the hospital with its facilities—under our care and observation, away from your job (or, perhaps, doomed), we wish to profit from your being available for some other research of great interest we are presently engaged in" ("Philosophical Reflections on Human Experimentation", Ethical Aspects of Experimentation with Human Subjects, *Daedalus,* Spring 1969, pp. 241–43).

comfort and dignity. He acknowledges that if an extraordinary treatment (such as use of a respirator) is stopped, that is *an action,* but it is "an 'invisible act' of omission." Morally, it is decisive that "the patient dies not from that act but from the underlying disease or injury." [37] The physician simply stands aside.

For Elkinton also, in caring for the dying, it is a matter of indifference whether usual or rare and untried or new treatments are at issue. "More than 20 years ago," he writes, "I was responsible for the care of a young woman in the end state of multiple sclerosis. She was in great pain and had widespread ulcerations over the surface of her body from which she developed a septicemia (infection of her blood stream). At that time a new antibiotic, penicillin, had just become available. With the agreement of the patient's family I withheld the penicillin and the patient died quickly—her suffering was relieved. Penicillin is an ordinary treatment today but I would still make the same decision." [38] Thus, the advancement of medical science and practice is not alone sufficient to transform elective into morally imperative treatments. So also said Dr. G. B. Giertz in the Ciba Symposium: "No step is taken with the object of killing the patient. We refrain from treatment because it does not serve any purpose. . . . I cannot regard this as killing by medical means: death has already won, despite the fight we have put up, and we must accept the fact." [39]

This is also the medical care that small children deserve. "I will fight for every day," writes Dr. Rudolf Toch of the Pediatric Tumor Clinic at Massachusetts General Hospital, "if I have even the slightest chance of doing something more than just gaining one more

37. J. Russell Elkinton, "The Dying Patient, the Doctor, and the Law," *Villanova Law Rveiew* 13, no. 4 (Summer 1968): 740, 743.

38. Ibid., p. 743, n. 4. Noteworthy also is the fact that Elkinton believes that a physician as a man should take into account the fact of age and the range of human activity in judging whether we should always oppose death. "Perhaps we have lost our perspective on death as a natural part of the life that has evolved on this planet," he writes. "Death is more natural for the old than for the young and middle-aged. A physician friend has told me of the occasion when, visiting his elderly, widowed, and very lonely father, the father suddenly collapsed with an arrested heart. The son began external cardiac massage—and then he stopped. It seemed to him that it was the right time for his father to die. My friend had the perspective of which I speak" (ibid., p. 750).

39. G. B. Giertz: "Ethical Problems in Medical Procedures in Sweden," in Wolstenholme and O'Connor, *Ethics in Medical Progress,* p. 145.

day. . . . On the other hand, I recall a youngster whom we recently had on the ward with osteogenic sarcoma, the lungs completely riddled with tumor, who had not responded at all to the most potent chemotherapy and for whom we really had nothing further to offer. I did not feel any compunction at all about not doing thoracenteses daily, keeping intravenous therapy going, etc. All we did was give her adequate sedation, and I think she rather peacefully slept away." In saying this, Dr. Toch expressed the general and continuous consensus of western medical ethics.[40]

However, the ethics of only caring for the dying which, as we have seen, was our traditional medical ethics, and which is still promulgated by theological moralists and many doctors, will be opposed, trivialized, and ridiculed by two opposite extremes. One of these extremes is the medical and moral opinion that there is never any reason not to use or to stop using any and all available life-sustaining procedures. The other extreme is that of those, including a few theological ethicists, who favor the adoption of active schemes of positive euthanasia which justify, under certain circumstances, the direct killing of terminal patients. The case for either of these points of view can be made only by discounting and rejecting the arguments for saving life qualifiedly but not always. In both cases, an ethics of only caring for the dying is reduced to the moral equivalent of euthanasia—in the one case, to oppose this ever; in the other case, to endorse it. Thus, the extremes meet, both medical scrupulosity and euthanasia, in rejecting the discriminating concepts of traditional medical ethics.

Proponents of euthanasia agree with advocates of relentless efforts to save life in reducing an ethics of omitting life-sustaining treatments to a distinction without a difference from directly killing the dying. Thus D. C. S. Cameron, former Medical and Scientific Direc-

40. Rudolf Toch, "Management of the Child with a Fatal Disease," *Clinical Pediatrics* 3, no. 7 (July 1964): 423. A sampling of articles by other medical writers in support of this point of view includes Naomi Mitchison, "The Right to Die," *Medical World* 85, no. 2 (August 1956): 159–63; John J. Farrell, "The Right of a Patient to Die," *Journal of the South Carolina Medical Association* 54, no. 7 (July 1958): 231–33; Frank J. Ayd, Jr., "The Hopeless Case: Medical and Moral Considerations," *Journal of the American Medical Association* 181, no. 13 (September 29, 1962): 1099–1102; Eugene G. Laforet, "The 'Hopeless' Case," *Archives of Internal Medicine* 112 (1963): 314–26; William P. Williamson, "Life or Death—Whose Decision," *Journal of the Medical Association* 197, no. 10 (September 5, 1966): 139–41; Aring, "Intimations of Mortality," pp. 137–52.

tor of the American Cancer Society, writes that "actually the difference between euthanasia and letting the patient die by omitting life-sustaining treatment is a moral quibble." [41] Dr. David A. Karnofsky, of the Sloan-Kettering Institute for Cancer Research, also vigorously defends continuous "aggressive or extraordinary means of treatment" to prolong life. Karnofsky acknowledges that "the state of dying" may often be protracted only by "expensive and desperate supportive measures," and that the patient may be "rescued from one life-threatening situation only to face another." He has heard the pleas of those who, "contemplating this dismal scene," beg the doctor to "let the patient go quickly, with dignity and without pain." This strikes him as the same as getting rid of the dying by any means: "Withholding of aggressive or extraordinary treatment can be urged and supported by state planners, efficiency experts, social workers, philosophers, theologians, economists, and humanitarians. For here is one means of ensuring an efficient, productive, orderly and pain-free society, by sweeping out each day the inevitable debris of life."

The medical imperative, in Katnofsky's opinion, is to apply one temporary relief after another, stretching the life of a patient with cancer of the large bowel to ten months, who would have died within weeks if any one massive remedy had not been used. To the question, "When should the physician stop treating the patient?" there can be but one answer: "He must carry on until the issue is taken out of his hands." [42] From the point of view of this medical

41. D. C. S. Cameron: *The Truth about Cancer* (Englewood Cliffs, N.J:. Prentice-Hall, 1956), p. 116.
42. *Time* magazine, November 3, 1961, p. 60. One reason Dr. David A. Karnofsky comes to this conclusion is that it is, for him, a function of medicine's scientific mission in fighting *disease*:

> The sense of mission . . . is diminished . . . [by] the view that the fight against cancer should not be continuously waged on all sectors.
> The achievements and triumphs that may occur in the fight against cancer will come from doctors who do too much—who continue to treat the patient when the odds may appear overwhelming—and not from those who do too little.
> The physicians . . . can learn a great deal from the study of these patients. . . . In facing every challenge, even if doctors usually fail, they are kept in training to handle the remediable situations more effectively. ["Why Prolong the Life of a Patient With Advanced Cancer?" *Cancer Journal for Clinicians* 10 (January–February 1960), p. 10]

There is strength in this argument, if it is not possible for the physician to combine ethics of univocal and relentless life prolonging, the moralists' notion of imperative and elective means is bound to seem a moral quibble, and such an outlook will be exceedingly suspicious of all talk of allowing patients to die and only caring for them. There are moralists who agree with this point of view, and who, in order to protect human life at all costs, would be very suspicious of vesting physicians with the right to make the balancing sorts of medical and moral judgments expounded in this chapter.

On the other hand, precisely the same objection will be brought against the flexibly wise categories of traditional medical ethics from the opposite quarter. This time the objection is raised by proponents of schemes of euthanasia or the direct killing of dying or of untreatable patients. Tribute should be paid to Professor Joseph Fletcher for in season and out of season having kept open the question of allowing to die in the minds and consciences of the public beyond the limits of the medical profession. Still, the fact that he is himself a proponent of euthanasia—he "almost" says "honest" or "straightforward" euthanasia [43]—has meant on his part a serious misunderstanding of the ethics of only attending the dying. He subscribes to this ethics, of course, in moments when he seems compelled to acknowledge that euthanasia is a nonproblem in our present society, and when he wants provisionally to endorse the more commonly shared ethics of allowing to die. But because this is for him a halfway house, he seriously misunderstands the positive quality of the nonconsequential "action" put forth in attending and caring for the dying, and he introduces some confusion by his use of the carefully wrought categories of this ethics.

---

both resolves: care for the *patient* and his struggle against the *disease*. The practice of patient-centered medicine must surely cut across Karnofsky's concerns, or at least dethrone them. Follows is an extreme statement of the opposing principle: "A physician-counselor . . . cannot be a good personal and confidential adviser representing the patient's best interests if his own allegiance is divided between the patient's good and the general good of medical science or the welfare of the race at large" (John C. Ford, S.J., and J. E. Drew, M.D., "Advising Radical Surgery: A Problem of Medical Morality," *Journal of the American Medical Association* 151 [February 28, 1953]: 714). Another medical article generally in support of never stopping treatment, however extraordinary, is Louis P. Pertschuk and Albert S. Heyman, "The Physician's Responsibility in 'Hopeless Cases,'" *American Osteopathic Association* 64 (February 1965): 618–19.

43. Bernard Bard and Joseph Fletcher, "The Right to Die," *The Atlantic Monthly*, 221, April 1968, p. 63.

There is a terminological problem to be settled one way or another at the outset. It is possible to use the term *euthanasia* with the meaning of the two Greek words of which it is composed: a "good death." Dr. Wasserman uses the word in this sense when he says, "The inevitability of death suggests that medicine's greatest gift to mankind could be that of euthanasia in its literal meaning, i.e., death without suffering." [44] By this he meant the practice of only caring for the dying, and he proposed the establishment of a program of "pre-mortem care," and training medical students not only as invincible conquerers who unhappily fail, but also in this positive aspect of their profession. While this is the literal and the original meaning of the term *euthanasia,* it has since and in modern times acquired a quite different meaning. This meaning, I suggest, is now unreformably the meaning or part of the meaning the term will have in current usage. It is better to invent terms of art such as *agathanasia* or *bene mori* [45] or *pre-mortem care* to convey the ethics and practice of only caring for the dying, if this is what is meant.

Of course, we can agree to use either convention. But there is evidence that efforts to use the term *euthanasia* with any other sense than the one it has in current usage, i.e., direct killing, do not fully succeed. If this is true, our terminological problem has substantive import for ethical analysis and the moral life. The writings of Joseph Fletcher are an instance. He wishes to subscribe both to an ethics of caring, but only caring, for the dying, and to euthanasia in its current meaning. He calls both these practices by the name of euthanasia. He then must attach to the term qualifying predicates. This leads to confusion and inaccuracy in his use of the carefully wrought categories of traditional medical ethics, which he uses as these qualifiers, and to a failure to grasp the positive quality of only caring for the dying.

Thus Fletcher permits himself to speak of a decision to only care for the dying as *indirect euthanasia.* We cannot move forward without flatly denying this concept to be true. There is only one procedure in caring for the dying that need invoke what moralists call the "indirectly voluntary." This is the use of pain-relieving drugs that may also debilitate a patient's strength and shorten his life, or

44. H. P. Wasserman, "Problematic Aspects of the Phenomenon of Death," *World Medical Journal* 14 (1967): 148.
45. Cavanagh: "Bene Mori: The Right of the Patient to Die with Dignity."

his dying. In this case, the justification is that relief of his pain is the "directly voluntary" action, while the administration of the drug shortens the dying process in only an "indirectly voluntary" way. What ones does directly and immediately is to help the patient in his insufferable pain. That he dies sooner is not the primary result. This case is a prism in which we can see the ingredients that must be present in a case for which the language of "direct" or "indirect" is at all appropriate. There must be two effects caused by the same action, whether these effects are relieving pain and shortening life, or, in conflict-of-life cases, unavoidably and foreknowingly causing the death of a fetus as the "indirectly voluntary" effect of action whose directly voluntary end is the saving of a mother's life.

Incidentally, the life-shortening effect of using pain-relieving drugs is not quite as clear as moralists sometimes assert. Prolonged suffering from extreme pain is also exceedingly debilitating; and it is not always clear whether to keep pain at bay or not to do so would be more effective in hastening the dying man to realms beyond our love and care. In any case, drugs are not given for that consequence. They rather express in objective service to the dying that we still care for them, and are affirmatively doing so.

It may be entirely appropriate to use the expression *indirect euthanasia* in the case of death-hastening pain-killers. But it is not at all appropriate to use these words to describe cases of ceasing treatments that prolong the patient's life, or withholding life-sustaining treatments altogether, which Fletcher lumps together under this rubric with positive acts of administering drugs which cause the double effect we have described.[46] This he does on the grounds that in these cases "death occurs through omission rather than directly by commission"; it is "not induced but only permitted." Fletcher calls this concept *"indirect euthanasia"* and his warrant for doing so, he says, is because "in some kinds of Christian ethics and moral theology, an action of this kind is called 'indirect voluntary.' "[47] This usage is entirely mistaken. Fletcher's is a *persuasive* use of language, not a convincing one. Writing primarily as a proponent of euthanasia

46. Joseph Fletcher, "The Patient's Right to Die," *Harper's*, October 1960, pp. 141–42.

47. Joseph Fletcher, "Dysthanasia: The Problem of Prolonging Death," *Tufts Folia Medica* 8 (January–March 1962): 30. This article and the one cited in the previous footnote are now reprinted as "Euthanasia and Anti-Dysthanasia," Chapter 9 of Joseph Fletcher, *Moral Responsibility* (Philadelphia: Westminster, 1967), pp. 141–60.

(current usage), he subscribes along the way to an ethics of only caring for the dying. By calling the latter "indirect euthanasia" his words, at least, gain the force of suggesting that this point of view is not quite as honest or forthright as "direct" euthanasia.

To insist that this usage confuses the carefully fashioned categories of medical ethics is no mere logomachy, since it is of first importance, in the characterization or description of actions to be morally evaluated, to make clear precisely this distinction between acts of omission and acts of commission.[48] The difference between only caring for the dying and acts of euthanasia is not a choice between indirectly and directly willing and doing something. It is rather the important choice between doing something and doing nothing, or (better said) ceasing to do something that was begun in order to do something that is better because now more fitting. In omission no human agent causes the patient's death, directly or indirectly. He dies his own death from causes that it is no longer merciful or reasonable to fight by means of possible medical interventions. Indeed, it is not quite right to say that we only care for the dying by an omission, by "doing nothing" directly or indirectly. Instead, we cease doing what was once called for and begin to do precisely what is called for now. We attend and company with him in this, his very own dying, rendering it as comfortable and dignified as possible.

In any case, doing something and omitting something in order to do something else are different sorts of acts. To do or not to do something may, then, be subject to different moral evaluations. One may be wrong and the other may be right, even if these decisions and actions are followed by the same end result, namely, the death of a

---

48. On the need for accurate characterization or description of actions before evaluating them, see Paul Ramsey, *Deeds and Rules in Christian Ethics* (New York: Scribner's, 1967), pp. 192–225. In his essay on "Elective Death," in E. Fuller Torrey (ed.), *Ethical Issues in Medicine* (Boston: Little, Brown, 1968), p. 147, Professor Fletcher further multiplies the concepts he uses in ethical analysis. He speaks of four sorts of euthanasia: direct voluntary, indirect voluntary, indirect involuntary, and direct involuntary. Under the last pair of terms, one allows to die or kills without the consent of the dying or by construing their consent. Under the first pair of terms, with the patient's consent he is killed or allowed to die. These may be better and more illuminating terms to use in ethical analysis; but it must be pointed out that by means of them one can say little or nothing about past moral reflection and cannot enter into helpful discourse with the meanings in past medical ethics. Fletcher's are *replacing* definitions.

patient. One need not deny that in the moral life commission and omission may sometimes be morally equivalent. Still, before we reach the individual case or the sort of cases in which to do and not to do are judged to be the same, we need to explore the possibility that to omit and to do may not at all be equivalent actions, and to ascertain the pertinence of this possibility for medical practice.[49]

What Fletcher has gained by an improper characterization of actions that allow a patient to die while caring for him—by calling them indirect voluntary euthanasia—is that, without abandoning the case he and many other moralists have made for only caring for the dying, he can the more readily succeed in apparently reducing the warrants for omitting medical interventions to the moral equivalent of the alleged warrants for acts of direct euthanasia. Here it is that he mounts the very same objection against an ethics of only caring for the dying as the one also affirmed by defenders of medical scrupulosity in the unending use of all available means. Many teachers, Fletcher writes, Roman Catholics and others, "claim to see a moral difference between deciding to end a life by deliberately doing something and deciding to end a life by deliberately *not* doing something." This, Fletcher writes, "seems a very cloudy distinction"; and he asks rhetorically, "What, morally, is the difference between doing nothing to keep a patient alive and giving a fatal dose of a pain-killing or other lethal drug?" Of course, as Fletcher goes on to say, the decision to do or not to do are both "morally deliberate." Who ever said they were not? Of course, "the intention is the same, either way"—meaning the end in view (and not bothering here to introduce the usage of the word "intention" in a considerable number of ethical writings where its meaning is *not* restricted to the end in view). Fletcher's whole case depends, then, on his next statement: "As Kant said, if we will the end we will the means." [50]

That, I suppose, is a statement from Kant's analysis of hypothetical imperatives, which are dependent on consequences; and it might be pointed out that Kant did not believe conditional imperatives to be at all constitutive of a truly moral life. One could argue that if one

49. For a discussion of the law on acts and omissions, see an article by George P. Fletcher of the University of Seattle Law School, "Legal Aspects of the Decision Not to Prolong Life," *Journal of the Medical Association* 203, no. 1 (January 1, 1968): 65–68.

50. Fletcher: "The Patient's Right to Die," p. 143.

wills the end he wills the means—but not just any old means. One could argue that it is ethical to will the end we have here in mind; for the strictest religious ethics "the desire for death can be licit." [51] One could say that there are different means—and differences between action and omissions that make room for properly caring actions—that may let the patient have the death he not improperly or even quite rightly desires. While it might be argued that the Kantian maxim applies to means necessary to secure a desired and desirable end, still where there are more than one means to this same end, to will that end leaves open the choice among means. A means may be right, another wrong, to the same end.

But to respond in this way would exhibit a considerable misunderstanding of the positive quality and proper purpose intended in only caring for the dying. It is true that death is now accepted; and it is no longer opposed. This makes room for appropriate caring actions which are means to no future consequence. These actions are fulfillments of the *categorical* imperative: Never abandon care! Perhaps they should not be called means at all, since they effectuate or hasten the coming of no end at all. Upon ceasing to try to rescue the perishing, one then is free to care for the dying. Acts of caring for the dying are deeds done bodily for them which serve solely to manifest that they are not lost from human attention, that they are not alone, that mankind generally and their loved ones take note of their dying and mean to company with them in accepting this unique instance of the acceptable death of all flesh. An attitude toward the dying premised upon mature and profoundly religious convictions will display an indefectable charity that never ceases to go about the business of caring for the dying neighbor. If we seriously mean to align our wills with God's care here and now for them, there can never be any reason to hasten them from the here and now in which they still claim a faithful presence from us—into the there and then in which they, of course, cannot pass beyond God's love and care. This is the ultimate ground for saying that a religious outlook that goes with grace among the dying can never be compatible with euthanasiac acts or sentiments.

We shall inquire in the final section of this chapter whether there can possibly be any significant further qualifications, modifications,

51. Gerald Kelly, "The Duty of Using Artificial Means of Preserving Life," p. 217.

or extensions of this requirement that we always care if only we care and if we only care for the dying. Before concluding the present discussion, however, reference should be made to the "special ethics" of Karl Barth. Barth provides us with an example of a theological moralist who, because of the great weight he places upon the sanctity of each human life and upon our human duty to respect and protect any life that God has valued, initially defends the practice of medical scrupulosity in never ceasing to try to save the dying. From this point of view he brings the same objection against main-line western medical ethics as comes from the opposite extreme: it is a muddle and a quibble, and moreover, for Barth, a dangerous quibble. In the end, however, Barth breaks away from this extreme and, because his mind is bent on following the lineaments of grace among the dying, he is driven to an understanding of care for the dying which at first he opposed. It is fitting to conclude with Barth because what he says in this brief section in his special ethics is enough to show that always caring and only caring for the dying arises from within the heart and soul of Christian ethics. This is not the property of Roman Catholic moralists alone—unless we mean to deny our common moral heritage which measures every requirement upon men by a relentless charity.

No theologian in the twentieth century has prosecuted more vigorously the meaning of respect for life and the protection of life than the Protestant, Karl Barth. The motif powerfully at work in Barth's analysis is that of a man who understands our fellow humanity in terms of Christ who was the man with and for other men with indefectable charity. Barth seeks in his "special ethics" to form and inform his thoughts by the degree to which God has from all eternity surrounded with sanctity all these nascent and dying lives of ours and alone knows their secret and destiny. In this outlook and according to this measure of cleaving to the life of a fellow man, it seems to Barth clear that one can "give up" the life of a sick or useless or horribly deformed person *no less* by "letting his life ebb away" than by "encompassing his death." [52] For this reason, the attempted distinction between directly intending the death and allowing to die completely collapses in Barth's view, because both are "deliberate

52. *Church Dogmatics* (Edinburgh: Clark, 1961) III/4, p. 426.

killing." He seems therefore to agree with medical scrupulosity and proponents of euthanasia that this is a muddled distinction that cannot be maintained. But it is in the face of divine charity seeking always to save life that it cannot be maintained, and so Barth's own view is at the opposite pole from euthanasiacs who are allied with him in ridiculing what he rejects.

It can hardly be said that this form of deliberate killing ("letting life ebb away") "can ever seem to be commanded in any emergency, and therefore to be anything but murder." The suggestion that a patient could be "helped to die," not directly but only in the form of mercifully not applying means for artificial prolongation of his life, seems to him to raise "tempting questions" which "contain too much sophistry" to be a form of obedience to the command to respect, protect, and save life. "The same truth" applies to "passive failure to apply the stimulants" in heart cases as to cases of "active killing." [53]

In all this, Barth mistakes the proposal of past moralists to depend on an ethics of "the well-meaning humanitarianism of underlying motive"—i.e., only on consequences subjectively, well-meaningly aimed at—and he correctly believes that "respect for life" knows more than that about right and wrong. He also fails to distinguish between declaring another life to be useless, and declaring a treatment to be useless. Then Barth comes to a breaking point, out of the same powerful respect for the dying man. Out of an unremitting effort to probe the ways in which human life may be sanctified, protected, and served, Barth's analysis brings him to this breaking point. This very concern raises the question

> whether this kind of artificial prolongation of life does not amount to human arrogance in the opposite direction, whether the fulfillment of medical duty does not threaten to become fanaticism, reason folly; and the required assisting of human life a forbidden torturing of it. A case is at least conceivable in which a doctor might have to recoil from his prolongation of life no less than from its arbitrary shortening. . . . It may well be that in this special sphere we do have a kind of exceptional case. For it is not a question of arbitrary euthanasia; it is a question

53. Ibid., pp. 427, 425, 427.

of a respect which can be claimed by even the dying life as such.[54]

There comes a time when "letting life ebb away" is *not* the same as "actively encompassing" a patient's death.

Thus love's casuistry brings Barth finally to the distinction between allowing to die and arrogantly using all the resources of medical science artificially to prolong dying. Out of respect for the dying life as such, there arises a fresh understanding of the forbidden torturing of it; and, of course, from this same source springs the awesome understanding of the forbidden taking of life.

It may be that only in an age of faith when men know that the dying cannot pass beyond God's love and care will men have the courage to apply these limits to medical practice. It may be that only upon the basis of faith in God can there be a conscionable category of "ceasing to oppose death," making room for caring for the dying. It may also be that only an age of faith is productive of absolute limits upon the taking of the lives of terminal patients, because of the alignment of many a human will with God's care for them here and now, and not only in the there and then of his providence.

It may be that it is quite natural that in an atheistic and secular age the best morality men can think of is to make an absolute of saving life for yet a bit more spatio-temporal existence, even when this is worked massively upon the dying as if death were only and always an unmitigated evil. It may also be that, paradoxically, a secular age is productive of equally powerful currents of thought toward the arbitrary taking of life for the sake of earthly good to come. If this has to be the conclusion of a secular age, then it is the root of many problems, since this would mean, as Barth suggested, that medical duty has become fanaticism. Or, alternatively, that medical duty becomes the engineering of the future of the species. Together, medical men and moralists need most urgently to renew the search for a way to express both moral recoil from any arbitrary shortening of life, and moral recoil from any arbitrary prolongation of dying. This was in fact the morality of the western

54. Ibid., pp. 425, 423, 427.

world until a scientific ethic inspired by a secular humanism took over and for the first time in our heritage began to draw the conclusion that whatever can be done should be done to ward off death. Since Christians believe that death and dying are a part of life and like birth no less a gift of God, they have not to wrestle with the Almightly with no holds barred for the dying man.

Two Possible Qualifications of Our Duty Always to Care for the Dying

A number of contemporary moralists have recently raised the question whether to assist a patient through his own "process of dying" may be justifiable. (Even liberal Catholics seem to have an aptitude for coming up with ideas like that!) We need now to examine these suggestions, and finally ourselves to ask whether there are any further possible qualifications or proper exceptions to our duty always to care for the dying.

Kieran Nolan, O.S.B., ponders whether, "if to use expensive means to add a few hours of life to a terminal patient is not in keeping with Christian charity, [it is] in keeping with Christian charity to allow a terminal patient to continue for months in such a condition without providing some positive assistance to the dying process." Fr. Nolan puts this forward as a question needing further exploration. He anticipates, however, that future serious moral reflection may eventually make "somewhat clearer how positive assistance to the suffering-*dying* is a matter quite different from euthanasia as the merciful relief of suffering when one is not dying." [55]

In a wide-ranging discussion with Dr. Robert White, neurosurgeon at the Cleveland Metropolitan General Hospital, the Rev. Charles E. Curran puzzled: "In the past, we have definitely placed great stress on the distinction between acts of omission and acts of commission. . . . Let me ask you, doctor, is there such a thing as the dying *process?* . . . Maybe death isn't an instantaneous thing. And if all you do is *hasten* the dying process, is this 'interfering with nature'? I'm not suggesting that we can justify such a procedure here and now, but we're not being true to our profession if we're afraid to ask ques-

55. Kieran Nolan, "The Problem of Care for the Dying," pp. 259–60.

tions." [56] Fr. Curran might better have asked: If all we do is *hasten* the dying process, is this not morally equivalent to no longer opposing the process of dying?

Thomas A. Wassmer, S.J., writes that "it can plausibly be asked just where the difference lies in accelerating the dying process by acts of commission as well as by acts of omission." And concerning the use of pain-relieving, life-shortening drugs, Fr. Wassmer states his opinion that "it is hard to see at times how the effect of death is not involved in the very intentionality of the administrator. It seems somewhat unreasonable to assert that a patient who is given such drugs in order to eliminate pain, although the process of death is going to be accelerated, is always unaware of this combined intentionality in the minds of his physician and family." [57]

The entire argument of this chapter affords some response to these suggestions.

1. Reference to the fact that, in keeping a patient comfortable by the use of pain-relieving drugs, shortening his life may be the meaning held and conveyed to him (because of the double intentionality in the act accompanying the double effect of the drugs) is surely a contingent possibility and not a really fundamental argument. One could as well say that in caring for the dying by giving the patient a glucose-drip "cup of cool water," he may get the idea that the physician is officiously trying to prolong his dying by the input of calories. If a patient knows enough about these procedures, or if he does not, he will likely receive them as *care*. The administrator of them knows they are objectively needed primarily for the patient's comfort, and subjectively it is easy enough for him to tell whether in the one case he is trying to kill or to hasten death (instead of giving a patient relief from pain) and whether in the other he is trying uselessly to prolong a patient's dying process (instead of caring for him in his dying).

56. "The Morality of Human Transplants," *The Sign,* March 1968, p. 26. The reference to "interfering with nature" is simply an obsession of Roman Catholic moralists—traditionalists opposing such acts and liberals generally favoring them in the war they are waging against "physicalism" in moral theology.

57. Thomas A. Wassmer, "Between Life and Death: Ethical and Moral Issues Involved in Recent Medical Advances," Symposium on the Medical, Moral and Legal Implications of Recent Medical Advances, *Villanova Law Review* 13, no. 4 (Summer 1968): 765–66.

2. Each of these authors addresses himself solely to the span of end-time described by the words "the process of dying" and to which the moral judgment "the dispensability of any and all efforts to save life" is applicable. If during this span of end-time there is no significant moral distinction to be made between omitting life-sustaining treatments in order to make room for caring and only caring for the dying, on the one hand, and, on the other, injecting a small bubble of air in his veins in order to kill him or hasten his dying or assist him in the process, then no such distinction can validly be drawn earlier in the case of the "living sick" (the seriously ill and the incurably ill not yet doing their own dying) who also may elect death. This, we have seen, is the meaning of nonimperative efforts to save life over and above omitting such means in order to make room for caring for the dying. In suggesting the possible collapse of the moral difference between omission and commission, none of these authors takes up the question of the patient who is "not bound to accept excessively burdensome means of prolonging his life unless the foreseen consequences of his dying are such as to make it his duty to live on." [58] When these authors do take up the question, they are likely to find that if the distinction between omission and commission is abrogated (or if the grounds for this in *care* is forgotten) in the case of patients in process of dying, it cannot be maintained in the case of the ill who are not yet dying.

3. In simply exploring and pondering the question whether in extending medical care to the dying there may be no significant moral difference between acts of omission and acts of commission to assist in the dying process, these authors are lost in the forest of the technical terminology of past moral reflection, and they neglect to stress what the omission was for. They have lost firm grip on the positive quality of an ethics of caring for the dying, and so their discussion of omission-commission turns out to be rather like that of proponents of medical scrupulosity who would extend unending efforts to save life, or that of proponents of euthanasia, when they undertake from either extreme to reduce the flexibly wise and grace-full categories of past medical ethics to a moral quibble. In caring for the dying, *we cease doing what was once called for and begin to do what is called for now*. The omission is only incidentally a "not doing," in

58. "Decisions about Life and Death," p. 27.

order positively to care, to comfort, to be humanly present with the dying. The call cannot go forth: abandon care!

It would be a defection from the faithfulness-claims of a fellow human being that his very own dying be blessed as an event in the human community to which we attend if the dying are hastened beyond the reach of our love and care. To "assist" the process of dying would itself be a sort of abandonment: an affirmative abandonment of the dying solely to God's care in *separation* from ours, a self-contradiction at the heart of Christian charity ceasing, by this act, from its works before released from the claims and needs of a still living fellow man.

Still, there may be possible qualifications of our duty to care for the dying even if, as I argue, the general moral species-term "to assist the dying process" is not one of them, or is too sweeping as a stipulation. This final question must now be addressed. There can be justifiable modifications of moral principles and rules, whether these are based on justice or fairness- or faithfulness-claims or on the moral importance of the consequences of actions. These qualifications or modifications, if there is good reason for introducing them, may be called "exceptions" to the principles or moral rules first subscribed to—since the word "except" or "unless" is usually used in formulating such modifications. A proper exception or "unlessment" specifies a type or class of actions having universalizable right-making features in which similar agents should act similarly. They in no sense weaken the original principle or moral rule governing in all cases except of the type mentioned in the exception. This will be the method of medical ethical analysis to be used in now asking: Are there any specifiable just and charitable qualifications of our duty always to care for the dying? [59]

59. See my essay, "The Case of the Curious Exception," in Gene H. Outka and Paul Ramsey, *Norm and Context in Christian Ethics* (New York: Scribner's, 1968). Thus, we could say: "Never kill, always protect human life, never hasten death but always care for the dying, *unless* one is a member of a group of men on reconaissance in jungle warfare or treking across a desert, and a 'buddy' is seriously wounded and cannot go on; he will be tortured to death or eaten to death by insects and wild beasts. All *may* choose to stay and die together, but there is no *obligation* that all should perish when only some can be saved. The mission should go forward for the sake of its important consequences, and there is no other recourse." Such a modification of the moral rule forbidding direct killing in no sense weakens that rule. It states in general terms the right-making features of a sort of situation, repeatable even

I suggest that there may be two such qualifications.

1. We may say, Never abandon care of the dying except when they are irretrievably inaccessible to human care. Never hasten the dying process except when it is *entirely indifferent to the patient* whether his dying is accomplished by an intravenous bubble of air or by the withdrawal of useless ordinary natural remedies such as nourishment.

A moralist cannot say whether or not there are cases falling under this justification of direct killing, or assisted dying. This would be for physicians to say. Still there may be actual, or if not there are supposable, sorts of cases in which the duty always to keep caring for the dying is suspended by their inaccessibility to any form of care or comfort. The permanently and deeply unconscious person is, so far as can be known, not suffering at all. An argument that he should be treated "mercifully" by being allowed to die or by being directly killed is misplaced. It is only the suffering of relatives that could be relieved. To do either of these things *for that reason* would be a defect of care for him—*if* this still makes any difference to him.

The proposed justifiable exception depends on the patient's physiological condition which may have placed him utterly beyond reach. If he feels no suffering, he would feel no hunger if nourishment is withheld. He may be alone, but he can feel no presence. If this is a true account of some comatose patients, then in this sort of case we have correctly located the point at which the crucial moral difference between omission and commission as a guide to faithful actions has utterly vanished. The condition of the patient renders it for him a matter of complete indifference whether humankind's final act toward him directly or indirectly allows death to come. He already is beyond our love and care. We must not, as Dr. Karnofsky supposed, carry on our medical efforts to save life until the issue is taken out of our hands. Still we must carry on our ministry of care and comfort and keeping-company with the dying until but only until *that* issue is taken out of our hands. This is not to secure charity's premature release. It would rather be the case that men may, consonant with char-

---

if never repeated, in which sort of case *alone* it may be permissible to kill a man (or leave him a gun with a warning that whatever happens he should save the final bullet for himself). To replace the ordinary word *exception* by the term of art *unlessment* might assist some theologians to think what they should mean about ethical judgments.

ity, take note of the fact that they have been released. Can we never say, This man is beyond earthly caring?

The sort of situation that may be covered and resolved by the present proposal in ethical analysis, if it is valid, are the cases of patients in deep and irreversible coma who can be and are maintained alive for many, many years. It has to be acknowledged, of course, that in making a human presence felt to the dying we should not lightly assume that the patient is not aware of the sound of human voices or the touch of a loved one's hand or his breathing nearness. But must it be assumed that this is always so? If there are cases of neglect and defect of care for the dying, there may also be not an excess but a now useless extension of care. Acts of charity or moving with grace among the dying that now communicate no presence or comfort to them are now no longer required. If it is the case that a wife is tragically mistaken when she takes twitches of the eyes to be a sort of language from her husband irreversibly comatose for seven years, or when she takes such reflex actions as the response of the lips to a feeding cup to be evidence of reciprocation and some minimal personal relatedness, then her care is now worthless. Indeed it is no longer care for him. It is no contradiction to withhold what is not capable of being given and received. If caring for the dying should stop, then the basic reason for a significant moral distinction between omission and commission is abrogated. The grounds for that were that we should cease to do something once called for in order to begin to do what is now called for in always only caring for the dying. Now care is no longer called for. Indeed no calls to the dying reach them, and no answering presence to presence. It is then a matter of complete indifference whether death gains the victory over the patient in such impenetrable solitude by direct or indirect action.

2. We might formulate the moral rule governing premortem care so as to include in it a second possibly justifiable stipulation. We could say: Always keep officious treatments away from the dying in order to draw close to them in companying with them and caring for them; never, therefore, take positive action to usher them out of our presence or to hasten their departure from the human community, *unless* there is a kind of prolonged dying in which it is medically impossible to keep severe pain at bay.

Again, it is not for the moralist to say whether there is this kind of dying. Persons dying from bone cancer may be the sort of case that would fall under this second qualification of the requirement that we always care for the dying and do nothing to place them more quickly beyond our love and care. If this is true of dying from bone cancer, or from some other specific disease, then at the heart of ordinary medical practice today there are cases of suffering-dying that should rather be compared to the injured, slowly dying man who must be left behind in jungle warfare or by lonely companies of men on ventures over deserts or fleeing from war zones, etc.[60]

One can hardly hold men to be morally blameworthy if in these instances dying is directly accomplished or hastened. The reasons are the same as those advanced in favor of the first stipulation: A patient undergoing deep and prolonged pain, who cannot be relieved by means presently available to use to care for him and make him comfortable, would also be beyond reach of the other ways in which company may be kept with him and he be attended in his dying—as much so, depending on the degree of his undefeatable agony, as the prolonged comatose patient. For the same reasons, this may be another place to locate an abrogation of the good moral reasons for distinguishing between omission and commission in our dealings with the dying.

Suppose that it were agreed that directly death-dealing or death-hastening actions are not inherently or always necessarily wrong. Suppose that it were agreed that, solely in the sort of cases we have discussed, to bring or hasten death would be consonant with caring for the dying. Suppose that it were agreed that the acts described would be no violation of charity; that instead these are qualifications that do no more than extend the meaning of caring for the dying so as to comprehend problematic cases. It would not at once follow that the moral rule of practice governing medical care should include these provisos; that the moral constitution of medical practice should

60. See note 59 above. Kieran Nolan, "The Problem of Care for the Dying" p. 259, suggests that patients dying of bone cancer may suffer unconquerable pain. It is difficult to say whether there is any pain that cannot be relieved by increasing doses of drugs, because pain studies are studies of subjective states. The best medical opinion seems to be that in hospital situations pain can always be suppressed. This may be done at great cost to the patient's strength, etc., and these large doses of pain relievers would not be administered if the cost of not doing so were not greater, from the patient's endurance of suffering. I think, therefore, that this second possible "exception" is a supposable class without any members. Cf. Beecher, *Research and the Individual*, p. 161.

admit these possibly justifiable cases of actively bringing or hastening death.

To say this requires an affirmative answer to the question raised already by an ethics and a practice of allowing to die. Can a doctor, we asked, admit that a patient is incurable while in the ethics of his medical mission never admitting that diseases are incurable? The question now is: Can a doctor and can medicine as a rule of practice admit that a patient is beyond earthly care, inaccessible to care, and so warrant as a practice positive actions that accomplish or hasten his death while not weakening medicine's life-saving mission? Would the doctors who are the moral agents in these exceptional acts of killing the dying, or acts that allow to die, be corrupted by them, and medicine's impulse to save be weakened? The medical imperative specifying that physicians never cease trying to find the cure or the relief (e.g., to the pain of bone cancer) which future patients need is more extensive and might have to be given preeminence over the humane moral judgments that could warrant bubbles of air for permanently comatose patients and dying patients suffering from undefeatable pain. The question of questions is whether both that imperative and these permissions (with appropriate actions) can dwell together in the same person and calling. Or must one be bartered against the other, and in practice the one weaken the other resolve?

Within the limits of the moral rules for extending care and faithfulness to the dying elaborated in this chapter, and within the strict limits of the "unless" we have appended to the categorical imperative that we keep covenant with them, I do not believe that we need fear any weakening of medicine's impulse to save life. Still no one should forget the judgment of the leading scholar of the Nazi medical cases: "Whatever proportion these crimes finally assumed, it became evident to all who investigated them that they had started from small beginnings. . . . It started with the acceptance of the attitude . . . that there is such a thing as life not worthy to be lived . . . its impetus was the attitude toward the non-rehabilitable sick." [61] It is of prime ethical importance that we be concerned about the care and protection of all men in societal and medical practices, and not solely with mercy in individual acts.

61. Leo Alexander, "Medical Science Under Dictatorship," *New England Journal of Medicine* 241, no. 2 (July 14, 1949): 44, 45.

4

The Self-Giving of Vital Organs:
A Case Study in Comparative Ethics

Am I My Twin Brother's Keeper?

In 1956, identical twin brothers, Leon and Leonard Masden, 19 years of age, presented themselves to the Peter Bent Brigham Hospital in Boston. Leon's only hope for life was a transplantation of a kidney from his healthy twin. In 1954 the Brigham Hospital had performed the first successful homotransplantation of a kidney in identical twins. In that case, however, the twins were adults, and their consents alone were sufficient to keep the operation from being found at law to be an act of assault and battery. In the case of the Masdens, both twins and both parents consented; indeed they urgently requested the operation. The relevant rule of law is that parental consent is controlling in regard to medical treatments of operations potentially beneficial to the child. In this case the removal of one of Leonard's kidneys seemed clearly to be of no benefit to Leonard—only to Leon. Under these circumstances, before proceeding, the surgeons sought a declaratory judgment from the Supreme Judicial Court of Massachusetts. Decisions of the Court in 1957 approved of the operation in the Masden case, and also in two cases of identical twins 14 years of age.[1]

The line of reasoning by which the Court reached an affirmative decision in these cases is remarkably like the present state of the question of homotransplantation of an organ from a living donor in Roman Catholic moral theology. Moreover, the main objections that have been brought against the declaratory judgments of the Massachusetts Court and suggested corrections of its reasoning look remarkably like the ethical justification of organ transplantation

---

1. *Masden v. Harrison*, No. 68651 Eq., Mass. Sup. Jud. Ct., June 12, 1957; *Huskey v. Harrison*, No. 68666 Eq., Mass. Sup. Jud. Ct., Aug. 30, 1957; *Foster v. Harrison*, No. 68674 Eq., Mass. Sup. Jud. Ct., Nov. 20, 1957.

from living donors that might be developed within the ambit of
Protestant ethics in some of its fundamental contrasts with Roman
Catholic moral theology. We shall look first at the state of the question within past Roman Catholic moral theology and then at the
decision of the Supreme Judicial Court of Massachusetts, before taking up the criticisms of that decision and the ethics of the donation
of organs that might be developed on Protestant grounds (and, of
course, on more radically reformed Catholic grounds).

The discussion among Catholic moralists revolves around the
meaning of the principle of "totality" in distinguishing between a
justifiable and unjustifiable "mutilation" or invasion of a person's
bodily "integrity." Man has the power but he does not have the right
to do anything he wants to his own body. His right is that of a
steward or administrator of his bodily life. It is a proper act of
administration for a part of the body to be sacrificed for the sake
of the whole. Individual limbs, organs, or functions are related
to a man's bodily life and health as parts to the whole. These
may be removed and functions permanently suppressed if this is
proportionately useful for the good of the whole.

But men are not "members" one of another in the sense that limbs
are members of the body. Man is a "whole" within the social
"wholes" to which he belongs. He is not a mere "part" of society. In
him there is "finality" and in society another "finality." His good and
the social good are not related as part to whole. Both are ends. Therefore the principle of totality is not governing when the question
is raised concerning what may be done to the bodily integrity of one
man, or what he may do to himself, for the sake of another or for
"society." The parts and functions of the body are destined, indeed
subordinated, to the good of the whole man *alone*. But men themselves are not similarly destined or subordinated to any social whole
alone. Every moral association of men—from the family to political
community—exists for the advancement of the general good of that
association and for the advancement of the good of each single "member" in particular.

Therefore, in the matter of familial donors or of "society's" need
for organs, the fundamental question to be raised is whether we can
or may or must presume the principle of totality, or a subordination
of part to whole, to be among the moral warrants for the transplanta-

tion of an organ from a living donor into the body of another. The principle of totality governs "self-mutilation for one's own good": this may be justified in those terms. But the principle of totality does not govern in a case of "self-mutilation for the sake of one's neighbor": this cannot be justified by appeals to the principle of totality. Indeed, were such appeals alleged to be the justifying reason for organ transplantation from living donors, both the supporting principle and the act to which it leads would be grave violations of man.

When moralists take up the question of the self-giving of organs, their first move is to bracket the entire discussion by firm and unanimous agreement that "no mutilation for the good of the neighbor, even a minor mutilation, can be justified by the principle of totality." [2] That principle means the physical subordination of part to organic whole. Any suggestion of such subordination should be decisively excluded from our understanding of relations among men, and no use should be made of organismic analogies in connection with the "moral associations" of men.

This is the correct interpretation of the apparent force of statements of Pius XI and Pius XII when these are applied to the self-giving of organs, provided their numerous allocutions are seen in historical perspective. Pius XI was mainly interested in condemning eugenic sterilization, and Pius XII was condemning the Nazi abuse of medical experimentation involving human subjects. The latter, in his address to the delegates to the Eighth Congress of the World Medical Association [3] seems deliberately to pass over the question of the self-giving of organs. Contemporary Catholic moralists, therefore, argue that what this body of teachings adds up to is that, while it may be justifiable on other grounds, organ transplantation from living donors cannot be justified by the principle of totality. This would imply between man and man a physical relation of part to whole, and nothing can be justified by such a totalitarian understanding of man's relation to the good of his fellow man or to his societies and their good.

It is worth remarking that it is not easy to rise above using the principle of totality to distinguish between justifiable and unjustifi-

2. Gerald Kelly, S.J., "The Morality of Mutilation: Towards a Revision of the Treatise," *Theological Studies* 17, no. 3 (September 1956): 332.

3. September 30, 1954, *Acta Apostolicae Sedis* 46 (1954), pp. 587–98.

able invasions of bodily integrity without actually falling below the
respect and protections and weakening the prohibitions which this
principle affirms. There is some danger in viewing as historically
bound these papal statements, and also the writings of physicians
and moralists on the Nazi medical experiments when these first came
to light. To understand the importance of refusing to make a man
merely a part of any totality, one should rather consider the question
in the light of a totality far better than the Nazi society and in the
light of well-designed experiments from which great good would
likely come for all mankind: would what was done still have been
wrong?

Similarly, the judgment that the self-giving of organs is not to be
justified by the principle of totality is not a small point, or one that
loses its force or disappears as we go on to seek for better reasons. It
remains a warning, always valid, that there are many refined and
subtle ways by which men may be encouraged or allowed to treat
themselves as parts only, or collections of parts, in the service of
medical progress or societal value to come. In terms of our vision of
man and his relation to community, there may be little to chose
between the blood and soil, organic view of the Nazis and the technological, "spare parts," mechanistic analogies of the present day.
The exclusion of the principles of totality from among the possible
justifications of organ transplantation from living donors permits, at
least, the negative conclusion that, if transplants are to be sanctioned,
"there need not be an intrinsic connection between the mutilating
act and the saving of one's life" [4] or obtaining a proportionate improvement in the health of one's body. The next move made by the
moralists in the matter of "self-mutilation for the sake of one's neighbor" is to base consideration of this question upon an understanding
of mutual relationships among men according to which men have
naturally an "ordinatio" (an ordering or ordination, *not* a *sub*ordination) one to another. There is a natural, moral bond to one's neighbor as to "another self"; neither one is superior or inferior to the
other. Still, from this it is not at once to be concluded that men may
rightfully permanently impair their bodies by organ donation for
the sake of another. A parity between oneself and the other self ex-
cludes *subordination* of one to the other. In addition there is what

4. Kelly, "The Morality of Mutilation," p. 336.

is described as a "commonly held principle that, in the same order of values, love of self takes precedence over love of neighbor." [5] Therefore because of the equality among men in their natural ordination to one another, it does not immediately follow that a donor can rightfully consent to give an organ to his "other self."

One might reach this conclusion by reflecting upon the slight though real impairment the donor of a kidney will suffer in comparison—in the same order of values—to the life and health that will be bestowed upon the recipient. Here, as we shall see, the moralists should have paused and thought through their conclusions in order— from the nature of the case and within the same order of values— to weigh the responsibilities that may be undertaken in fidelity one to another, and to consider how one possible act may be limited by other like dues. However, because the moralists have been concerned to rebut the general presumption against self-mutilation, they have usually not so reasoned. Instead, they have argued that a man may rightfully consent to the removal of an organ (which does not, like blood or skin, replace itself) provided he is aiming at a higher order of values than the physical organ given and received. Just as in sacrifice of life in general one really prefers his own good of a higher order, i.e., the *bonum virtutis*,[6] to the good of life itself, so also in the self-giving of organs one seeks a higher benefit than that which is given away.

This justification of organ donation amounts to a reinterpretation of the principle of totality in terms of the "moral wholeness" of the donor rather than a rejection of that principle. The good of the donor's total being (and not, of course, simply his physical life or health) warrants the sacrifice of a physical part. "Perhaps the principle of 'helping thy neighbor,'" one Catholic moralist argues in a recent article, "is not so distinct from, but is an amplification of the principle of totality—of the totality of all the dimensions and not just the physical requirements of man." Here the appeal is to "the subordination of the physical perfection (of the donor) to *his own* perfection of grace and charity. . . . This would expand the notion of the total person (psychological and spiritual, as well as physical) beyond that which was originally envisioned in the 'principle of

5. Ibid., pp. 337, 341.
6. Ibid., p. 341.

totality.' " Thus, some degree of physical harm is permitted in view of the spiritual benefit. "The *donation* of an organ out of love for others may be just as necessary to the conscience of the donor as undergoing any surgical operation for his own benefit." This would justify the self-giving of an organ as an application of the principle of totality expanded to encompass "wholeness" or spiritual health. Just as particular organs are subordinated to the finality of the organism, the organism and its parts are, in turn, subordinated to the spiritual finality of the person himself. This line of reasoning seems in the end to be comparable to the justification of contraception in terms of "the *totality of family values,* out of a spirit of solidarity and love for the greater whole, the family." [7]

So said—in only slightly different language—the Supreme Judicial Court of Massachusetts in its declaratory judgments in the 1957 identical-twin kidney transplant cases. Some readers may wonder whether the court and the moralist in attempting to rise above the traditional use of the principle of totality in distinguishing between justifiable and unjustifiable "self-mutilation" do not come dangerously close to falling below it by making men members one of another in a moral solidarity that—in future, if not in the case in question—affords too little protection of each individual against invasions of his physical "integrity" for the sake of foreseeable benefits. Such readers are likely to be of the opinion that the Massachusetts Court permitted battery by departing from the rule of law that makes parental or any other consent controlling only in case of expected benefit to the child to be operated on and by invoking instead a concept of identical-twin "solidarity."

Instead of criticizing the Court, we shall examine the line of reasoning it followed in search of benefits to accrue to the donor, and the remarkable similarity of this to the foregoing justifications of the self-giving of organs proposed by some Roman Catholic moralists. Then we shall take up the argument of critics of the Court who hold that consent alone (on the part of parents with their minor children judged competent to consent) should have been sufficient without the allegation of benefit to someone other than the recipient. This would seem a more charitable way to donate an organ at risk of harm.

7. Warren Reich, *Medico-Moral Problems and the Principle of Totality: A Catholic Viewpoint* (Washington, D.C.: Veterans Administration Hospitals, 1967), pp. 34–36, 40.

In the Masden case a psychiatrist testified that Leonard would suffer "grave emotional impact" if he was not allowed to give a kidney and his brother Leon died. Judge Edward A. Counihan, Jr. found that the donor, 19 years of age, understood the possible consequences of the operation and was competent to consent to it. He further declared:

> I am satisfied from the testimony of the psychiatrist that grave emotional impact may be visited upon Leonard if the defendants refuse to perform this operation and Leon should die, as apparently he will. . . . Such emotional disturbance could well affect the health and physical well-being of Leonard for the remainder of his life. I therefore find that this operation is necessary for the continued good health and future well-being of Leonard and that in performing the operation the defendants are conferring a benefit upon Leonard as well as upon Leon.[8]

The benefit conferred upon Leonard was more "the prevention of possible detriment" than it was the "conferring of a possible gain." In this respect the Massachusetts Court's opinion was clearly more negative than the position of the moralists which we have examined. For the latter the benefit to the donor is a positive spiritual attainment through the manifestation of a concrete love of neighbor at some risk to oneself.

One may remark at this point that the "detriment" or emotional trauma to be prevented was itself a product of the launching of the experimental procedure of transplanting the organs of living donors and perhaps of "overselling" the therapeutic value of such transplants, even between identical twins, in 1957. The recipients in the case of the 14-year-old Huskey and Foster twins both died some months after their operations. In retrospect one might ask whether the donors in all three cases made a mature and informed consent to *an investigational procedure,* and whether it was not medical practice and our society that made them vulnerable to trauma from possibly not being allowed to save a brother's life. In short, our medical ethos may have created strong pressures toward self-mutilation that run ahead of actual benefits. In that case, the prevention

8. This and other references are from William J. Curran, "A Problem of Consent: Kidney Transplantation in Minors," *New York University Law Review* 34 (May 1959): 891–98.

of detrimental impact upon refused donors would be no excuse.

Now that kidney transplants are more therapeutic than investigational, and familial donors are still better than cadaver organs, the
protection of a member of the family from undue psychological
pressure to give an organ to save the life of another is a well-
established concern of the medical team. An inwardly reluctant or
outwardly pressured "volunteer" will, if detected, be rejected on
"medical" grounds without disclosing the real reason to him or to
other members of the family. It is therefore pertinent to ask whether
in the investigational stage of these procedures volunteers have always been sufficiently protected from the societal sources of the "emotional impact," itself factitious, of refusing, or not being allowed,
to "save life." This would seem a crucial question, especially in the
case of identical twins, who notoriously have an intimate solidarity
with one another and a corresponding difficulty in growing up to an
adequate sense of separate personal identity. Was the detriment prevented in these cases an actual misuse of the twins' too great and as
yet immature part-whole identity?

We can have only the highest admiration for the sensitivity of
kidney transplant surgeons in dealing with living donors—while
noting their reserve in justifying and doing a procedure which is
likely to receive more enthusiastic endorsement by moralists and
the general public, who are likely to suppose that saving life is the
only value and that "love" settles everything. On the one hand, for
example, Jean Hamburger and Jean Crosnier affirm that "it is impossible for a physician who has witnessed the love and generosity
of a father or mother who insist calmly that one of their kidneys be
given to their child not to bow before the dignity of this wish." These
authors report "the emptiness and desolation of a mother, whose
offer of a kidney for her child was refused," who feared she had not
insisted enough; and—perhaps more importantly—"the immense
satisfaction that persists in many familial donors in spite of the
death of the recipient." [9]

At the same time, these authors are remarkably reserved about
securing the benefits of this therapy. Physicians should yield to the
slightest contrary wish. "A refusal of therapy in the face of death,

9. "Moral and Ethical Problems in Transplantation," in Felix T. Rapaport and
Jean Dausset (eds.), *Human Transplantation* (New York: Grune and Stratton, 1968),
pp. 40, 39.

if fully thought out and reached in a free fashion should be respected and not be considered an act of suicide." This also means that, in the sort of case we are considering where the benefit conveyed could indeed be great, "the strong emotional ties which are so frequent between identical twins are not a sufficient reason to transplant all cases where one of the twins is in terminal uremia." In short, in familial donors, "the offer of a kidney by a brother or sister may just be a statement of courage; this is not necessarily a bad point of departure for this type of venture, but it must necessarily be considered with a wary and critical eye." [10] In other words, consent to such an operation out of "love" or the "benefit" of avoiding a donor's suffering is only the beginning of the question whether the gift should be accepted or solicited. Familial donors have only the advantage that, in the opinion of these authors, nonfamilial donors are so frequently pathologic that they should be refused.

To mankind's great good fortune, medical ethics is not a *gessinnungsethik*; it is not solely or even mainly an ethics of inner motive; love or a will to do good settles little of medical importance. Physicians are exceedingly sensitive to the fact that "for the first time in the history of medicine a procedure is being adopted in which a perfectly healthy person is injured permanently in order to improve the well-being of another." [11] This, at the very time theological moralists are busy entirely dissolving the protections of past teachings on self-mutilation. Physicians are rather more concerned about the integrity of the flesh—even when they adopt a procedure that makes a well person ill for the sake of making another well. They do this with ambiguity of conscience over the unmitigated conflict between the medical care both patients need.

In 1962 a 23-year-old woman with total kidney failure was considered for a transplant from her twin sister, who was quite willing to act as a donor. While tests were being made and dialysis used to prepare the ill twin for the operation, she suddenly died in convulsion. Subsequently in 1967, the healthy twin developed urinary incontinence following a cesarean section for her first baby. Her case and treatment is on record and described in detail.[12] Significant to

10. Ibid., pp. 39, 41, 39.

11. Francis D. Moore, "New Problems for Surgery," *Science* 144 (April 24, 1964): 391.

12. "Ethics for the Use of Live Donors in Kidney Transplantation," Annotations, *American Heart Journal* 75 (May 1968): 711–14.

note is the judgment of the medical doctors concerning this series of events: "We, at any rate, feel thankful that this patient was not used as a kidney donor, although at the time this was planned, we did not think that there was any ethical objection to the use of an identical twin as a kidney donor."

Moreover, physicians are alert to the fact that the personal values they help to make secure are to be found only within the ambience of fleshly existence. They know that psychological wholeness is deeply imbedded in the physical life and in the security of the fortress of the body. They are troubled not only by the risk to the health of the donor but also by the risk to the mental well-being of the actual donor, the solicited donors, and their families. On this there is counterevidence to that adduced by Hamburger and Crosnier. "I know," one writer states, "of a patient's brother who declined to donate his kidney—with resultant severe emotional trauma; I know of another family torn apart by a mother giving a kidney to her child against the wishes of the husband and father. Such psycho-social complications occur in many difficult clinical situations but never more so than in this one of transplantations of organs." [13]

In view of a child's inability to give an understanding consent to damage to himself, an exaggerated estimation of the benefit to be conferred may constitute an environmental pressure for self-mutilation upon twins or siblings. Because of this, Professor David Daube would have the law prohibit the use of children as donors of organs. "The likelihood of a trauma," he writes, "will be greatly lessened if the law leaves not the shadow of a doubt that a transplantation is here out of the question: the case will then be no different from where a twin dies from pneumonia—bad enough, but with no scope for offer of a sacrifice, disappointment or self-torture." Children should on no account be donors, he believes, and "there should be no cheating by maintaining, for example, that the child would suffer a trauma if he were not allowed to give his twin a kidney or whatever it might be." If medical progress and our news media have imposed on the child the possibility that he may suffer detriment if a kidney of his is not used in an effort to prolong the life of a twin or brother, then the advantage taken of sibling or twin solidarity should be

13. "Moral Problems in the Use of Borrowed Organs," editorial, *Annals of Internal Medicine* 60, no. 2 (February 1964): 312.

counteracted by the law's prohibition. No trauma could occur if the law leaves no doubt. "If the law were 100 per cent certain that up to the age of, say 17½, the operation would not be allowed, then no doubt could exist," and consequently no detrimental sequelae, at least, none beyond the loss of a brother.[14]

It is noteworthy that the age of mature consent to the self-giving of organs picked by Professor Daube would have included the Masden twins, who were 19, but not a number of the other identical-twin transplants performed at the Peter Bent Brigham Hospital. The surgeons said they would not perform a kidney transplant operation on a well identical twin below the age of 12 or 14. "When identical twins of very youthful age (children under 12) were presented for the question of transplantation, it was necessary for the doctors of the hospital to say 'No'—despite possible legal approval . . ."[15] This proves that *at some point* one has to stand against the self-mutilating pressures of a medical ethos that holds out great benefit to come to the ill twin child. One has to render his death, as Professor Daube suggested, simply the loss of a brother, by *in practice* forbidding the invasion of the body of the well twin or sibling in order to try to save the ill.

The State of the Question in Roman Catholic Morals

Critics of the Massachusetts Court say that it should not have created for itself a "very sticky 'benefit' problem" in reaching the decision that the operations should be performed. In place of direct therapeutic benefit to the healthy twin the Court put putative psychological benefit. It might have rested its affirmative decision on the healthy twin's consent alone, and it should have done so. The justice presiding at each hearing determined for himself by questioning the donor twin whether or not that twin was intelligent enough to understand the nature and consequences of the operation and fully and freely consented to it. He determined the validity of

14. David Daube: "Transplantation: Acceptibility of Procedures and the Required Legal Sanctions," in G. E. W. Wolstenholme and Maeve O'Connor (eds.), *Ethics in Medical Progress: With Special Reference to Transplantation* (Boston: Little, Brown, 1966), pp. 198, 203.

15. Francis D. Moore, *Give and Take: The Development of Tissue Transplantation* (Philadelphia: Saunders, 1964), p. 79. William J. Curran and Henry K. Beecher ("*Experimentation in Children,*" pp. 77–83) choose 14 as the minimum age for a minor to consent to nonbeneficial research; then, astonishingly, they suggest 7 years or older as the age of competence to give an organ to a member of a child's immediate family!

that consent. That determination, it is pointed out, was as difficult and as technical as the justices' decision concerning the "grave emotional loss" the healthy twin would suffer if the sick twin died without an attempt to save him by transplantation.[16] Thus, it is argued that the prevention of detriment *to the donor* obscures the one sufficient ground for the legality of the self-giving of organs by living donors. A free and informed consent having in view a calculable benefit *to the recipient* should have been the grounds. This, of course, is the chief legal justification used in cases of familial donors of kidneys who are adults.

It can be argued that moral reasoning should take this same line, if indeed we are to reach the conclusion that the self-giving of an organ is a justifiable mutilation. A possible justification of organ transplantation from living donors that might be developed within the ambit of Protestant ethics would rest the matter upon charitable consent alone; the benefit aimed at would be the benefit to the recipient, not the donor's own higher wholeness.

Since I shall presently draw out this contrast between the state of this question in some past and recent Roman Catholic moral theology and the ethical justification of the self-giving of organs that may be more amenable to Christians who are (instructed) Protestants, it is only fair to point out that some Roman Catholic moralists manifest that their treatments of this question are finally controlled, formed, and informed by the *agapé*-love (will, consent) of the giver. Fr. Gerald Kelly, S.J., for example, wrote concerning the views of past moralists that "whether they are still in the realm of immutable principles when they say that personal welfare is the only reason justifying serious self-mutilation is open to serious doubt. It seems to me that this is rather a practical principle, formulated with a view to ordinary cases, and patient of reformulation."[17] This line of reasoning must, indeed, be reformulated, he points out, in order to account for the fact that "all moralists would undoubtedly permit a cesarean section, or even an hysterectomy, if necessary for the welfare of the fetus."[18] These are "mutilations" which, we are supposing, may not be necessary to save the life or serve the health of the

16. Curran, "A Problem of Consent," pp. 894–95.
17. "The Morality of Mutilation," p. 342.
18. Ibid., p. 338.

mother. The benefit is solely or primarily to the unborn child, and yet the operations invade the physical integrity of the woman's body and may impair her health and functions as seriously as the loss of one of two healthy kidneys.

The risk accepted by a healthy donor of a kidney has been estimated to be the same as the likelihood of death or harm if one drives 16 miles to and from work each day.[19] The fact that this is a real even if slight impairment can be seen by remembering that donors also drive automobiles. So Fr. Kelly seems to conclude that when it is a question of saving another's life, there is no need to bring up the sticky problem of personal benefit or the attainment of a higher wholeness. It is significant that Kelly's article was published the same year—1956—in which the Masden case was brought up in Massachusetts. Already had he gone beyond the reasoning of that Court and beyond past moral analysis in strongly suggesting that a charitable and graceful consent should be sufficient to warrant self-mutilation for the sake of one's neighbor.

Nevertheless, there remain characteristic differences between Roman Catholic moral theology and a Christian ethics developed instead upon Protestant grounds which are likely to be revealed in the way each treats the question of the warrants for the self-giving of organs by living donors. This contrast should be noted, to the merit and demerit of each.

In the Catholic tradition, charity is an infused theological virtue which finds itself in continuity with "nature," confirms our experienced bonds of life with life, and elevates and perfects us in our existing direction toward God and toward life with and for our fellow man. This, theoretically, could give ground for now treating a child as charitable, communitarian, in its nature as a human being and for externally disposing of the child for the good of others in medical experimentation or organ transplantation. At the same time, an adult may be regarded as by nature charitable, in such fashion that organ donation would be taken to be a natural social obligation on the giver's part; and so the receiving of a needed organ would

19. Or an additional 8,000 miles a year. John P. Merrill, "Letters and Comments," *Annals of Internal Medicine* 61, no. 2 [August 1964]: 356. This is not a negligible risk. "Sooner or later a volunteer donor is going to die as a result of giving a kidney to someone else" (William J. Kolff, ibid., p. 361).

be listed among men's natural rights. Or familial society could be the group norm made overriding over the embodied being of one of its members.

Such could be the fruit of sanctifying the continuities of nature or social togetherness by a baptism of infused charity. Nowhere is this clearer among the premises and in the structure or outlook of Roman Catholic moral theology than in the recent volume of essays by—if I may use the term—some of the most liberal of contemporary moralists. There in an essay on "The Principle of Totality in Moral Theology," in which Martin Nolan, O.S.A., Professor of Moral Theology, St. Patrick's, Rome, prosecutes (as do the other authors) a war of overkill against the "physicalism" that was so prominent a feature in the writings of past Catholic moralists.[20] It is noteworthy that these writings do not alter by a hair's breadth the continuity of grace (love) and "nature," of charity and the perfection of the self with others, which is the most fundamental premise or insight upon which Christian ethical reflection proceeds in the Catholic tradition.

Nolan argues against preoccupation with man as a psychophysical totality, against a view of man which holds that his totality is confined to a "limited space," against "physicalism" in treating questions having to do with man's "integrity," against the conception that the wholeness of man is an "island existence" confined to the body or "a cage or network already existing in God's mind, a blueprint to which each person must comply." Such views would render God's creation "brutally material." Instead, in proper theological perspective we should understand man's totality always in terms of his ultimate finality. This means a "perfect totality not yet achieved," an envisioned "vast cosmic totality." Man is always *in via,* marching through the dark of time toward the dawn of a vaster totality," "the consummation of all in communion," a "rimless totality that fulfills." [21] A more expanded notion of the principle of totality would be impossible to conceive, and this notion is brought directly into relation with the mundane questions of medical experimentation and organ transplantation.

In via, there is continuity over the entire terrain between this

20. Charles E. Curran (ed.), *Absolutes in Moral Theology?* (Washington, D.C.–Cleveland: Corpus Books, 1968), pp. 232–48.
21. Ibid., pp. 237, 238, 239–40, 248.

"limited physical area of space" and men's final membership one with another and with God in a "rimless" communion. In this Nolan's purpose is a laudable one: he wishes to break out from the state of the debate among Catholic moralists over the self-giving of organs. It is not only that this debate has been rather evenly divided between proponents and opponents of the medical procedure of using living donors. More importantly, the arguments have been an "embarrassing" stand-off between those who would "barter" charity to totality and those who would "barter" totality to charity. "The 'conservative' held that totality confined charity, while the 'liberal' saw the hard edge of totality softened in the surge of charity." The only course left open is to "retain both principles to the theological end," [22] which means "the dawn of a vaster totality" or a membership one of another that only fulfills.

Some readers may wonder whether, in attempting to soar so eloquently above the traditional understanding of totality in distinguishing justifiable from unjustifiable self-mutilations, and whether, in trying to go beyond the rather plodding efforts of past moralists to reason about both the requirements of the integrity of man's bodily life and the requirements of charity, Fr. Nolan may not be in danger of falling below the respect and protections these views afforded. On the one hand, he writes that a man's bodily life and organs are not to be disposed of "arbitrarily." The test seems to be the total good of one's own person in achieving his destination toward rimless communion. This standard means, at least, that "the person must remain in the gift of himself: should he deliberately give over in suicide the life that he holds in gift from God, or diminish his possibilities for self-giving by maiming himself, he is acting contrary to his own personhood and thus too contrary to God's law." [23] In this there seems to be some reflection of the "limits" imposed upon charity (if such they should be called) by the integral life of the embodied person.

On the other hand, however, there seem for Nolan to be no limits of any consequence. He writes that "the 'extent' of physical or psychical self-gift in experimentation or transplantation is no longer to be measured in terms of what is merely physical or psychical

22. Ibid., p. 243.
23. Ibid., p. 241.

integrity." This being so, one may *not* "eliminate the possibility of giving oneself as a person even if it involved *maiming* oneself, for example, *by giving two eyes*." In which case, the integrity of the life of all who bear flesh (*sarx*) may have to be saved from our contemporary moralists (and some scientists) by the medical profession as a whole, who rightly would refuse to perform any such operation. There may be some dangerous consequences of the battle against mere "physicalism" that could follow from such an aspiring attempt to dissolve the entire creation into the continuous direction of mankind toward God. It may be possible for us to believe by faith that in heaven "one might give himself to the larger perfecting reality in every member and function that he himself is," while yet giving oneself "as a whole person to be fulfilled, not to be eliminated." But continuous anticipations of that heavenly totality are apt to yield either no medical ethical guidance or the worse earthly sort of advice.[24]

My purpose, however, is to point out what happens to charity when this is understood as an infused virtue that finds itself at home with, and only perfects, a man's natural quest for life in another. On our way (*in via*) toward that vast communion of One with all which fulfills, we find ourselves performing lesser acts of charity which fulfill. From the fact that everything exists in total relation to God, it follows that whatever exists that is not God is "totally relative"; and this means, writes Fr. Nolan, that "the innermost core of all creaturehood is utter relationship." If the human person is "utter relationship," he is "a vast emptiness to be filled." [25] In seeking to fill his own "vast emptiness" the human person "overflows the narrow limits of material existence" and "breaks the bonds of matter that anchor him to the dust of his origins."

This may be a telling point in the war against the alleged "physicalism" of past moral theology. The price paid for this vic-

---

24. Ibid., pp. 243, 239. It should in fairness be said that Nolan's appeal to a transcendent wholeness provides a limitation upon the action of the State that was formerly afforded by the inviolable physical integrity of the individual. "No inferior totality of grouping," he writes, "such as the State, can subordinate the person to itself or make the least demands on what constitutes the person" (p. 243). Still the donor himself and the medical profession are a moral association of men that seem not to be subject to much limitation.

25. Ibid., p. 238.

tory, however, is that the human person not only breaks the bonds of physical existence in quelling the emptiness that is the hallmark of his finitude by faith and love toward God. He also overflows the narrow limits of personhood by seeking to fill his own vast emptiness through love for another person as his "other self." Himself only "utter relationship" with no or no other "innermost core," he is bound to seek himself in all that he does or gives of himself. "He empties himself of self to receive." Men have "the need to love, to be whole." And when Nolan says that "the total good of the whole person" is "achieved in self-gift," [26] everything depends on whether the gift (and the recipient) or the achievement of wholeness is in view. I judge that his chapter must be read as a restatement of the "sticky benefits theory" in justification of the self-giving of organs.

This position was also restated by Dr. J. E. Murray in the Ciba Foundation Symposium when he interpreted the principle of totality to mean that "spiritual good is better for an individual than material good and even though the donor has lost something materially he has gained something spiritually which is greater." [27] The difference between this and the declaratory judgments of the Massachusetts Court is only that the verdicts of the latter were based on psychological benefits (or the prevention of psychological injury), while the moralists appeal to what they call "personal" or to "spiritual" benefits. Both are strange apologies for the donation of organs.

Transimplantation as a Single, Uninterrupted Action

Another approach would be to relate donor and recipient more closely together societally by an analysis of transplantation as a curative process. The two operations involved in the self-giving of organs

26. Ibid., pp. 238, 246, 240.

27. In Wolstenholme and O'Connor, *Ethics in Medical Progress*, p. 207. And by Dr. George E. Schreiner: "If giving a kidney is for his spiritual or psychiatric good, and this is recognized as part of the total person, it seems to me that the particular mutilation becomes quite permissible under the extension of the principle of physical totality to the totality of a spiritual person" (ibid., pp. 130–31). So also Dr. Jørgen Voigt of Copenhagen, reporting his experience of living donors: "In some cases, it has been of such great psychological significance for an individual to have volunteered as a donor, that it would be a great pity for the individual concerned if his offer was rejected. I consider that somatically and mentally normal adult persons should have the right to decide so much concerning themselves" ("The Criterion of Death, Particularly in Relation to Transplantation Surgery," *World Medical Journal* 14 [1967]: 144).

may be described as one composite procedure of "transimplantation" terminating in therapy for the needy patient. Thus, Professor David Daube advocates "viewing the whole transaction from the start with the living donor to the finish—which, one hopes, is some relief at least for the recipient—as one composite, curative transaction." He regards "the two operations in the transplanting transaction as a unitary, positive, curative process." This view may profitably be compared with a recent, excellent essay reconstruing the meaning of the ancient "rule of double effect." The author, Cornelius J. Van der Poel, C.S.SP., Professor of Moral Theology, St. Mary's Seminary, Norwalk, Connecticut, likewise contends in regard to transplantation of organs from living donors that "the excision is only willed insofar as it makes the future implantation possible. The implantation gives the *human* meaning to the excision." [28]

I fear, however, that some contemporary moralists display a relatively lesser concern over the grave question of making the excision in well persons in human acts of "transimplantation" than do a great many physicians and others who are deeply engaged in discussions of medical ethics. Professor Daube, for example, immediately says that "if we emphasize this curative, positive aspect of the business, the consent of the donor is not enough. . . ." Two additional tests must be pressed: "First, there must be no other way of achieving the curative end—no other way actually available . . . [Second] the plight of the prospective recipient must emerge as heavily outweighing the danger and loss incurred by the donor." [29]

28. Daube, "Transplantation," pp. 194, 208; Cornelius J. Van der Poel, "The Principle of Double Effect" in Charles E. Curran (ed.), *Absolutes in Moral Theology?* (Washington, D.C.–Cleveland: Corpus Books, 1967), pp. 186–210, n. 33 on p. 299. This essay is controlled by the author's use of "indirectly voluntary" to include *both* "the means to and the concomitant effects of human action"; these are alike "regretted but unavoidable aspects of the total act," and are willed "only because and insofar as the totality of the act demands them" (n. 28 on p. 299).

29. "Transplantation," pp. 194–95. Daube's chief interest is to reinterpret medical "invasions" of the body generally as curative and not as assault and battery made legal by consent. "An operation should be treated as a positive, beneficient, admirable action from the outset, not as a lawful infliction of harm"—just as we do not construe marital intercourse as rape authorized by virtue of consent (ibid., p. 193). Daube wishes to replace the "assault-consent" principle with a "positive good" approach in forensic medicine, and incidental thereto to give moral warrants for transplant surgery. This at once requires him to recognize in the totally curative action of "transimplantation" this "novel and unique feature: the role of the donor fits into no

By contrast, some moralists are likely rather more readily to take consent "in its directedness toward God" to be sufficient. There is room, of course, for both of Daube's tests in Van der Poel's account, but the stress is taken off them. If the moralist's justifications of the self-giving of organs were taken with utmost seriousness, by prospective donors and physicians alike, the moral reason and impulse to move entirely beyond the acceptance of living donors to the use of cadaver organs alone would be weakened or removed.

Van der Poel campaigns against (1) assigning decisive importance to the "physical structure" of actions, and against (2) understanding the two effects of an action as "independent entities rather than as one human action" to be evaluated, or as "independent responsibilities," "two human activities in one and the same human act." He does not want "one effect viewed as a completely independent human act in itself . . . to be weighed against the other effect, also viewed as a completely independent human act in itself." [30] No doubt this opinion holds as a formal matter regarding the rule of double effect where the two effects terminate in the same human body, e.g., therapeutic action that sterilizes. But when the two component parts of the composite action of "transimplantation" each terminate in the bodies of different persons, the foregoing language is likely to introduce some questionable stresses and consequences. The two "termini" in transplantation are each one human life. Doubtless the excision is not a "completely human act in itself" to be weighed against implantation as another "completely independent human act in itself." Doubtless this is one composite human activity to be evaluated.

But we do have here "two human activities" and "responsibilities" within the same complex procedure. The first—the excision—terminates in an impairment of the body of one person. It makes a well person ill.[31] To say this is *not* to assign excessive importance to the physical structure of actions. It rather assigns proper *human* im-

---

orthodox category" (ibid., p. 194). For Daube, it remains problematic how we can say that this is a lawful infliction of harm. Some moralists, if I do not misunderstand them, are rather more eager to find an orthodox category of religious ethics in which the role of the living donor nicely fits.

30. "The Principle of Double Effect," pp. 187, 188, 189, 193.

31. Canon G. B. Bentley in Wolstenholme and O'Connor, *Ethics in Medical Progress*, p. 185.

portance to the body and its welfare or impairment. The second human activity, including the first, terminates in a bodily curative procedure performed upon the needy patient. If the first is "physicalism," the second is also. Neither is. Both aspects of transimplantation are performed upon men in the only place they are to be found, namely, in the flesh. The impairment of the donor may not be evil in any moral sense of the word, as Van der Poel contends, and this action may receive its moral determination finally from its totally curative purpose and effect. But the bodily impairment of the donor is not "just a physical occurrence."

We should flatly reject Van der Poel's appeal that we "avoid viewing the physical harm in the donor as an *independent* disvalue which is to be compared with the other value of charity." Of course, the harm to the donor and the cure of the recipient are values of the same order to be compared. Charity may justify composing these two consequences into the complex procedure I have called "transimplantation." It is also true that to compare the harm to the donor with charity would be to compare values of a different order. All this can be said while saying that physical harm to the donor is an independent disvalue (it, too, results from a human activity and responsibility) in the calculations of charity as it goes about doing its curative work. Of course, it is the whole human action that is voluntary, and the cure is willed in itself while the harm is willed only in relation to that purpose.[32] Of course, *"in the means* the act of the will is concerned with the goal." But *in the means,* in this case, moral agents are also concerned for the man who is harmed by the excision. It is altogether too bland, weak, dangerous, and erosive of the medical resolve to cease eventually the acceptance of living donors for Van der Poel simply to say "the *physical* effect may not be disregarded as if it had no value," or for him to call the excision of an organ from a living human being an "intermediary stage" [33] or a merely physical part in the structure of the curative action.

It is far better to speak of two termini in this complex curative action, of two human activities and not one only, of the proportion-

32. "The Principle of Double Effect," pp. 197, 198.
33. Ibid., pp. 200 (cf. p. 205: "the end determines the human meaning of the means"), 201, 206–207.

ing of bodily harm to life-saving at the same rank of values sacrificed and gained, and of the supravaliance of charity in ordering one of these human activities to the other. In any case, applicable moral principles and rules governing medical practice or transplant surgery are not likely to come down from above—from "the totality of society and its welfare in its proper directedness . . . towards a union with God," from "the relation of the human action toward human existence and dignity," from "the *human* quality of the total action" as "community-building, and not destructive," or from simply replacing human concern for living donors with "the ultimate moral criterion" of "the community-building or destroying aspect of the action." [34] On these terms, it is hard to see why living donors should ever be deprived of opportunity for their proper directedness toward God and community-building by the exclusive use of cadaver donors when this becomes equally curative medically. Those are "orthodox categories" in which it is made to appear that making a well person sick, or harming him, is something other than a novel and unique feature of medical practice, and one that should be rapidly made transitional even if meanwhile it is justifiable.

The State of the Question in a Possible Protestant Position

From the standpoint of Christian ethics within the tradition of the Reformation, however, charity (agapé) is a free act of grace—first in God's gift of himself in love to man, and then in man's gift of himself in love to neighbor. By miracle God was manifest in humankind; by miracle also a Christian can and may and must and will become incarnate on the neighbor's side of the human equation. This free act of love, however, is not thought to be continuous with men's natural disposition to seek their own highest good as this is now desired or known, nor does self-giving aim to establish and perfect such continuity. While our bodily existence and the integrities of twinship or of familial society are the conditions of the possibility of covenants of utmost faithfulness among men on earthly pilgrimage, these elements of dust from which we are created do not by nature bind us to such covenants. The latter are free actions as one goes with grace among the equally needy. Gifts

34. Ibid., pp. 192, 196, 204, 207.

are not rights to be claimed or duties to be imposed; the giver is
not manifesting what should naturally be done, nor is he out of the
continuities of life with life pursuing his own wholeness with that
of another.

A Protestant who is properly instructed and whose conscience has
been formed in terms of the overruled discontinuity between God
and man, between self and other, or between giving and receiving,
is likely to wince when he hears the meaning of love for neighbor
expressed in terms that seem entirely natural to Catholic moralists.
He might reply in statements that paraphrase those of Martin
Luther: they do not good who do it from a servile and mercenary
principle in order to obtain personal fulfillment; they are rather
numbered among the wicked who, with an evil and mercenary eye,
seek the things of self even in God and in relationship with their
neighbors; take heed not to do good in order to obtain some benefit,
whether temporal or eternal, material or spiritual; both alike are
pleasure-seeking, while Christian love counts not rimless totality as
a thing to be grasped; true faith is effective in love which seeks the
neighbor's good alone and not the self's compensation, fulfillment,
or wholeness; self-giving acts should not be done under the false
impression that through them you are to come into cosmic communion; this would in fact be a godless presumption and perversity
and a godless addition to the self-giving of organs, that personhood
and a higher spiritual wholeness is to be sought through such donations; yet Grushenka's onion,[35] or an organ given away, will not
break under the load of its service to others; you have nothing more
to do than to go about your business and serve your neighbor, living
in utter relationship to God by faith and in utter relationship to
your neighbor through love; that is a right holy life and cannot
be made more wholly; therefore, do nothing in life except what you
see is necessary, profitable, and salutary to your neighbor; the
Christian faith issues in works of the freest service cheerfully and
lovingly done, with which a man willingly serves another without
hope of rewards in another order of values, and for himself is satisfied on this earth with the fullness of God's love and with the fullness and wealth of his faith.

It therefore looks as if a possible moral justification of organ

35. Dostoevsky, *The Brothers Karamazov* (Modern Library Giant edition), pp. 367–70.

transplantation from living donors that might be developed within the ambit of Protestant Christian ethics would not need to resort to any "sticky (psychological or spiritual) benefits theory." A reasonable secular transcription of this is the appeal solely to a free and informed consent on the part of the donor. A demerit of this outlook should also be noted. A justification of the self-giving of organs developed on Protestant grounds, precisely because of its freedom from the moorings of self-concern, is likely to fly too high above concern for the bodily integrity of the donor, higher than one finds in even the most "liberal" Roman Catholic thought. (Here again the physicians may have to save us from the moralists—because of their respect for the embodied life they know, and, I would add, the only life any man knows.)

It is, therefore, important to mention a "counterargument" within the structure of Protestant ethics insofar as this has been more profoundly Biblical than past Catholic moralists. Biblical authors not only speak of love to God and neighbor. They also hold a very realistic view of the life of man who is altogether flesh (*sarx*). God is in heaven, man is on earth. God is enthroned upon the praises of men, but these are the praises of men who are of the earth earthy, who for the glory of God made known among them can drink the wine of gladness during the season granted them for creaturely existence and in the face of the death of all flesh. No one who has been consciously formed by Biblical perspectives is likely to be beguiled by notions of the person whose origin actually is a Cartesian dualism of mind and body; nor will he yield to the enchantment of mystical, spiritual notions of unearthly communion with God and fellow man. The world of thought that comes closest to replicating the Biblical understanding of man's existence as flesh is that of physicians when they are discussing the "definition" of death (and so of "life" also), or when they are pondering with great reserve whether they should in a given instance perform the composite operation of excising a kidney from one embodied soul and implanting it in another embodied soul.

It is therefore necessary for us to come to terms with traditional Jewish ethics, which throughout expresses this concern for man's embodied existence and joyfully affirms the integrity of the flesh—including, indeed, powerful respect for the body after death. For all the important differences in detail, traditional Jewish medical ethics and traditional Catholic medical ethics have manifested a common concern for the integrity of man's bodily life. What other life is there, we may ask, known to men or medicine or moralists? In principle, Protestant ethics should have this also among its premises— perhaps more than most, because of the Biblical motifs which should be fully at home with us. From this point of view, one must ask of any Christian, who today without any hesitation flies into the wild blue yonder of transcendent human spiritual achievement while submitting the body unlimitedly to medical and other technologies, whether his outlook is not rather a product of Cartesian mentalism and dualism, and one that, for all its religious and personalistic terminology, has no longer any Biblical comprehension of joy in creaturely life and the acceptable death of all who are flesh.

A Meditation on Medicine's Ministry to the Flesh

I shall conclude this deliberately inconclusive inquiry by reference to a case of the self-giving of an organ by a living donor that has not yet occurred. The case is a fictitious one, invented for discussion in a seminar on Religion and Law whose participants were law students at the University of Texas and divinity students at the Presbyterian Theological Seminary in Austin, Texas.

Many months ago the 15-year-old son of Mr. Roger Johnson was admitted to a Houston, Texas hospital for tests to determine the cause of his generally debilitated condition. Use of the latest available diagnostic techniques and equipment eventually led to the conclusion that the lad was suffering from a progressively deteriorating congenital condition of the valves of the heart. The prognosis communicated to the distraught Mr. Johnson was that his son could not live past the age of 20, and that there was no known treatment for the malady with which he was afflicted.

At first Mr. Johnson tried to resign himself to his son's plight. Then he began to brood and think of the pleasures and joys of adult life which he, at the age of 42, had already known, but which his son would never know. The more he thought of this, the less willing he became passively to accept the doctors' verdict. Finally he thought of a means by which his son's life might be spared.

His plan, which he communicated to a physician friend, was an uncomplicated one. In light of the success of recent heart transplant operations with unrelated donors and donees, he reasoned, there must be a high probability that a transplant of the heart of a genetic relative would be successful. Accordingly, he would simply donate his own heart to his son. He had lived a full life, he said, and he could leave his son well provided for financially. His wife had died several years earlier, so that complication was not present. His own parents had no rightful claim to his continued life. He asked his friend's aid in finding a physician who would perform the operation. Not without considerable misgivings, his friend complied, eventually finding a heart surgeon eager to attempt the transplant of a heart from a healthy and related donor not *in extremis* at the time of the operation.

In the course of preparation for the transplant, elaborate precaution was taken to ensure that the son would not know the real nature of the proposed operation. He was told simply that a transplant operation on his heart was to be attempted in the hope of prolonging his life, and he agreed to try it with full knowledge that death could certainly result if the try were unsuccessful. In reality, of course, it was contemplated that Mr. Johnson's heart would be removed from his chest while he was under general anaesthesia and that it would be transplanted in the chest cavity of his son.

When the date of the scheduled operation arrived, the father went to the son's room, affectionately wished him good luck, and returned to his own room to be prepared for his own operation. He was eventually placed under general anaesthesia, and taken to a special operating room to await the transfer of his heart to an oxygenating and circulating "heart-lung" machine.

He is in the operating room now, and the surgeon is scrubbing. You are chief of staff of the hospital in which the operation is to take place. You had no prior knowledge of the planned operation, but this is frequently so. A worried nurse has brought you word of the planned operation on this occasion. You have power to stop the operation. Should you do it? Why or why not? Discuss fully. (Assume that you will not be punished by society, whatever decision you reach.)

This case, or one like it, will happen one day. Psychologists will testify that from the donor's point of view the giving of his heart is a rational sacrifice, not the choice of a warped or guilt-ridden mind. They will testify that the donor's request qualifies as a free and informed consent, and if need be that he will suffer grave psychological impact if not allowed to give his heart to save his son's life. Thus, the self-giving of hearts may well meet the test of consent alone, if this is the necessary and a sufficient right-making feature of such situations. If need be, the self-giving of hearts can also meet the "prevention of detriment" test—the detriment of suffering a son's death judged to be more unbearable than one's own—or it can meet the "spiritual benefits" test.

Then the crucial question raised will be: Are a person's consent or his spiritual or psychological wholeness the only right-making considerations to be taken into account in deciding such a question? Are violation of a person's consent or violation of his felt need for spiritual or psychological wholeness the only wrong-making features? Are these the only ways to violate a man, or for him to do impermissible violence to himself? Is anything left of the notion that a human being *has* (or better, *is*) a bodily integrity, and that out of the respect due also to this there are some actions that must be judged to be wrong—even when they are embraced by a free and informed consent and even when the self-giving of a heart is deemed the only way to avoid intolerable sorrow and may (for all we know) give promise of spiritual benefits in the age to come, and —what is more important still—is the only way successfully to oppose for a time the death of a beloved son?

One will hear quite a fluttering in the dovecote of the moralists. "Conservatives" will for a time wage a battle of the barricades. They will argue that an act of direct self-killing, or killing of another, is morally wrong even if done in a sacrificial spirit and even if it is reasonably related as means to the extrinsic end of saving another man's life. They will argue that the self-giving of an unpaired vital organ is not to be compared to the sacrifice of life incidental to heroic attempts to save a person from drowning or in battle, nor to be compared to the act of "jumping from an overloaded lifeboat," which has intrinsic to the act itself (as thus described) two effects, one the lightening of the boat and saving the lives aboard (this good effect is intended and directly done) and the other, that one's own life will foreknowably and certainly be lost (this evil effect is intended neither as means nor as desired end, nor is it—like removing one's weight from the lifeboat to save life—directly done). They will argue that "to make dashing into the burning house parallel with having an organ cut out for someone else's benefit you would have to suppose that burning off the rescuer's leg was the necessary means of achieving rescue." [36] In the case of the self-sacrifice of life by the self-giving of a heart they will argue that "the analogy which was proposed with jumping into the sea to save a child is to be taken with a grain of salt. In the jumping case, no doctor bound by the Hippocratic oath is in a curative capacity deliberately depriving a man of an organ"—an unpaired vital organ such as the heart. "A surgeon must not open up a healthy man for a glove unless he himself left it there on a previous occasion." [37]

Liberals will reply that this is quibbling. They will call for descriptions of human acts that always terminate in the person, if we are properly to appraise the morality or immorality of human actions. In this instance, the whole action of the self-giving of a heart begins with taking this vital organ from the father and ends in its implantation in the son and the saving of his life. How could that be wrong, or anything less than praiseworthy? To this a proper rejoinder is that—however we express the matter (as two acts related as means to end, or as two parts of the same human act of saving a person's life)—there are two termini, each ending in a human being, killing one, saving the other. Cries of "physicalism" will not be to the point (as they are in reducing to indifference whether, for sufficient reason, a man is sterilized directly or indirectly), since the only human life we know to respect, protect, and serve in medical care is irremediably physical, and presented to us with its moral claims solely within the ambience of a bodily existence.

This, however, will prove to be a losing battle of the barricades.

36. Bentley in Wolstenholme and O'Connor, *Ethics in Medical Progress*, p. 19.
37. Daube in ibid., p. 195. Professor Daube is a legal scholar, of Jewish background, not a Catholic moralist.

Those moralists will be crowned victors who say that in the self-giving of a heart the donor prefers his own perfection of grace and charity, subjecting his physical organism to the finality of his person; who approve of acts transcending physical life itself, having in view a real and calculable benefit to the recipient; who would free man from the brutal materiality of his island existence in the limited physical space of the body into a vaster consummation of one with all in communion; who, after hesitating a moment over the donor's self-abolition of further possibilities of creaturely self-giving, may not be able to rule out the possibility that such a sacrificial self-destruction is an expression of the giving of oneself as a person to be fulfilled in that utter and transcendent relationship of persons who are spiritually members one of another in God; who as Protestants affirm that a man of faith free from self-concern has nothing more to do than to go about his business in untrammelled service of his neighbor; who cannot exclude the self-giving of hearts from among the works of the freest service cheerfully and lovingly done, although this breaks all bonds with the dust of man's origins and with joy in the life of the flesh and the acceptance of the death of all who bear flesh, however dear they are.

The evidence for predicting that this is the view that will win out is the gradual South Vietnamization of the Western moral heritage in the approval given to the recent acts of self-immolation, and the performance of some of these acts among us. These acts have been sanctioned because subjectively they showed admirable courage even though the suicide was directly done as a means to an extrinsic end. The saving of the life of a loved one is surely an equal or a higher cause in which to enlist human devotion; and, in the case we are supposing of the self-giving of hearts, the good to come will be more certain to result than was the case in some or most or all of the acts of self-immolation which were "demonstrations" out of hope that was on the edge of despair over the cause for which they were done.[38]

The reason for the predictable victory in the coming age of the self-giving of hearts of what will undoubtedly be called the "liberal"

38. The question of the morality of conscientious self-immolation was treated briefly by the present writer in *The Just War: Force and Political Responsibility* (New York: Scribner's, 1968), Chapter 19, pp. 468–69, 471–72.

point of view among moralists—Catholic and Protestant—is another matter. The reason will be that the aspiring and unquestionably religious language we have reviewed will simply baptize the Cartesian mentalism and dualism of mind (soul, person) and body that is endemic to the modern mentality and an epidemic afflicting almost all contemporary outlooks. Our culture is already prepared for technocratizing the bodily life into collections of parts in which consciousness somehow has residence for a time, and for calling by the name of "the direction of mankind toward God" what can better and exhaustively be described in secular terms as the onward thrust of technological progress. Therefore, the use of hearts from living donors can come to be regarded as a proper administration or stewardship of a man over his organic life. The contagious dualism of modern culture has already placed him, as a spiritual overlord, too far above his physical life. To most of us a part of the body or the bodily life as a whole is already only a thing-in-the-world, not to be identified with the person.[39]

Meantime physicians will remain the only Hebrews, and, inarticulately, the only classical moralists. Among doctors the human life that is to be respected, protected, cured, or cared for means an integrated and mutually sustaining whole of vital functions. This is the operative meaning of life—of life that has sanctity—whatever else doctors may believe or think they should believe about the "soul." It is true that when there was need for a greater supply of undamaged cadaver organs physicians began to discuss the "updating" of death and revisions of the procedures for determining that death has occurred. Some part of the motive for this concern for better stating when donors had died may have been the suspicion

39. Professor John Batt of the University of Kentucky Law School gives many a delightful scenario of where we are going with our morally unbounded biological technology in an extraordinary article entitled, "They Shoot Horses, Don't They?: An Essay on the Scotoma of One-Eyed Kings," UCLA *Law Review* 15, no. 2 (February 1968): 510–50. He rightly traces this home to the bloodless rationalism and dualism of the present age and the absence of any true sense of the body. In other words, we are a culture disposed to be "brutally spiritualistic" precisely in our applications of science. He incorrectly (or at least too simply) accounts for this as the result of the cultural influence of Christianity. As a consequence the only corrective he can see is in an "Eros-centered vision," jurisprudence, justice to the body, etc., drawn from various sources (underground—because of the prevailing rationalism with its mentality favoring "invasion" and "control" of the psychophysical organism).

that, on hitherto accepted definitions of life and death, they were "killing" their own patients who were near death from heart failure before making them "alive" again by transplant therapy. It is true also that, before the proposal of the use of hearts from living donors came to be considered a real option the doctors had begun to use "spare parts" transplant therapy as a form of preventive medicine, replacing organs at the first signs of wear and tear and no longer waiting until patients were in the last stages of heart failure and transplantation the only alternative to imminent death. Nevertheless physicians will not in that day be found willing even to discuss the proposition that a man be killed in order to save the life of another, any more than the students in the seminar in 1967 found doctors willing to take seriously their fictitious case. If they are, men will have achieved this unspeakable thing: a medical profession without a moral philosophy in a society without one either.

The grounds for making that last, seemingly extreme statement is simply this. I have discovered only one physician who, in allowing the self-giving of organs by living donors, proposes merely this additional test: "in all cases the advantage to the recipient has to be greater than the disadvantage or danger to the donor." [40] Other physicians say that, in respecting the desire of one person to risk his life for another, the doctor must "be sure that the risk to the donor is very much less than the probability of success to the recipient." [41] And, as we have seen, Professor Daube requires that the plight of the prospective recipient and his probable objective benefit from the gift of an organ "heavily outweigh" the danger and loss incurred by the donor.

Now, if the benefit conveyed to a recipient and the loss incurred by the donor were equal, then a justifiable act of "transimplantation" would signal the fact that the organ "belongs" as much to the one as to the other. These would be interchangeable parts between interchangeable personal embodiments. If the benefit conveyed has to be only a little bit greater (Revillard), then justifiable "transimplantation" signals the fact that the organ "belongs" only a little bit more to the donor than to the recipient. These are not quite

40. J. P. Revillard, in Wolstenholme and O'Connor, *Ethics in Medical Progress*, p. 202.
41. Jean Hamburger, in ibid., p. 357.

interchangeable parts, but nearly so. The integrity and welfare of the donor's personal embodiment has the edge of action.

If, however, to justify making a well person ill for the sake of making another person well requires that the risk to the donor be very much less (Hamburger) or that the objective benefit heavily outweigh (Daube) the loss to the donor, then the physical integrity of the donor is considerably respected as an independent value and responsibility even while warranting "transimplantation" for the sake of another.[42] If care for the donor barters bodily integrity against charity and limits charity by "totality," then the moralists will have to make the most of it!

The truth is that this is the only way to conceive of charity as the action of creaturely men, of men of flesh, and not as the action of disembodied spirits. It is the only way men can manifest the fact there are limits to their *refusal* to accept the death of a dear one in the flesh. Bodily integrity must be a norm operating in the assessment of the morality of the self-giving of organs, even if it is outweighed. When one thinks on it, if the only relevant categories were those of some of the moralists which we have reviewed, there would be no grounds for refusing "transimplantation" in cases in which the advantage to the recipient is much less than the disadvantage or danger to the donor, or in which the benefit of the gift of an organ is even trivial in comparison to the danger and loss the donor wishes "charitably" to incur. Then one is on the way toward justifying the self-giving of hearts or livers from living donors as a curative practice in medicine. It is to be hoped that physicians to a greater extent remain Hebrews in their treatment of human beings and in the factors they weigh in estimating what would be a reasonable sacrifice.

After these reflections on the question of the self-giving of vital organs from several ethical points of view, we can return to the

42. One way to hedge against the loss of a vital part would be to "borrow" a paired organ on some "lend-lease" arrangement. Then if or when the recipient died the organ would be quickly returned to the person to whom it belongs, against the day when he might need it. Macabre as this may sound on first hearing, such an arrangement would at least keep clear the fact that the donor suffers mutilation as a man, not benefit, and that there are limits normative for men of flesh who would remain in the gift and who would remain answerable to God and man by their lives. *Lending* organs would keep clear whose man the organ is, whose "self/not-self" it is.

facts in regard to kidney-transplants—the paired organ that is at issue. Data from the renal transplant registry as of July 1967 discloses a 55 percent *five year* survival rate among 41 transplants between identical twins. Although the data for 1968 were not available to the author in time for inclusion, it was anticipated in 1967 that the results in 1968 would exceed significantly the record of the previous year. Through the fall of 1967, 1187 transplants had been recorded. The donors were living and related in 47.8 percent of the cases and unrelated in 52.2 percent. Cadaver donors were utilized in a total of 41.4 percent. (If these figures seem confusing to the reader, so are they to the present writer.) Important to note is the fact that the best results can still be obtained from living related donors. The four-year survival rate of transplants from parent donors is approximately 50 percent; that from sibling donors is slightly higher; that from cadaver donors 15 to 20 percent. A 95 percent one-year survival rate has been attained by Dr. Thomas E. Starzl. His results and the fact that recipients who survive two years have a greatly improved chance of continuing to do so, suggests that long-term survival after kidney transplant will greatly improve. The report from which these figures are taken concludes: "It is thus apparent that renal transplantation is rapidly reaching the period when it can be considered a clinical procedure for treatment of patients with fatal renal diseases. . . . If a one-year survival rate of 85% to 95% can be achieved with reasonable regularity in a number of centers, these results will be significantly better than the results of surgical treatment of many types of cancer at the present time".[43]

While a cancer operation terminates in one person and the transimplantation of a kidney terminates in two persons, the foregoing figures seem to offer the opportunity of a reasonable sacrifice. Since related donors are still needed, it is to be hoped that they have the strength of grace to move with freedom among the dying, and not from compulsion, societal expectation, or a servile spirit, and to live with the unforeseeable consequences of an act of self-giving once performed. There is, however, no avoidance of measuring the costs/ benefits. Moralists, meantime, should learn to follow the lineaments

43. *Status of Transplantation 1968*, A Report by the Surgical Training Committee of the National Institute of General Medical Sciences, (Bethesda, Md.: National Institutes of Health, November 1968), pp. 43-44.

of the physicians' reasoning when they let themselves be the moralists they are while undertaking the unique medical procedure of impairing one patient in order to heal another. Otherwise, medicine's ministry to the life of flesh and the work of charity could exhaust itself in taking and the self-giving of vital paired organs. There would then be no sufficient reason to go on to the next chapter.

5

Giving or Taking Cadaver Organs for Transplant

There is a great and growing need for organs to be used in transplant therapy. Two main proposals have been put forward for making the organs of patients who have died more accessible to the surgeons. Each in different ways would revise by statute the common law tradition and past case law concerning who has the right to dispose of dead bodies. The first proposal is for the "routine salvaging of cadaver organs" in hospitals—no affirmative consent required from anyone. The second is the Uniform Anatomical Gift Act, drawn up by a special committee chaired by Professor E. Blythe Stason of Vanderbilt University, and adopted by the Commissioners on Uniform State Laws on July 30, 1968.

Less than a year after this uniform law was proposed, 20 states had passed Anatomical Gift Acts. In another state, a statute awaited only the governor's signature. The legislation had passed one chamber of the legislatures of 9 additional states, and had been introduced in an additional 16. Thus, by the end of 1969 more than a majority of the states were expected to have enacted the Uniform Anatomical Gift Act or one of its previous tentative drafts.[1] This is a remarkable record, never approached before in the history of attempts to encourage uniformity in state laws.

Thus, the *giving* of organs, not the *taking* of them, is likely to be the practice in the United States. However, Dr. Theodore Cooper, Director of the National Heart Institute, estimates that the potential need for hearts might require using as donors one out of every three persons between the ages of 15 and 64 who die of causes other than heart disease or cancer.[2] Shortages in the supply of blood, skin, and corneas often occur despite appeals for donors. Under certain circumstances, one can imagine that the premortem (and post-mortem)

---

1. *News About Uniform Anatomical Gift Act*, (New York: National Transplant Information Center, United Health Foundations, 150 Fifth Avenue, May 1969).

2. *New York Times*, September 15, 1968. By May 1970, Uniform Acts had been adopted in 48 jurisdictions including the District of Columbia.

giving of organs may not meet the need, and that the Uniform Anatomical Gift Acts will prove to be but a stop halfway on the road to the routine use of the organs of all who have died. The routine salvaging of organs is the practice in designated hospitals in France; a proposal to this effect is current in Great Britain; and a number of physicians and lawyers in this country strongly defend this alternative.

The practice in regard to autopsies presents many of the same issues, and the same alternatives. If the relatively routine obtaining of signatures on forms consenting to autopsies in our large medical centers and teaching hospitals proved insufficient, there would be strong pressure toward the adoption of the Swedish practice, and that of a number of other countries, where everyone who dies in a hospital is autopsied unless he has previously objected to the procedure. Autopsies needed for the advancement of medical science are analogous to the need for organs in transplant therapy in that in either case we have the same two main options: to provide for these needs with or without the giving of positive consent.

We therefore need to examine carefully these two alternatives to see what is at issue between them. Since both the routine salvaging of organs and a man's right and power to donate his organs premortem would place limits upon the rights of the surviving spouse and the next of kin to dispose of the body, we must also enquire what was the human and moral meaning of that earlier legal tradition and medical practice which these proposals seek in radically different ways to change.

One purpose of the Uniform Anatomical Gift Act is to sweep away the inadequate provisions of existing donation legislation. Its authors do not believe that an extension into this field of the testamentary disposition of property, medical examiner and coroner statutes, unclaimed body statutes, or autopsy statutes can meet the unique demands of organ and tissue donation while also adequately protecting competing interests. A separate act is needed. Another purpose is to sweep away "the antiquated principles of the common law" [3] and

3. Alfred M. Sadler, Jr. and Blair L. Sadler, "Transplantation and the Law: The Need for Organized Sensitivity," *Georgetown Law Journal* 57, no. 1 (October 1968): 31. See also A. M. Sadler, B. L. Sadler, and E. Blythe Stason, "The Uniform Anatomical Gift Act," *Journal of the American Medical Association*, 206, no. 11 (December 9, 1968): 2501–06.

of past case law giving, under some or most circumstances, prevailing right of disposition of the body to surviving spouse and next of kin. The act is "based on the belief that each individual should be able to control the disposition of his body after death without having his wishes frustrated by anyone, including his next of kin." Therefore, the Act grants authority to "[any] individual of sound mind and 18 years of age or more [to] give all or any part of his body for any purposes specified in [the Act], the gift to take effect upon death." [4] This provides a premortem donation authority not found at common law or unambiguously in case law to date.

Prior donation by the deceased will prevail over any objection of next of kin. An easily carried card will serve as a valid mechanism of gift. At the same time, the donor's final wishes are respected in that means of repudiation or amendment are readily available, including oral deathbed revocations. His expressed wishes will prevail, and only his *expressed* wishes. If he made no positive gift, no organs will routinely be taken. If the deceased expressed no wish and registered no gift, however, the next of kin are enpowered to consent to postmortem donation of the organs of his body if they wish to do so; and to avoid conflict, the Act specifically creates six classes of donating priority among them.[5] In the case of postmortem donation by kin, consent may be made by telegraphic, recorded telephonic, or other recorded message.

Where the Uniform Anatomical Gift Act gives effect to an individual's positive consent that organs of his body be used for transplantation, the proposal for routinely salvaging cadaver organs would give effect only to his negative objection or expressed wish that they be not so used. If he did not say, "Nay," the "Aye's" have it!—i.e., the needs of others for efforts to be made to prolong their lives by organ transplantation. Public policy shall dictate that organs not

4. Sadler and Sadler, "Transplantation and the Law," pp. 18–19; Uniform Anatomical Gift Act, Sec. 2(a).

5. Theoretically, the wishes of one or more members of a deciding class could fail to be consulted. At Sec. 2(b), the Act authorizes a member of a kinship group to give all or any part of the decedent's body "in the absence of . . . actual notice of opposition by a member of the same or of a prior class." Perhaps an affirmative obligation should be placed on the doctor to secure the consent of all members of the deciding kinship class—unless in practice this will be done anyway.

expressly withheld by their former "owners" will be placed at the disposition of medical practice. A recent article [6] defending this procedure for obtaining cadaver organs seems chiefly concerned to enact the "objectives of the community," "the preferences of society." "Whether a person should be permitted to order disposition of his body," the authors say, "depends upon what objectives the community has." But then, to give effect to a person's desires is "one of the strongest preferences of society." That statement discloses the political philosophy and the source and warrants for individual rights on which this article is premised. In view of the need for organs, a person should at least be able to donate his kidneys or other organs at death and not have his wish vetoed by spouse or next of kin. However, since on this philosophy the community's objective in providing organs may be overriding (as are the necessities of criminal investigation into cause of death) even if he does not want to give them, "we must face the question"—if a person forbids the use of his organs—whether these desires of his should prevail and "whether he ought to have the right to deny life to another."

Somewhat reluctantly, it seems, Dukeminier and Sanders, the authors of this article, stop short of concluding that objections of the decedent should not prevail. "Any system for salvaging cadaver organs must provide a mechanism whereby either the donor or the next of kin can object to the procedure. If it did not do so, grave constitutional questions respecting the freedom of religion might be raised." Moreover, it is not necessary to jeopardize these freedoms in order to secure sufficient organs. The procedure of using the suitable organs of all who have died should simply be made routine by law and in hospitals, and if routine it will become accepted and few objections will be raised. Where expressed consent to the gift is neither required nor sought, ordinarily the expressed refusals will be few, and the yield of organs routinely harvested will be more than would ever be expressly donated. Thus the need can be met without overriding anyone's objection. The change in law and in practice should be based on four principles:

6. Jesse Dukeminier, Jr. and David Sanders, "Organ Transplantation: A Proposal for Routine Salvaging of Cadaver Organs," *New England Journal of Medicine* 279 (August 22, 1968): 413–19. Subsequent unannotated quotations are from this article.

Removal of useful cadaver organs is routine practice; leaving them to putrefy is unusual.

Removal of organs is performed under conditions that do not burden the bereaved persons with the problem.

The donor may object during life to removal of his organs after death, and the objection is controlling. If, however, the donor expressly agrees to the use of his organs after death, his next of kin has no power of veto.

If the donor neither objects nor expressly assents, his next of kin may object to removal any time before the organs are removed, and the objection is controlling. This principle should be included in order to obviate any constitutional problem regarding freedom of religion.

These principles effectively shift the burden of action from the gift to the refusal of the gift of a cadaver organ.

Indeed, this is the cardinal difference between these two proposals: who shall have the burden of action? The Uniform Anatomical Gift Act would encourage the giving of organs, while the proposal to salvage organs routinely shifts the burden of action to the person who did not want his organs removed, or to the kin who do not want a decedent's organs removed. The great advantage of routine salvaging operations is that the great majority of the "donors" are such only technically. Their giving is only a taking. If this law were enacted, persons would not be real donors. The giving of organs would proceed from inaction, from failure positively to refuse the "gift." Such, indeed, is the intent of the proposal. Before, the rule was that bodies be buried intact; the exception was that consent might transmit an organ for use in transplant therapy. The proposal is that "the legal rule should favor removal of cadaver organs and preservation of life; the exception should permit objection and decay."

It is notable that the defenders of each of these alternatives use much the same language in characterizing, argumentatively, the opposing point of view. Dukeminier and Sanders believe that to ask someone whose relative is about to die for his kidneys would be "a ghoulish request" (while salvaging would have minimum or no impact on the bereaved relatives). They think it "macabre" if we become a society of people walking around with little cards saying we have donated our organs at death to so-and-so. Dr. R. Y. Calne, Professor of Surgery, University of Cambridge, and a supporter of Lord Kilbrandon's proposal that routine salvaging be enacted into British law, has written that "a computer register of the names and addresses of objectors which could be consulted by telephone" along with legislation providing for the routine taking of organs "would be a significant advance from the point of view of obtaining satisfactory cadaveric material and would shield recently bereaved relatives from a distressing interview." Dr. Calne's view is not that the request is under these circumstances "ghoulish"—but simply that "in the majority of cases relatives would prefer not to go into these details." [7]

In the Ciba Symposium, Dr. H. E. deWardener, of the Charing Cross Hospital Medical School, London, reacted to the premortem *giving* of organs in exactly the same vein as Dukeminier and Sanders to the Uniform Anatomical Gift Act. "I think this scheme of yours is odious!" he said. "You are going to educate people, which means a lot of publicity, with newspapers asking people to think about letting organs go after they are dead. They have to carry little cards when they are in the hospital saying—'I have donated . . .' This is a terrible state of affairs." [8] In a rejoinder, Sadler and Sadler defend the premises of the Uniform Anatomical Gift Act by saying that "it would be more macabre and unacceptable to allow any surgeon to remove an organ or tissue upon death without having an obligation to give notice to anyone. It is difficult to imagine public acceptance of such a proposal." And they write that "to obtain permission for the removal of an organ for transplantation is not ghoulish; it demonstrates respect for the wishes of others concerned. Not to be told of such practices or to be informed only after the fact would indeed be ghoulish." [9]

7. R. Y. Calne, "The Present Position and Future Prospects of Organ Transplantation," *Annals of the Royal College of Surgeons of England* 42 (May 1968): 289–90. The bill introduced in the British Parliament in March 1968 to legitimate the routine salvaging of organs would permit relatives to object only on the grounds "that the deceased during his lifetime had instructed otherwise," while Dukeminier and Sanders would permit next of kin to object on any grounds.

8. In G. E. W. Wolstenholme and Maeve O'Connor (eds.), *Ethics in Medical Progress: With Special Reference to Organ Transplantation* (Boston: Little, Brown, 1966), p. 160.

9. Sadler and Sadler, "Transplantation and the Law," p. 28–99, n. 138. These authors question the constitutionality of a statute permitting routine salvaging ("whole-

Before attempting to adjudicate between the organized giving and routine taking of cadaver organs for transplant, we need to understand the values that were preserved and the interests protected by the legal tradition that gave controlling voice to spouse and next of kin, and which both of these proposals are designed measurably to qualify. Originally, of course, burial was under the jurisdiction of the ecclesiastical courts; such matters did not come before the common law courts.[10] The way this "judicial restraint" was expressed was to say that there were no "property rights" in a dead body. This meant that neither a man himself before death nor anyone else after his death possessed any right of ownership in a commercial sense in his body. This states what was meant to be denied; it does not yet tell us what was affirmed in our past legal tradition and practice in regard to dead bodies. It is important to take note of these values if the interests which were protected by lodging right to the body in spouse and next of kin are to be significantly qualified either by the organized premortem (and postmortem) giving or by the routine taking of organs. There may be real threats to the sanctity of human life and to the human community, as much from restricting what was affirmed (the duty to give decent burial) in our past legal tradition as from attributing to anyone what was denied by the common law (property in the body in the common commercial sense).

What was affirmed became clear as the secular courts assumed responsibility for the disposition of dead bodies formerly belonging to the ecclesiastical courts. This was expressed in the doctrine of "quasi-property right" to a body; but that strange expression means nothing until we ask of the legal decisions what was meant to be conveyed by it. The right was "quasi" in that possession for commercial purposes was still denied to any claimant (the man himself or his kin). It was a sort of "property" in that possession for a certain human and familial purpose was assigned and legally protected. The latter was the positive human value and interest at stake.

---

sale removal") of organs not simply as a possible abridgment of religious freedom but also as a violation of due process of law.

10. For the following exposition, I rely on Allan D. Vestal, Rodman E. Taber, and W. J. Shoemaker, "Medical Legal Issues in Tissue Homotransplantation," *University of Detroit Law Journal* 18 (1954): 171–94; *Medicine and the Law* 159, no. 5 (October 1 1955): 487–92; and on Carl E. Wasmuth and Bruce H. Stewart, "Medical and Legal Aspects of Human Organ Transplantation," *Cleveland-Marshall Law Review* 14 (1963): 442–71.

"There is a duty imposed by the universal feelings of mankind to be discharged by someone towards the dead; a duty, and we may also say a right, to protect from violation; and a duty on the part of others to abstain from violation; it may therefore be considered as a sort of *quasi* property." "Although . . . the body is not property in the usually recognized sense of the word, yet we may consider it as a sort of *quasi* property, to which certain persons may have rights, as they have duties to perform towards it arising out of our common humanity." "The person having charge of it [the body] cannot be considered as owner of it in any sense whatsoever; he holds it only as a sacred trust for the benefit of all who from family or friendship have an interest in its period." [11] So said one of the hinge cases in American law. There exists in the next of kin of a deceased person a qualified property interest in trust for burial.[12] The entire meaning of possession of the body is that it holds the possessor to a "sacred trust." [13] "Greatly to its credit," therefore, as another decision expressed this issue, "England and the United States have always considered the decent burial of the dead as of more importance than the payment of debtor claims." [14] The door to property in bodies in a commercial sense was paradoxically barred and bolted by the doctrine of quasi-property!

If it is held that a body cannot be detained or sold as security for the payment of a debt,[15] the question now being raised is whether it can be detained and its parts taken (or sold?) for the sake of transplantation efforts to prolong the lives of others. It does not matter whether this is called property right, quasi-property, or something else. The issue is the "sacred trust" that possesses the family of a deceased man. The question is what social interests should be made to override that one. It is now the case that when society's needs require it—in compelled autopsies in criminal investigation, and pursuant of the provisions of an insurance contract—the sanctity and immunity of dead bodies and the wishes of next of kin must give way.

11. *Pierce* v. *Swan Point Cemetery*, 10 R.I. 227, 237, 238; n. 107 at 242, 243; 227 (1872).

12. Walter F. Kuzenski, "Property in Dead Bodies," *Marquette Law Review* 9 (1924): 19.

13. *Pettigrew* v. *Pettigrew*, 207 Pa. 313, 56 Atl. 878, 64 L.R.A. 179 (1904).

14. *Long* v. *Chicago, R.I. and P.R. Co.*, 15 Okla. 512, 514, 86 Pac. 289, 290 (1905).

15. *Regina* v. *Francis Scott*, 2 Q.B. 248, 114 Eng. Rep. 47 (1842); *Jefferson County Burial Soc.* v. *Scott*, 218 Ala. 354, 118 So. 644 (1928).

The question is whether the unique need for cadaver organs is another such instance. Then the question is: How shall the sacred trust of kinship be modified?

This is enough to make clear that in sweeping away "the antiquated principles of the common law" (Sadler and Sadler), it would at least be possible to sweep away much else besides. It is also enough to show that Dukeminier and Sanders display an inadequate comprehension of the human and moral meaning of the references in past legal tradition and case law to "property" and "quasi-property" in a decedent's body vested in his family. " 'Property' is whatever claim to an object the courts choose to protect," these defenders of the routine taking of organs declare. "To say there is no right to dispose because there is no property in a cadaver is simply to say there is no right to dispose because the court refuses to recognize such a right." [16] This is to assert a legal positivism and the omnicompetence of legislatures and courts in making and unmaking legal rights. Factually, of course, this cannot be denied. Remembering, however, that the rights legally recognized in the past were founded upon familial duties and sacred trusts arising out of our common humanity and from respect for the dead, we may question whether legislatures or courts are omnicompetent to make and unmake legal rights without violating real human interests, concerns, and values. This is what was meant by saying that "a dead body belongs to no one and is therefore under the protection of the public" [17]—under the protection of our legal tradition, which both of the proposals we are considering would change in significantly different ways.

None of the foregoing is meant to settle the choice between the organized giving and the routine taking of organs. Far from it, since both alternatives can be defended as in different ways and degrees protecting these ancient rights and dues while providing for new moral claims that have arisen with transplant therapy. Nor has the foregoing been meant to suggest that we should not move to one or the other of these alternatives. To the contrary, my purpose has simply been to lift up to view what is humanly and morally at stake when or as we move to revise significantly medical and social practice in regard to the dead, and change the law that in the past accorded

16. Dukeminier and Sanders, "Organ Transplantation," p. 414.
17. *Foster* v. *Dodd* 3 Q.B. 67, 77 (1867).

meaning to the fact that a man had died from the human community
by providing that the very body he was when alive be given decent
burial according to the wishes of the fellow men who were closest to
him in life. On balance it seems to me that our decision should favor
the organized giving over the routine taking of cadaver organs for
transplant. Yet if one glaring defect in the Uniform Anatomical Gift
Act is not corrected by the legislatures enacting state statutes, it seems
to me that the predictable social and human consequences could be
such as to render the routine use of the suitable organs of all who
die in hospitals in the absence of objection from them or from kin
the preferable one of the two alternatives.

Initially, both proposals we are considering take some getting used
to; and behind our sentiment and habitual feelings there are important points at issue. Yet I think that it cannot be denied that the requirements of respect for the deceased and decent burial of his body
in the company of family and friends are consistent with either the
decedent's premortem and controlling gift of his organs of the routine taking of them in the absence of any objection to this being
done—provided only that the body handed over for burial is not
visibly mutilated.[18] It is true that we ought not to begin to think of

18. The Uniform Anatomical Gift Act requires simply that "the donee . . . shall
cause the part to be removed without unnecessary mutilation" (Sec. 7 [a]. It is arguable,
of course, that a bill requiring affirmative donation does not need to say that the
body handed over for burial shall not be "visibly mutilated." That would be encompassed by the premortem or postmortem consent of the persons concerned. This is a
desirable provision, however, in a bill instituting the routine use of the suitable and
needed organs of all who die in hospitals. It is included in the British bill ("provided
that such removal shall not disfigure the dead body"). This point is not mentioned by
the American proponents of this procedure.

Professor David Daube seemed unusually insensitive to the need for this provision
if we are to adopt the routine taking of organs. "Never mind about disfigurement,"
he said. Once the law mentions that, people will be "put off" and "the door is open
to pointless litigation." I say "unusually" insensitive, because Daube was alert to the
human significance of disfigurement of the living in the course of transplantation.
While the gift of a kidney involves greater immediate risk to the donor, the possibility of his serious future illness and death, and a lesser prospect of lasting success
for the recipient, than the gift of a cornea by a living donor, yet people give kidneys
and not corneas while alive. The reason for this, Daube believes, is "the noticeability
of the loss of an eye"; our "deep-rooted aversion to the sight of a person whom we
have rendered less than whole"; the offense to "our sensibilities to have in our midst
a man we have deformed" (In Wolstenholme and O'Connor, *Ethical Issues in Medical
Progress*, pp. 192–93). The removal of a cornea may not be as serious disfigurement to

our bodies as an ensemble of parts left behind, like old clothes, to be given away or taken or—worst of all—sold. We are the bodies we live, while we bodily lived in our clothes and our houses. Proper respect for the body is irremovably a part of respect for the sanctity of the life of all flesh. It is true also that when it may be technically possible to use 17 of the organs from the body of a single decedent, we would come into an order of magnitude that might severely burden a proper celebration of death and remembrance of the deceased by his family in face of his premortem donation or the routine taking of all these "parts."

It is true, finally, that death is an event that takes place in a family and in the community of one's friends. One ought not wholly to disagree with those legal cases in which the wishes of spouse or next of kin have prevailed over some of the wishes decedents have expressed. This is just one more exhibition of the fact that the law favors the living over the dead within the limits of their proper discharge of the sacred duty to respect in ways meaningful to them the body that was lived and is now all that remains among them. That the kin ought always to obey the decedent's premortem rational will contrary to the respect they actually find it possible to render in disposition of his body remains, for me, a profoundly unpersuasive proposition. In any case it is a product of an unearthly dualism in our understanding of the life and death of all flesh, and does not spring from any outlook of the religions of the West. Since death is an event that takes place within the company of the family, I would hope that premortem donation of organs will be, so far as possible, familial decisions, as burial is, and not in actual practice individualistic decisions made controlling by law.

Still I think that we can begin with the judgment that neither the giving or the taking of cadaver organs (according to the proposals that have been made) is inherently wrong or should never be done. Then why favor the organized giving over the routine salvaging of cadaver organs for transplantation?

----

a dead body as it is to a living man. Still, if as Professor Daube believes a body is not nothing and its burial in a human community is a sacred duty of those who have concern for its period, visible mutilation would seem to be a needed prohibition in a bill routinely taking the suitable and needed organs of all who die in hospitals before handing them over for burial.

Before answering that question, let it be said that there is something a little macabre about 7 out of 10 of us or a predictable 80 million Americans [19] becoming a nation of card-carrying precadavers. Behind the gruesome feeling that this arouses, there is a real danger that the organized giving of organs will only erode still more our apprehension that man is a sacredness in the biological order (where else?), and our respect for men of flesh who are only to be found within the ambience of bodily existence. Here the metaphors in use today are exceedingly revealing. "Reconstructive" surgery. Surgical "plumbers." Biological "carpentry." "Spare parts." The "artificial man." Biological "engineering." Genetic "tailoring." The "management" of the future of the species. "Embryonic farming"—a veritable "orchard" of limbs, kidneys, hearts, lungs, livers, etc., all grown to order and perfectly compatible with the recipient.[20] And, just think, it used to be fashionable to regard St. Augustine's imagery as unconscionably degrading of man, when he spoke of sexual intercourse as a man "plowing a field" or "sowing his seed"! One may sentimentally prefer pastoral imagery to that of an overweening technology. But what has to be said is that man has no homeland, humanism and morality no future, when man is reduced to either. If we wish to avoid being inundated by either horticultural or engineering metaphors, that will depend in great measure on the recovery of a proper sense of the integrity of man's bodily life, as against the Cartesian dualism and mentalism of the modern period which rejoices without discrimination over every achievement or intervention or design which shows that the body is only a thing-in-the-world to be subjected to limitless control. So we ought not to proceed without pausing to reflect that men who powerfully sense that they are composed of spare parts may be on the way to themselves becoming interchangeable parts composing a larger whole— everyone a useful precadaver.

Still, after that somber interlude, I think we should conclude that to foster the organized giving of cadaver organs is preferable to the routine use of organs by hospitals; and that this is in itself choiceworthy as a matter of public policy and medical practice. There are

19. Gallup Poll, *New York Times*, January 17, 1968.

20. This last prospect is mentioned in an article by Fred Warshofsky whose title, however, is "Spare Parts Surgery," *Today's Health,* June 1965, p. 72.

two reasons supporting this verdict. The first is that the wish to exercise a more ancient wisdom concerning the body ought not to be specially burdened. Jewish people or Jehovah's Witnesses or anyone else holding religious objection, or persons without religious philosophy having deeply felt opinions in this matter, should not have, in hours of grief and suffering, to protrude those objections against the whole edifice of a hospital practice which routinely goes on without their wills. It is one thing to be a minority voice in a society of other consenting voices. It would be another thing to be a minority in a society in which, without voice, one may routinely become a "donor." [21]

The second reason is a related but more positive and encompassing one. A society will be a better human community in which giving and receiving is the rule, not taking for the sake of good to come. The civilizing task of mankind is the fostering, the achievement, or the shoring up of consensual community in general, and not only in regard to the advancement of medical science and the availability of cadaver organs in efforts to save the lives of others. Civilization means living our consensual communities, not living in communities in which consent and refusal go on, just as surely as we live our bodies, not in them. The positive consent called for by Gift Acts, answering the need for gifts by encouraging real givers, meets the measure of authentic community among men. The routine taking of organs would deprive individuals of the exercise of the virtue of generosity. If, as is said, the young rarely think about their own deaths or about giving their organs upon death, then they should be constrained and enabled to do so by the institutions and practices and laws we enact. To become partners in proved therapies, or joint adventurers in proving therapies, could be among the most civilized and civilizing things young people can do. The moral sequels that might flow from

21. Professor Daube's formulation of the routine practice went a long way toward mitigating this objection, because he would require hospitals to take cognizance of the objections of religious groups and not only to abide by individual refusals. "I think one could now aim at legislation," he said, "which would make available a corpse for therapeutic or scientific use, if the deceased expressed a wish, not revoked, in this direction or, in the absence of such a disposition, if he did not express a contrary wish, if he did not belong to a group normally opposed to such availability, and if his next of kin does not immediately express a contrary wish" ("Transplantation: Acceptability of Procedures and the Required Legal Sanctions," in Wolstenholme and O'Connor, *Ethics in Medical Progress*, pp. 191–92).

education and action in line with the proposed Gift Acts may be of far more importance than prolonging lives routinely. The moral history of mankind is of more importance than its medical advancement, unless the latter can be joined with the former in a community of affirmative consent. Where Sadler and Sadler say, in the subtitle to their article, "The Need for *Organized* Sensitivity" (italics added), the moral emphasis is rightly placed by them upon "The Need for Organized *Sensitivity*." [22]

At one point, however, the framers of the Uniform Anatomical Gift Act faltered—or so it seems to me—and fell well below the premises and principles that had guided their work. This was when they came to the question of "Remuneration for Donation." [23] Acknowledging that there was considerable sentiment against this in the commission, the uniform bill "does not specifically provide for this prohibition." The apology for this omission is that "the draftsmen . . . believed it improper to include an absolute bar to commercial relationships and concluded that this would best be handled at the local level, by the medical community." It should be pointed out that other matters equally well decided at the local level are nevertheless included in the Act. Moreover, at what level the matter should be handled, and by whom, is not the issue to be raised. The question is what we are to think about leaving the door open to monetary remuneration and commercial relationships in this field; and what lead, if any, the commissioners meant to give on this matter to the framers of public and medical policy on the local or the state level.

This is left quite ambiguous. On the one hand, it was pointed out

22. Additional rebuttal of the routine taking of organs is given in Alfred M. Sadler, Jr., Blair L. Sadler, E. Blythe Stason, and Delford L. Stickel, "Transplantation—A Case for Consent," *New England Journal of Medicine* 280 (April 17, 1969): 862–67. These authors point out that if only premortem or postmortem objection is made prevailing, and not positive consent, "the burden actually remains with the responsible surgeon to assure himself that no objection has been raised either by the deceased himself before death or by the next of kin after death. To absolve himself of this burden adequately would require an inquiry tantamount to obtaining consent itself." There would have to be a national "registry of objections" to ensure the physician against law suits. To this we may add that under the Uniform Anatomical Gift Act a responsible surgeon must bear the burden of assuring himself that there is no objection or conflict within the deciding class of next of kin.

23. Sadler and Sadler, "Transplantation and the Law," p. 30.

that "words such as 'gift,' 'donation,' and 'donor' strongly imply a non-profit transaction." On the other hand, it is said that "the use of professional donors for blood transfusions and blood banking may well foreshadow a similar occurrence in the transplantation area." One of the states cited as in its existing statutes prohibiting donations to "profitmaking concerns" (Mississippi, where the donation of tissue is viewed as a "contract") does not exclude monetary remuneration from among the considerations that might lead a man to enter into such a contract with nonprofit institutions. In fact, the Mississippi statute restricts the revocation privilege that can be exercised at any point during the lifetime of a contracting party by the rather un-savory even if necessary stipulation: "provided, however, that if any such person has received any monetary consideration for entering into the contract he shall repay such consideration to those from whom he received it, in full, plus 6% interest from the date of the signing of the contract." [24] Until, that is, his attempted deathbed oral revocation!

This is a matter that should not be left open or ambiguous, whether it is to be decided by the medical profession or by law, at the local or at the state level. The analogy with commercial donors of blood tissue and commercial blood banks is not a good one. Most of the difficulties over maintaining standards for donors and blood have arisen in the case of commercial transactions. But this is a small point, and I suppose it can be corrected. The main point is that blood tissue is not qualitatively the same or quantitatively of the same magnitude as the present and future unique need for cadaver organs. Blood and skin are replaceable tissues, from living donors; other needed organs are not replaceable. In the future these may be needed in great numbers.

We should copy quite another practice that is used in obtaining blood tissue. As is well known, an individual who freely gives blood can himself freely receive. When himself in need, he can get blood without paying for it. This sometimes includes members of a donor's family. This practice of giving and receiving, not buying and selling, is the one that should be extended to other tissues. With this analogy we could also address one of points made earlier: since death is an event in a family, the premortem giving of cadaver organs ought also

24. Sadler and Sadler, "Transplantation and the Law," pp. 30–31, 45.

be if possible a familial or shared decision. So also families that shared in premortem giving of organs could share in freely receiving if one of them needs transplant therapy. This would be—if workable—a civilizing exchange of benefit that is not the same as commerce in organs. The question to be raised is whether in medical practice and public policy there ought not to be an absolute bar to the premortem sale of vital, irreplaceable organs, and to their postmortem sale by surviving spouse or kin. The commission was of uncertain mind concerning this question.

The issue seems to me to be one that can be resolved in one way only. If we mean to call upon and call forth positive consent to supply the unique need for cadaver organs, this consent should not then be coerced or tempted by money. The aim of the Uniform Anatomical Gift Act was to free a man's premortem decision to give his organs from possible frustration after his death by the contrary wishes of his spouse or next of kin. Unless the door to monetary gain as the reason for such a premortem decision is barred, the title of the freedom accorded him will be "property right in his body in a commercial sense." Greatly to our discredit, this will make anticipatory "payment of debtor claims" of more importance than the decent burial of the dead among the poor. Clearly it is possible by statute to make a person the sole administrator of what happens to his body or organs after death for the purpose of gifts without making him the owner of it for commercial purposes. If we allow a person to dispose premortem of his organs, we ought not (for the protection of his own sense of the dignity of his bodily life) go so far as to reverse the common law principles entirely and allow him commercially to "dispose of that which after his death will be his corpse." [25]

As concerns the surviving spouse and next of kin, the purpose of the Uniform Anatomical Gift Act was to enable these persons to give consent to the use of a decedent's organs in transplant therapy, if need be by quick, recorded telephonic communication. Unless the door to monetary remuneration is barred, the name of the freedom and right accorded these persons will be "ownership of the body for commercial purposes." No longer will this be a "quasi" property right in the bodies of the dead, but full property rights for commercial purposes—at least in the body's 17 potentially usable organs and

25. *William* v. *Williams,* 94 Ch. Div. 659 (1882).

tissues. No longer will survivors "possess" the body for a sacred trust that possesses them, namely the right and duty to give decent burial, to which have been added the clear right and perhaps the duty to give organs of the decedent, as another sort of sacred trust, to prolong the lives of others. Instead, survivors may have gained a lucrative asset in the body.[26] How lucrative will depend on supply and demand, the maldistribution or fortunate location of potential donors and needy recipients, the wealth and social status of recipients, the strength of their will to live, and the cunning of family members when they give telephonic consent.

I do not say that these consequences will take place, but that unless the door to commerce is effectively barred, in practice and at some level and by whatever means or authority, there is no reason why they could not do so. Genuine consent to make a gift which shapes the Gift Act throughout cannot be replaced at any point by pro forma "giving" with gain in view without in principle opening a hole in the entire scheme. Through this opening could flow some very unsavory practices. Then, learning from an actual and growing disrespect for the body the meaning of respect for it, civilized men might yearn for the restoration of some of the "antiquated principles of the common law" that were too hastily swept away.

If giving is better than routinely taking organs to prolong the lives of patients needing transplants, then it must also be said that routinely taking them in hospital practice would be better than for us to make medical progress and extend treatment to patients by means of buying and selling cadaver organs. That society is a better and more civilized one, I have said, in which men join together in a consensual community to effect these purposes, than a society in which lives are saved routinely, without the positive consent and will

26. "Reduction of the decedent's final hospital bill might be a useful means of acquiring the next-of-kin's consent." "If the value of the kidney were includible in the gross estate and if it qualified for the charitable deduction, many cadaver kidneys would be made available for transplantations. The kidneys would be given to avoid paying estate taxes on one or both of them." These possibilities are explored with at least speculative approval by David Sanders and Jesse Dukeminier, Jr., "Medical Advance and Legal Lag: Hemodialysis and Kidney Transplant," Reflections on the New Biology, *U.C.L.A. Law Review* 15, no. 2 (February 1968): 391, 393. Additional vistas open before living potential donors: governments might assess the increasing value of their property in their bodies while alive; or upon the gift of a kidney, count that as a capital gain.

of all concerned to do so. It must also be said, however, that a society would be better and more civilized in which men are joined together routinely in making cadaver organs available to prolong the lives of others than one in which this is done ostensibly by consent to the "gift" but actually for the monetary gain of the "donor." It would be better to know that hospitals use all the suitable organs of the patients who die there, if they are needed and if no one objects to this practice in his own case or that of a loved one—it would even be better to learn this too late for all one's feelings to be fully respected than to know that the bodies of any of our fellow men have been reduced to the property of another, or that the so-called "consent" to premortem or postmortem organ donation was coerced or tempted by commercial gain. If this prospect is a remote one, still it should be removed altogether.

We cannot too strongly oppose "the potentially dehumanizing abuses of a market in human flesh." [27] We cannot do too much to promote that consensual community which must undergird medical practice in the future. Then may be fulfilled the words of Dr. Francis D. Moore, when he said that tissue transplantation (itself often called into question) may in point of fact give "an entirely new meaning to human generosity as living persons or families of those recently dead make free donations of tissue for the assistance of others." [28]

27. J. Ledenberg in G. E. W. Wolstenholme, *Man and His Future* (Boston: Little, Brown, 1963), p. 268.
28. Francis D. Moore, "Ethics in the New Medicine," *The Nation* 200 (April 5, 1965): 361, and *Canadian Hospital* 42: 90.

6

A Caveat on Heart Transplants

In the Prism of a Far Away Case

The case of "Mrs. G. L. (PBBH 3M330)" at the Peter Bent Brigham Hospital in Boston during April–May 1958 is one of the most remarkable in the entire 50-year history of research and the development of organ transplantation. By this time it had been shown that the surgical procedure of kidney transplant in animals and man could be accomplished, and that the new organ as such would do its job. The antagonism which "individuality" arouses against foreign tissue had been identified and studied. Identical-twin kidney transplants had been proved as a therapy earlier in that same decade. Then in 1958 Mrs. G. L. became a coadventurer with medical science in the most important of all the "irradiation experiences." The experiment was one in which the physicians sought to "batter at the barrier" of "self/not-self" rejection. After an injury of some sort a kidney was removed from Mrs. G. L. because of massive hemorrhage. A day or so later it was discovered, because there was no urinary output, that she had been born with only one kidney. At that time dialysis on the artificial kidney was available to tide her over, but daily or intermittent dialysis of patients with total kidney failure was not yet practicable. In this sense, it can be said that there was no other hope for Mrs. G. L. than the procedure the physicians tried.[1]

A procedure was outlined for her that had never before been tried in the human being. Mrs. G. L. lay on a stretcher about 19 feet from

1. The following account is taken from Francis D. Moore, *Give and Take: The Development of Tissue Transplantation* (Philadelphia and London: Saunders, 1964), pp. 80–90. Since many days passed while decision was made for the solution of her problem—days in which she improved immensely in her physical state on hospital dialysis—a layman can only ask whether in 1958 trial of intermittent dialysis was not as likely to prove successful as the total body radiation that was tried. In raising this question with hindsight, perhaps one should expect a negative answer from the physicians then.

the portal of a two-million electron-volt X-ray source so that her whole body was exposed to the X-ray beam, and was given whole-body irradiation to the extent of 600 roentgen units. Although this had never been tried before, "it was hoped that the precise dose was just right, so that her own antibody defenses against bacteria would not be depressed too much." There was known to be a very delicate balance of survival, and "we knew her defenses against infection would be lowered to a very dangerous level."

Shortly after the irradiation was complete, the patient was given 36 billion bone marrow cells from 11 donors. This was done because the patient had received a *lethal* amount of radiation to her whole body. "This bone marrow *had* to live in order to permit survival of the patient." Mrs. G. L. had "a very large and devoted family" and several of the donors of bone marrow were her brothers. A young child undergoing a hydrocephalus operation permitted a "free kidney" to be used, i.e., one necessarily removed in the course of that patient's operation. Just before the kidney graft, Mrs. G. L. received another 170 million bone marrow cells from the hydrocephalic child whose kidney was used. The graft was implanted in Mrs. G. L.'s thigh, where its condition and functioning could be kept under constant observation.

The design was a " 'beachhead' concept of grafting: bombardment first with [lethal] irradiation, then a shore party of bone marrow cells to prepare the way for the main invasion by kidney." In other words, first there was what the older theological moralists called a massive "mutilation" of the patient's "self/not-self" immune response (a mutilation justified, of course, if it is to save life). Then the cellular factories of her damaged bone marrow were to be replaced by cells that might later recognize the kidney graft as "self." For this reason 11 donors of mixed bone marrow were used, and then cells were borrowed from the child who also "donated" the kidney. In this experiment there was a sort of "circular relationship": the bone marrow cells had to survive in the new host so as to permit the new host to survive the damage that made it possible for the bone marrow cells to live at all. The "invasion" of the kidney had to be preceded by a battering down of Mrs. G. L.'s immune response and its attempted replacement (by means of the bone marrow "transplants") by one having a greater receptivity to the kidney that was poised to come later. Dr. Francis D. Moore also describes the procedure that was used as trying to float a "cork cargo in a bottomless ship." If you get the cork cargo in place, the ship will float; but the ship needs to float (or be somehow made to float) while you are engaged in placing aboard the cork cargo!

"The graft lived but the patient died"—this was the result for Mrs. G. L. Every day up to 15 or 16 postoperative days the transplanted kidney made urine of better chemical quality. But "the balance of survival had tipped over the wrong way," and finally, 32 days after irradiation, the patient died. "The kidney appeared to survive," Dr. Moore writes, "but the patient could not withstand the effects of irradiation despite her courage throughout this perilous course." The consequences for medical progress and future benefit to other patients were, nevertheless, significant. The fact that the graft survived, although Mrs. G. L. had been so severely radiated that she could not be saved, held open the prospect that some gentler and more specific immunosuppressive regimen might be found. If Mrs. G. L., having received a lethal dose of radiation, had at the same time been able to summon from the depths of her body cells enough antibody to reject the kidney, then it would have appeared that no useful method of suppressing immune response was likely to be found. Organ transplantation might have been seriously delayed or stopped in its course, except for the survival of Mrs. G. L.'s kidney.

In the foregoing account, reference was made to Mrs. G. L.'s great courage throughout the perilous course on which she embarked with her doctors. Reference was also made to her brothers' devotion. Whether her courage or their devotion, however, are altogether to be admired depends on whether or not these human qualities were called forth by an illusion that the patient herself would benefit. Whether the physicians ought to have admired that courage and devotion depends on whether these virtues were enlisted by an informed and free consent to an experiment of possibly great benefit to future patients and to mankind generally, but quite unlikely to help Mrs. G. L. Otherwise, her courage and her brothers' devotion were not as fully human as they might have been; these qualities would then have been used for the purpose of research. Pity as a response on our parts to the case of Mrs. G. L. would then seem more appropriate than admiration—and for more reasons than that she died.

I do not mean to suggest that Mrs. G. L. did not herself elect that an investigational trial be made in the case of her own dying, or that the doctors left standing any degree of illusory hope that her life might be saved. The contrary may have been the case. Dr. Francis D. Moore, from whose book I have taken the case of Mrs. G. L., makes quite clear his own view concerning the morality of homo-transplantation: "it is not enough to tell the patient that 'there is no other hope.'"[2] The patient must join in the decision. If, however, the patient is not fully informed that a procedure is experimental, he joins in some other decision—perhaps a decision which in desperation he hopes will have greater likely or possible therapeutic benefit to him than the physicians have any right to hold out. The patient, then, if he dies, dies without dignity; he was not accorded respect as a participant in the trial that was made.

This case occurred only ten years before transplant surgeons began cardiac replacement. Yet it seems far away when measured by the progress that has since been made in organ transplantation. In the perspective of the case of Mrs. G. L. we can perhaps free ourselves from unqualified endorsement of every one of these accomplishments and better discern the chief caveat that should be raised about the 1968 and 1969 heart transplants. At least, we ought to be able to sort out the elements that enter into making an ethical decision concerning cardiac replacement in a given case. If these operations are to be deemed investigational trials, then the ethics governing the manner in which they should be carried out is the ethics of medical experimentation involving a human subject. If, however, these operations are a legitimate form of treatment, or a mixture of treatment and further trial, then some would hold that the judgment concerning their permissibility (or the sort of patient-consent that needs to be obtained) is significantly changed. We shall examine this experiment-therapy distinction as it applies to heart transplants. Then we shall turn to the assumption that heart replacements are therapeutic, or are to be located at some point along a spectrum between experiment and treatment that admits of no sharp disjunctions.

The upshot of this will be to argue that the patient's consent has still to be sustained or enabled to be free to say "no" to transplant therapy. "When we move . . . in the explanation of alternatives to such desperate measures as kidney or liver transplantation, it is evi-

2. Moore, *Give and Take*, p. 166.

dent that the hopes of the surgeon, the fears of the patient, and the inborn optimism of youthful science combine to push the patient onward." [3] This can produce a terrible coercion upon men. If in cases of cardiac replacement, it is not enough to say, "There is no other hope," what more is there to say? Since all agree that we should not now begin to replace defective hearts as a matter of preventive or palliative medicine, what can be the meaning of the American Medical Association's statement in its *Ethical Guidelines for Organ Transplantation* that "the physician should be objective . . . in disclosing known risks and possible hazards, and in advising of the alternative procedures available" [4] in the case of end-stage heart disease, or the end-stage of the disease of liver or other unpaired vital organ? What other explanation of alternatives is there to talk over with the patient so that he can share in the decision?

In such last-ditch therapy (or therapy plus experimental trial) the options would seem to be reduced to accepting a heart transplant or an immediate death—between, on the one hand, a radical attempt to stay alive by choosing to "die twice," now and a little "indefinite" time later and, on the other hand, a comparatively more acceptable death. This is an exceedingly important point in regard to heart transplants and other ways medical science has given us of not dying. Dying is not only physiological, it is also a psychological matter. Unless an interval of choiceworthy human living can, by radical surgery, be set between a person's "first dying" of an end-stage illness and his "second dying" after that remedy finally fails, then the patient passes from desperation to desperation, or is simply maintained within the constant, comparatively assured presence of his own death. The acceptance of death never meant the unrelieved savoring of it.

Unless the hopes of the surgeon-investigator and the desperation of patients are to conspire to push them onward, a renewal of the notion that death may be electable, fostered and held in common by surgeons and patients alike, would seem to be the only way to sustain a covenant of free men between them. This requires a frank discus-

3. Francis D. Moore, "Therapeutic Innovation: Ethical Boundaries in the Initial Clinical Trials of New Drugs and Surgical Procedures," Ethical Aspects of Experimentation with Human Subjects, *Daedalus*, Spring 1969, p. 511.

4. *Ethical Guidelines for Organ Transplantation*, E. G. Shelley, Chairman of the Judicial Council, adopted by the House of Delegates of the American Medical Association, June 1968.

sion of the possible acceptability of death over the chances of life, or the kind of life the surgeons can realistically promise. Unless this "alternative procedure" is fully explored and weighed, then the desperation of patients and the interest surgeons rightly have in performing remedies, however radical, and in pushing back the frontiers of transplantation therapy must always prove overriding—certainly not against the wills of their patients but still without their choices being fully free and fully human. This, I confess, would require a sea-change in the attitude toward death in our culture, and the adoption by physicians of a rather more "priestly" and therefore more human relation to their patients, and of a less triumphalist attitude toward death.

Heart Transplants as Investigational Trials

The Board of Medicine of the National Academy of Sciences issued a statement which, it seems to me, exactly described the heart transplants performed in 1968 and 1969, and at the same time points to the chief moral assessment to be made of these operations.[5] The transplantation of hearts "cannot as yet be regarded as an accepted form of therapy, even an heroic one," the Board said. "It must be clearly viewed for what it is, a scientific exploration of the unknown." This means that "the primary justification for this activity in respect to both the donor and recipient is that from the study will come new knowledge of benefit to others in our society." The Board rightly emphasized the responsibility this places upon the investigator to make sure that he has a design and the equipment to record the maximum useful information from such an operation, and to make this information available to the scientific community. The Board also pointed the surgical investigator to another aspect of his responsibility to donor and recipient alike. "The ethical issues in-

5. "Cardiac Transplantation in Man," Statement Prepared by the Board of Medicine of the National Academy of Sciences, *Journal of the American Medical Association* 204, no. 9 (May 27, 1968): 805–806. On December 4, 1968, the American Medical Association adopted a set of guidelines for heart transplant cases which also states that heart implantation "must be regarded as investigative." The AMA urged that the use of the operation be "restricted to patients for whom there is no other means of therapy offering a life-sustaining prognosis," and that the procedure should not be extended "to patients in whom it might be regarded as palliative or preventive rather than life-saving." *Journal of the American Medical Association* 207, no. 9 (March 3, 1969): 1704–05.

volved," it stated, "are a part of the whole complex question of the ethics of human experimentation."

The chief ethical principle governing in medical investigations is that they shall proceed only after an informed and free consent has been obtained. This means that donor and recipient alike must consent to heart transplant as a scientific exploration from which may come new knowledge of benefit to others in the future, and not primarily as a present form of therapy, even a heroic one. It is this canon of loyalty between physician-investigator and patient-subject—and not any other that I can think of—which may have been violated in some or many, if not all, of the heart transplants to date. Admittedly, there are gray areas in determining which is which. Still there is good reason to say (as did Dr. William Likoff of the Hahnemann Medical College at Dartmouth) [6] that "today renal transplantation is more therapeutic than experimental" while "liver and heart transplants . . . must be considered more experimental than therapeutic." In liver and heart transplants, then, the donor (and his family) and the recipient are more subjects than patients (and should be so treated), and the surgeons are more scientific investigators than physician-friends.

The purpose of an experiment is fulfilled either by success or by conclusive failure; by either indifferently. The purpose of treatment, however, is fulfilled only by success. Granting that there can be debate about how much possibility of success is required for a procedure to be deemed "therapeutic," surely just any possibility of success would not be sufficient. How therapeutic or how successful, the investigation aims to find out. It is a troubling situation when (as

6. William Likoff, "A Perspective for Considering the Moral, Legal and Ethical Problems Arising from Advances in Medical Science," *Villanova Law Review* 13, no. 4 (Summer 1968): 739. The list can be indefinitely extended of those who agree that experimentation with human beings is the ethical context in which to evaluate the morality of cardiac replacement today. "Cardiac transplantation cannot be considered as a therapeutic measure. Rather, it is at best an experimental procedure, fraught with all the perils that characterize a hazardous clinical trial" (editorial, "On Cardiac Transplantation," *The Pharos*, April 1968, p. 72). "The ethical principles of human experimentation . . . apply with particular relevance to transplantation" (Delford L. Stickels, "Ethical and Moral Aspects of Transplantation," *Monographs in the Surgical Sciences* 3, no. 4 [1966]: 268). ". . . purely experimental . . ." (Lyman A. Brewer III, "Cardiac Transplantation: An Appraisal," *Journal of the American Medical Association* 205, no. 10 (September 2, 1968): 691–92).

Dr. Likoff pointed out) "the public has not been trained to recognize the difference between clinical investigation and proven treatment." The difficulty is that the responsibility for telling which is which must be lodged with the physician-investigator. The public cannot train itself to recognize this difference—thus enabling donors and recipients to consent to heart transplants as investigations if they wish to do so—in the face of newspaper releases that almost daily tell them otherwise.

The fact that patients are in desperate need of therapy must also be taken into account. It is not enough, as we have seen, to tell a potential recipient that "there is no other hope." "The surgeon," Dr. Michael T. DeBakey urges, "must scrupulously guard against taking inadvertent advantage, for purely experimental purposes, of the eagerness of a desperately ill patient to consent to almost any procedure suggested." [7] How is the surgeon who is both physician and investigator going to do this, or be constrained to do so?

Recipients of borrowed hearts should not be tempted to consent to a trial under the impression that it is a more hopeful procedure than it is, or under the impression that it is as yet a procedure primarily for their treatment. Nor should they be barred from fully voluntary participation in the experimental stages of a treatment that may later be of great medical significance. In order better to ensure that this does not happen, at least one of the committees set up to draft statements about the social and ethical issues in transplantation seriously considered the suggestion that the physician to whom a patient may give consent be quite independent of the surgeons doing the transplantation. This procedure would keep the functions of physician-friend separate from those of the physician-investigators. Not only prospective donors but prospective recipients of borrowed hearts and their freedom to decide for themselves should be protected from the persuasive powers of transplant surgeons. This suggestion—if effective in that direction—had much to recommend it, if these surgical teams are today primarily engaged in research trials.

The suggestion is only a variation of Guttentag's idea that there should be a "physician-friend" to attend a "patient" who is also a

7. Michael T. DeBakey, editorial, "Human Cardiac Transplantation," *Journal of Thoracic and Cardiovascular Surgery* 55 (March 1968): 449.

research "subject," separate from those interested in experimentation for the development of a therapy.[8] Perhaps this division of powers and responsibility would help to ensure that a patient can soberly estimate the, as yet, secondary worth of a transplant as treatment in his own case or, if he wishes, can give informed consent to participation in an operation that is still primarily experimental. This would be to locate the 1968 and 1969 heart transplants where they most properly belong: under the ethical principles governing medical research involving human subjects. The presumption that desperately ill patients always are willing to consent to measures that have any possibility of success, or ones not yet known to cure or not yet proved to promise a significant extension of their normal lives, is often a false presumption; and if false, it is a violent presumption. It is often also a false and violent presumption that donors and their families meant to consent to give organs for anything less than a life-saving practice of medicine. If so, the violation has its beginnings in a failure to find out whether they would agree, recipients and donors alike, to become partners and coadventurers with the doctors in a surgical trial that was not now or not yet a significant life-saving practice.

To separate the responsibilities of physicians to a dying patient who is a prospective donor from the responsibilities of physicians to a needy recipient has as its purpose the exclusion of the possibility, however remote, that the prospective donor may be neglected or his death hastened for the purpose of making the needed organ accessible to the transplantation surgeons. This rule of practice has evolved from within the medical profession itself, and was not externally imposed. The suggested practice—which also expresses the concern of doctors themselves—of keeping the physician who counsels a dying patient who needs organ replacement and who may obtain his consent entirely separate from the surgeons who are testing heart transplantation would have as its purpose the protection of that patient's freedom to choose a desperate remedy for an already desperate situation, or to choose it not—or to choose it simply as a service that can finally be made of his likely dying. This way, to elect to "die twice" can be a noble act and not one of desperation.

8. Otto E. Guttentag, "The Problem of Experimentation on Human Beings: II. The Physician's Point of View," *Science* 117 (February 27, 1953): 207–10.

It would also seem that the way to secure donors would be to enlist them premortem or their families postmortem in a medical investigation, and not leave them uninformed about what it is they are consenting to. Dr. James J. Nora, a member of Dr. Cooley's heart transplant team, said, "Initially, we had a big flood of donors because we were doing so well, but donor families got discouraged because so few patients survived beyond a few weeks or months." [9] Who —the donor families or the doctors or the press—was responsible for this discouragement? How much better it would be to create a consensual community of patients, donors, and doctors knowingly engaged in a medical trial, not under the illusion of practicing therapeutic medicine!

To oversell a procedure leads inevitably to reaction against it, and to its devaluation. This is the case whether we have in mind the publicized worth of heart replacement today, or the publicized power of papal excommunication in the Middle Ages. The medical profession needs to listen attentively to words people use, in their ordinary meanings, when they speak about what they have been doing in giving and receiving hearts. Mrs. Virginia May White was overheard by her family to say, while watching a TV news report concerning heart transplants, "How marvelous to give someone a chance to live." Upon her accidental death a few days later, her husband and children quickly agreed that her heart could be transplanted at the Stanford Medical Center into the chest of Mike Kasperak, a 54-year-old retired steel worker, who died 15 days later. Kasperak's wife told reporters that she urged her husband to "go ahead, don't waste any time; I want you alive and with me." [10] Helen Krouch, of Patterson, New Jersey, told her parents while in perfect health, "If I could save someone's life, I would do it. If I knew I were going to die, I'd like to die that way." Upon her death or while dying, she was, as a consequence of this statement, moved so that her heart could be implanted in Louis Block at Maimonides Medical Center in Brooklyn, N. Y. Thereby she may have contributed to the advancement of medical science and the benefit of future patients, but she did not accomplish what she said she was willing to do for Louis Block.

Do we not have in these expectations the true explanation of why

9. *New York Times,* March 1, 1969.
10. *New York Times,* January 8, 1968.

the "big flood of donors" ended in a trickle when it became apparent
that heart replacement was only an investigational procedure in human beings, with predictably small life-prolonging results? To have
described the procedure, in season and out of season, as investigational only would have meant the creation of a consensual community of heart donors, heart recipients, and transplant surgeons acting
in a spirit of fully informed partnership in behalf of medical progress. If not a flood, the donors might have come forward in a more
continuous stream or brooklet.[11]

The same indiscriminate and vernacular talk about saving "life"
can be cited from the families of patients who have died. Thus, Ann
Washkansky, the wife of Louis Washkansky, the first human being
on whom heart replacement was tried (experimentally, in this case,
surely), said after his death, "I know the doctors did everything possible to save my husband's life." [12] And Dr. Adrian Kantrowitz of
the Maimonides Medical Center in Brooklyn, feelingly described his
patient, Louis Block, as "a brave and courageous man whose only

11. Admittedly, the number of operations attempted might have been fewer. This
could well have been a better way to advance the experiment and world-wide exchange
of the knowledge gained. It would certainly have dampened the atmosphere of show-
manship and gala international and intercity competition which has afflicted this
clinical surgical trial from the beginning. Among medical writers, John Lear of *The
Saturday Review*, January 6 and February 3, 1968, was from the beginning most critical
of this aspect of heart transplantation. Among physicians, Dr. Irving H. Page of the
Research Division of the Cleveland Clinic Foundation made these and other criticisms.
See his article on "Instant Reporting" in *The Saturday Review*, February 3, 1968, and
"The Ethics of Heart Transplantation: A Personal View," a paper read before the
National Congress on Medical Ethics sponsored by the American Medical Association,
Chicago, October 5, 1968, and published in the *Journal of the American Medical As-
sociation* 207, no. 1 (January 6, 1969): 109–113.

12. *New York Times*, Dec. 22, 1967, reporting Washkansky's death of pneumonia
18 days after surgery at Groote Schuur Hospital, South Africa. While this patient
would certainly have died anyway, "it is a perfectly logical assumption to say that
Louis Washkansky's life was shortened by this transplant rather than prolonged by
it" (Dr. George Schreiner, as reported in *The Lexington Leader*, February 8, 1968).
Moreover, an experiment can be a success even when the patient dies, as in the case
of Mrs. G. L. and the first heart transplant. This raises a basic question about the
way in which these successes are reported, which the public takes to mean something
quite different. "Is it right to emphasize that the transplanted kidneys [or transplanted
hearts] were functioning fully at the time the patient died from a pneumonia that
was almost surely contributed to by the requisite immunosuppressive therapy? This
kind of publicity may be unavoidable, but again it lacks perspective and it is certainly unfortunate in that it raises false hopes" ("Moral Problems in the Use of Borrowed Organs," editorial, *Annals of Internal Medicine* 60, no. 2 [February 1964]: 312).

real opportunity for life was through this procedure." [13] This sounds remarkably like praising Mrs. G. L.'s courage and the devotion of her brothers—praise that was not necessarily misplaced, but a tribute that raises decisively the question whether in these cases of heart replacement the patient shared nobly in a decision to join in a clinical trial from which he himself would likely not benefit, or was left with the hope that there was real opportunity of life for him. Most physicians who have commented on the ethics of last-ditch therapies, not to say the ethics of medical experimentation, agree that it is not enough to say, "There is no other hope." These references to saving "life" raise decisively the question whether the "more" that was left silently said to these patients was not precisely the illusion that the proposed heart replacements held real promise to therapeutic value for them.

In face of numerous statements by official and semiofficial committees of scientists and physicians that cardiac transplantation should be regarded as yet as no more than investigational, it is difficult for a layman to believe that the day will not come when a relative of some deceased patient will bring suit for therapeutic malpractice against a transplant surgical team. Would not such a plaintiff have on his side the testimony of a large segment of the medical profession, if he can show that the patient did not consent to an experimental trial? The fact that no one has brought such a complaint is itself testimony to the fact that subjects trust their researchers as patients do their physicians. Whatever the legalities may be, confusion of these two relations is exceedingly likely to lead, morally, to a violation of the covenant between the man who performs and the man who is the subject in clinical surgical investigations.

This brings us to the question whether the foregoing caveat on heart transplants can be restated on the assumption that heart replacement is a type of treatment, as some believe.

Heart Transplants as Treatment, Elective Only

A minority of the medical profession affirm with conviction that heart replacements now are treatments, not investigations having in view the development of a future treatment. Not surprisingly, the strongest voices in support of this thesis are those of the heart trans-

13. Ibid., January 11, 1968.

plant surgeons. After only four attempts to transplant the human heart had been made, Dr. Christiaan Barnard declared (at a meeting of transplant specialists from across the nation in the VIP room at Chicago's O'Hare International Airport) that "on the basis of our experimental work and the work of other investigators, we decided that we must now consider heart transplantation as a therapeutic procedure. It is not an experiment that we perform on someone who is otherwise dead—but a form of treatment we offer seriously ill patients." [14] To credit that statement, made so early in the heart era, one would have to reject the general assumption that, despite the work of investigators on animals or on other organs in humans, the step from animals to man must always be regarded as a further step in research having unknown consequences. Perhaps more to be credited is the conclusion drawn by thirteen surgeons assembled at the Cape Town Conference on Heart Transplants in July 1968: "In the spirit of extreme optimism and goodwill, the panelists reviewed the heart transplants performed to date and concluded that transplantation is no longer an experimental procedure. For the patient at end-stage heart disease, it has become an effective therapeutic measure to prolong and improve his life." [15]

A more balanced viewpoint holds that there is a large gray area between the extremes of pure research and proved treatment, and that along the spectrum from one to the other it is difficult to say that a given procedure is primarily the one and secondarily the other. "The question of whether a medical procedure has reached that stage of acceptance to be deserving of the label 'therapeutic' rather than 'experimental,' " write Sadler and Sadler, "frequently comes down to nothing more than an exercise in semantics. There is no litmus paper test. We believe the therapy-experiment dichotomy is best viewed as a continuum ranging from routine procedures at one end to investigative procedures, involving 'normal volunteers' or 'normal controls,' at the other. While with the former, the risks and benefits of the procedure are well known and the reason for its use is to benefit the patient directly, with the latter, the new procedure is applied to a healthy, 'normal,' person with the intention of gaining

14. "Medical News," *Journal of the American Medical Association* 203, no. 3 (January 15, 1968).

15. "Minutes of the Cape Town Meeting," as told by Dr. Denton A. Cooley to Judith Ramsey, senior writer, *Medical World News,* August 9, 1968, p. 23.

important medical knowledge." A procedure performed upon the dying, such as the first heart transplant, in the opinion of these authors, may be "a blend of both." "While the knowledge to be gained from the operation, whether it be a 'success' or a 'failure,' would be invaluable in subsequent operations, no one could deny that to Louis Washkansky and the doctors involved, the operation represented the lone hope for a prolonged life, all other reasonable alternatives having failed." [16] Much the same is the view of Dr. Francis D. Moore.[17] Every surgical operation is an experiment in bacteriology, and a dose of digitalis or an aspirn is an experiment in pharmacology. But when we move to "entirely new treatments for critical illness, we pass from smooth sailing into choppy waters." In the choppy waters of last-ditch investigational therapy, "the doctor can no longer tell his patient the chances of success or failure because he does not know them himself—nor can he minimize the risk."

Let us therefore assume that the 1968 and 1969 heart replacements were in this sense treatments. They were the "lone hope" of prolonging the life of the patients. On the first interpretation, we concluded that for participation in these investigations to be fully human the consents of recipients and donors alike should primarily have been solicited and given to engage as a partner in human experimentation. On the present view, the question is how we are to weigh the therapeutic worth of heart replacements to date. If the investigational aspects of the heart transplants were merely extensions of the usual patient-physician relationship in last-ditch therapy, this does not abrogate the moral principles implicit in the covenant of man with man under these circumstances. It merely alters the terms. If it is not enough to say that a heart replacement is the "lone hope," we still have to ask the meaning and limits of acceptable persuasion in order to preserve and cherish the freedom and humanity of end-stage heart patients in covenant with the living, and especially with those who proffer them help.

If heart transplants are not primarily experimental, if they are

16. Alfred M. Sadler, Jr. and Blair L. Sadler, "Transplantation and the Law: The Need for Organized Sensitivity," *Georgetown Law Journal*, 57, no. 1 (October 1968: 7, n. 8.

17. Francis D. Moore, "Ethics in New Medicine: Tissue Transplants," *The Nation* 200 (April 5, 1965), pp. 358–62, and "Ethics in New Medicine," *Canadian Hospital* 42 (June 1963): 87–90.

"treatments we offer seriously ill patients," if they are investigational therapy, we still should appraise their worth as treatments and support the freedom of these patients to appraise their therapeutic worth to them. I shall argue that the caveat on transplants stated above does not need to be significantly changed even if these operations should be classified as treatments and even if there is an admixture of research/treatment purposes. The 1968–1969 transplants were, if anything, more choiceworthy because of investigational benefits to come, had these benefits been the principal terms of the "contract" between the participants, than if they were mainly therapeutic or were chosen as treatments. This conclusion must follow from an evaluation of the quantity and the quality of their benefits as treatments. I shall further argue that heart replacements are now and are likely to remain irremediably "extraordinary" measures and at most elective only. If they become "ordinary" treatments in the physician's sense of "customary," they are likely to remain "extraordinary" in the moralists' sense (see pp. 120–23, above). That is to say, ethically no man need choose to live when he can live only by making himself patient to these procedures or choose the way of life they make possible. Of course, he may do so.

First, a quantitative appraisal of the treatment value of heart replacements, i.e., the length of days or months of additional life likely for any recipient. One way of reporting the statistics at any given time communicates a built-in unintended "deception" that was bound in the end to be seen through by the general public, potential donors, and recipients alike. Thus, on September 28, 1968, the *New York Times* could correctly report that of 11 operations performed by Dr. Denton Cooley at St. Luke's and Texas Children's Hospital in Houston, six patients were still living. That strongly implies a choiceworthy treatment-value for a new last-ditch therapy: 6 out of 11, a decimal point more than half, but still a good proportion. Poorly hidden by these statistics is the question how many of the six were shortly going to join the dead. If enough *new* heart transplants continue to be performed, the statistics will keep on showing that only slightly fewer patients have died than are still alive. But this tells us little or nothing about whether for an individual patient heart replacement is a way of staying alive. In a "Year's Report Card" on heart transplants, Harold M. Schmeck, Jr., science writer for the *New York Times,* stated that of the first 99 operations the world over, 59 had died but 40 were still alive. Those seem like odds any end-stage heart patient might choose, but they are also odds that any reasonable man knows to discount. Behind these figures was the "grim," "blunt" fact that, besides Dr. Philip Blaiberg, only 9 patients of the 99 in the whole world had lived more than *three months* following heart replacement.[18]

This is not to use retrospective data for the purpose of present or prospective moral analysis. The data could have been reported at any time during 1968 by the formula used in renal transplant statistics. In the case of kidneys we are told that the four-year survival rate of transplants from parent donors is approximately 50 percent. We are told that the four-year survival rate from sibling donors is slightly higher, that the four-year survival rate from cadaver kidneys is between 15 and 20 percent, and that a 95 percent one-year survival rate has been obtained by Dr. Thomas E. Starzl.[19] The same could be indicated for heart transplants. Take, for example, the "Year's Report Card" showing that of 99 heart transplant patients in the whole world, nine had lived more than three months. That figures to be approximately "10% *three month survival rate.*" The two-month survival rate would have been higher, and the four-month, six-month, etc., survival rates lower. One needs to know such estimates, whether he is going to commit the gambler's fallacy (of concluding anything about an individual case from general statistics) on the gloomy or the bright side of the prospects. "10% three month survival rate" is a quite different and more revealing figure than "40 out of 99 are still alive" to take account of if one is pondering whether it is worthwhile to give or receive a heart. For this reason, to agree to this procedure would seem to be a more reasonable decision if the operation were regarded as investigational than if it is claimed to be primarily a treatment.

To summarize, we need to consider a table of length of survival, cause of death, and of the patients still living out of 16 Houston heart transplant cases reported by Dr. James J. Nora, Dr. Denton A.

18. December 8, 1968.
19. "Status of Transplantation 1968," A Report by the Surgical Training Committee of the National Institute of General Medical Sciences (Bethesda, Md.: National Institutes of Health, November 1968), p. 43.

Cooley, et al., in May, 1969.[20] Patient No. 1 in the above table was undoubtedly Mr. Everett C. Thomas, who was first implanted in

TABLE 1. Clinical Experience with Cardiac Transplantation

Case No.	Date of Operation	Age (Yr)	Sex	No. of Rejection Episodes	1st Rejection Episode Began	Survival	Cause of Death
1							
a	5/2/68 (1st Operation)	47	M	2	8 days	200 days	—
b	11/21/68 (2d Operation)	47	M	1	Immediately	3 days	Rejection
2	5/5/68	48	M	0	—	3 days	Infection
3	5/7/68	62	M	0	—	8 days	Pre-existing diseases
4	5/21/68	54	M	2	50 days	145 days	Rejection
5	7/2/68	46	M	6	6 days	149 days	Rejection
6	7/20/68	58	M	0	—	181 days	Living
7	7/23/68	57	M	3	13 days	170 days	Rejection
8	7/29/68	49	F	1	11 days	55 days	Infection
9	8/18/68	5	F	1	5 days	8 days	Rejection
10	8/19/68	50	M	1	5 days	68 days	Infection
11	9/15/68	1 (2 mo)	F	0	—	14 hr	Pulmonary insufficiency
12	10/25/68	52	M	1	23 days	85 days	Living
13	11/5/68	50	M	1	5 days	7 days	Rejection
14	11/9/68	55	M	0	—	48 days	Infection
15	11/16/68	50	M	1	7 days	63 days	Living
16	11/29/68	54	M	1	6 days	13 days	Rejection

20. James J. Nora, Denton A. Cooley, et al., "Rejection of the Transplanted Human Heart: Indexes of Recognition and Problems of Prevention," *New England Journal of Medicine* 280, no. 20 (May 15, 1969): 1079–85. I do not know what to make of the fact that Dr. Cooley (whose views of the treatment-value of heart replacement are strong, and are cited above and below) was among the authors of this scientific article, which concluded with the words: "Human cardiac transplantation is still an investigative procedure with minimal clinical application. . . . If cardiac transplantation is going to have wide clinical application in the future, new methods will have to be devised for overcoming poor histocompatibility matches" (ibid., p. 1085).

May 1968, who survived to leave the hospital and take a position in a bank *nearby*, but who had to be implanted again in November 1968, and who died three days later. The report of his death after the second graft went on to say that, as of that date, 44 of 87 persons who had received heart replacements were still alive. Significantly, the report also went on to say that of these only 6 had lived beyond six months.[21] The latter is the grim fact that is beginning to seep into the consciousness of recipients as they ponder whether this operation is as yet wholly choiceworthy as a form of treatment, and of donors who may have thought to give their hearts upon death to save someone else's life.

Notable in the above table is the fact that (1) only 3 of 16 patients were still alive at the time of the report, for 181, 85, and 48 days, respectively; (2) two had died of other causes than a failure of the therapy itself, which still must try to float cargo in a bottomless ship, one a baby who died because of pulmonary insufficiency and the other a 62-year-old man (the oldest in the series) of pre-existing diseases; and (3) eleven died of causes related to the treatment itself. Those who did not reject the graft, died of infection; those who did not die of infection, rejected the graft. In either case the cork cargo was not quite in place. The surgeons are obviously trying to walk a narrow ridge between the assault upon the body's integrity, and its resistance to foreign invasion, too much or too little. This seems to a layman to be a perfect description of an investigational procedure still in course and one not yet to be recommended as treatment.

But we need to probe behind the semantics of those who were willing to term the 1968–1969 heart replacements *treatments*. What, quantitatively and qualitatively, is meant by this? Are the rest of us bound to agree or likely to agree with this estimation? Of one of his patients who died—a Houston housewife, Mrs. Beth W. Brunk— Dr. Denton Cooley said, "The happiness and contentment we were

21. The *New York Times*, November 24, 1968. This figures to be approximately 7% six-month survival rate for all the world's heart transplant patients as of that date. *Cardiac Replacement: Medical, Ethical, Psychological and Economic Implications*, a report by an ad hoc task force on cardiac replacement, National Heart Institute, October 1969, presents an analysis of 134 heart transplant patients to July 1, 1969. It is fair to point out that this study—later than the information available in the text above—states at one point that as of that date "25 percent had lived at least six months" (p. v).

able to give her for a period of six or eight weeks justified the operation as therapy." [22] I assume this means that *if* Dr. Cooley had known that only six or eight weeks more of contented hospital life would be given Mrs. Brunk, he would nevertheless have performed the operation as therapy for her. This tells us how much and what sort of success Dr. Cooley would require for a procedure to be properly considered therapeutic. We do not know, and can reasonably doubt, whether Mrs. Brunk would have been of the same opinion, or that these were the sober terms of her own consent. We do not know that she would have judged six or eight weeks of hospital life worth the costs to her and to her family or worth the social costs. (The hospital costs of patients waiting for transplants are, I understand, borne by them, while the cost of the operation and subsequent treatment are provided from other sources—probably under the heading of "research"—and to date are not borne by the recipients.) On the other hand, we do not know whether she might have given her dying as a partner in the exploration of the unknown and for the perfecting of a future therapy that for herself in its present stage may not have been a treatment worth choosing.

At a conference in New York City in late February 1969, Dr. Cooley is reported to have said that "we're taking dying people and prolonging life, and improving the quality of those lives." He charged that some among the medical profession and many in the public at large "have become faint-hearted too soon, in the face of a few initial defeats." [23] The defeats, of course, are not few. Plainly, Dr. Cooley sincerely believes that an extension of life for six or eight weeks or more is worth choosing at these financial and personal costs. He also deems that to be a successful treatment of a seriously ill patient because of the quality of physical well-being secured for the patient for such a period of hospital existence. More, of course, is hoped for; but still heart replacement would be deserving of classification as a useful therapy if only on these limited

22. The *New York Times*, September 29, 1968.

23. *Washington Post*, February 28, 1969. If the operations are investigational procedures, there is much to be said in favor of the pioneering work of kidney transplant surgeons in the early days and the heart transplant surgeons in ours. There can always be debate about when to pass from animals to man. Without pioneers while this question simply *is* debatable, pure scientists might be still working exclusively on mice and monkeys and dogs.

terms. I for one find it incredible that Dr. Cooley is not adding to treatment value the additional weight of the value of ongoing research. Still we must take him at his word.

Then, it simply must be said that this is not what ordinary mortals usually mean by a life-saving and life-enhancing treatment. Heart replacement, as Dr. Francis D. Moore said of kidney dialysis, may be "a way of staying alive" (for a predictably short time, in the case of heart transplantation); it is, however, "hardly a way of life" [24] and ought not generally to have been proposed as such in recent months.

In another way, difference in word meanings may lead an ethical physician or members of the public astray. When some physicians say that a new radical therapy promises to extend the life of a patient "indefinitely," [25] they mean "unpredictably." Such a physician would be minimally satisfied (while hoping for more) by any length of days that is somewhat more (or maybe longer) than present prognosis or by any available alternative treatment. A member of the public hears him promise more, and this conspires "to push the patient onward" into investigative therapeutic surgery, perhaps without exercising full freedom of human decision that this is a good thing for him to do.

If it is said that other major surgery, e.g., in some cases of cancer, offer no more extension of days than heart replacement at present, then the caveat applies to both as treatments. Both are, morally, extraordinary remedies and at most elective only. It is not imperative that anyone choose them. It would be strange if palliative heart replacement came to be acceptable or customary precisely at a time when some palliative cancer surgery is more and more deemed to be "not indicated." Whether heart transplants are viewed as treatments or located at some point on the experiment-therapy continuum, patients should be helped to be free in appraising the actual worth to them of the length of life or the way of life promised by heart replacement. They should not by their desperation be

24. Francis D. Moore, "Ethics in the New Medicine," p. 359.

25. For example, in introducing Mrs. Haskell Karp, who was to read her poignant, personally drafted appeal over national TV for a heart donor, Dr. Cooley said calmly and simply that the mechanical heart could maintain Mr. Karp for only a few hours or days and that he hoped for a human heart so that the patient could be prolonged in life "indefinitely."

pushed onward toward the operation as the one "lone hope" of survival. To say "there is no other hope" does not mean that there is no other *choice*. Men as men need not choose survival under any or all conditions. Faced with some sorts of elective life, death may become more electable still and more consonant with human dignity.

Under the heading of the quality of life, we have to consider also the assault upon a patient's bodily integrity, his fortress against infection. He will continue to have to walk a narrow ridge between too much and too little, and by postoperative medication keep himself steady on course between "rejection" and "infection." That is to say, he will never be "normal" again. While this is also true following other sorts of major surgery, some patients—given full comprehension of the way of life they are choosing—may not want to elect the quantity and quality of life available only by suffering this major body "mutilation" and all that it entails.

"Heart swaps" and the intensity and isolation of the measures that must be taken have now been shown to be a definite threat to a patient's mental balance, even after psychological screening. Donald T. Lunde, psychiatrist and consultant to Norman Shumway's transplant team at Stanford, reported these findings to a meeting of the American Psychiatric Association in Bal Harbour, Miami Beach, Florida, May 7, 1969.[26] Any patient must now place possible psychotic outcomes beside the pictures of other patients at home or riding bicycles,[27] when he is weighing whether and how to go on living. He may be weighing whether to die of heart disease or to be at risk of becoming or dying psychotic. "As this kind of surgery becomes more routine," Dr. Lunde predicted, "the psychiatric complications will continue to become more common." Some of the "episodes" reported were fear of feminization upon receiving a woman's heart; the delusion of a 45-year-old man that he was 20, the donor's age; delusion and belligerency because the doctors seemed disembodied masks out to poison the patient. These are not, to psychiatrists, unexpected results. Sufficient explanation is to be found in the "mentally punishing procedure" including liberal

26. *New York Times*, May 8, 1969; "What Does a New Heart Do to the Mind?" *Medical World News*, May 22, 1969, pp. 17–18.

27. Picture of Robert C. McKee, implanted August 21, 1968, the longest surviving of six living patients who have received transplants at Stanford, in the *New York Times*, April 24, 1969.

amounts of prednisone, the linkage of "self-image" with "body-image," the "mind-taxing effect of an open-heart procedure," and the "mind-wearing effect of long confinement under intensive care" during which the patient is approached only by masked persons.[28]

These things are set down here not for their scare effect, but simply because the foregoing so well describes an "extraordinary" measure to prolong life. The quantity and quality of life expected, the massive impact of the entire procedure upon patients during and after surgery, all this tells us what more must be said besides "there is no other hope" if men are to be free in their living or in their dying. Principal among the considerations negating the choice-worthiness of electing a number of radical surgeries is the experience of "dying twice," unless an interlude of significant human living is set between the experiences of facing one's end-time. Man does not live by protraction alone. This, along with the costs, the extent and regimen of the remedy while it is being endured, the burden of living with permanent injury to one's self/not-self bodily integrity, etc., gives ground for saying that, however customary or routine heart replacements may become, they are likely to remain, morally, and from the point of view of the patient and of a humane physician, irremediably "extraordinary."

For seriously ill patients the banner of freedom from being coercively pushed onward by inner desperation and outer constraints has written on it the words of the traditional moralists: "*Extraordinary* means of preserving life are all medicines, treatments, and operations, which cannot be obtained or used without excessive expense, pain, or other inconvenience for the patient or for others, or which, if used, would not offer a reasonable hope of benefit to the patient." [29] Such remedies are not mandatory upon any patient's choice, or imperative to be done to save the life of any man, unless he affirmatively chooses them by a participatory consent that is adequately informed and free of overriding desperation. To make room for that decision, to seek and strengthen it, is the beginning and the foundation of care for an end-stage patient.

For the rest, I grant that the banner of human freedom in such

28. *Medical World News,* p. 18.
29. Gerald Kelly, S.J., *Medico-Moral Problems* (St. Louis, Mo.: The Catholic Hospital Association, 1958, 5th printing, 1966), p. 135. See pp. 118–24 above.

patients is not likely to be unfurled, or their choice to live by the means available or to die be made effectual, unless culturally we recover a religious sense that death is not an evil that ought always to be opposed. If it is not possible for modern men, when the one "lone hope" is gone, to believe that this is not the end of hope, perhaps we might share the conviction of Socrates, who said, "Now it is time that we were going, I to die and you to live, but which of us has the happier prospect, is unknown to anyone but God." [30] That outlook, too, might save men and doctors today from the triumphalist temptation to slash and suture our way to eternal life.

30. Plato, *Apology*, 42.

7

Choosing How to Choose: Patients and
Sparse Medical Resources

In an earlier chapter we saw that from one point of view modern medical progress can be described as the achievement of more and more treatments that are irremediably "extraordinary," i.e., elective only, never or rarely imperative, from the point of view of the patient or of a humane physician. Since so many of these therapeutic measures are also costly and in short supply in comparison with health needs at any given time or place, the physician faces the ethical dilemma of how to choose among medically eligible patients. If the disease is fatal and the means of remedy sparse, the question is: Who shall live and who shall die? Since some choice must be made, we need to ask whether there is any line of moral reasoning that will clarify how this decision should be made. In these cases of life or death, how shall men choose from among several ways of choosing? This is the main issue to be taken up in this chapter.

There is, however, a broader question concerning the distribution of sparse medical resources facing the medical profession and medical practice generally, and our society at large. With sufficient resources of money and personnel, any one or more remedy could be extended to all in need. But not all remedies can together be effectively extended in the social practice of medicine in this day of extraordinary treatments. Since health needs are almost by definition unlimited in any given society, and since the health needs of the world as a whole are infinite, choices must somehow be made among them. How shall sparse medical resources be allocated? Which needs should be given priority in medical practice and medical institutions generally? Beyond this, there is the question of the priority that should be given to medical needs among the many social causes having valid claims upon a nation's resources. Ideally, any one of these could be satisfied, but not all at the same time or in no order of priority. The needs of men (of which health is only one) are certainly unlimited; and, by comparison to the felt-needs or demand, the supply of the resources of any society are irremediably sparse. There is no avoiding this question of choosing societal priorities. We must choose how we shall go about choosing and ordering our medical and societal goals.

We shall begin with the first, more dramatic question of how we should choose how to choose who shall live or die. The larger questions of medical and social priorities are almost, if not altogether, incorrigible to moral reasoning.

In 1967, the Gottschalk Committee estimated that up to $237,000,-000 would be needed in 1975 to provide dialysis for about 18,000 patients and kidney transplants for more than 4,000 patients. These estimates assumed no change in the criteria for accepting patients, but the committee also predicted that in the future many more than the estimated number of patients would be considered medically acceptable. At the same time the Gottschalk Committee advocated a nationally financed program of kidney transplants, calculating this to cost an average of $13,300 per operation, plus $200 to $1,000 yearly for follow-up costs.[1] In California alone it would cost $10,000,000 a year to offer dialysis to all reasonably suitable cases of renal failure.[2]

The Burton Report, sponsored by the Office of the Surgeon General, estimated the cost of a "total push" program covering 50,000 *new* end-stage kidney patients each year to be $701,000,000 in the first year, $1,043,000,000 in the fifth year, and in the fifteenth year between $1,816,000,000 and $2,702,000,000 (in which year there would be an estimated 179,401 patients on chronic dialysis or transplanted). It therefore recommended accepting only the "ideal" candidates out of the total number of patients with end-stage kidney disease, i.e., 6,000 to 8,000 new patients a year.[3] That would eliminate well over 80 percent of the patients who need either dialysis

1. *Report of the Committee on Chronic Kidney Disease,* submitted to the Director of the Bureau of the Budget, September 14, 1967, pp. 20, 27, 69.

2. David Sanders and Jesse Dukeminier, Jr., "Medical Advance and Legal Lag: Hemodialysis and Kidney Transplantation," in Reflections on the New Biology, *U.C.L.A. Law Review* 15, no. 2 (February 1968): 364.

3. *Kidney Disease Program Analysis.* A Report to the Surgeon General, Benjamin T. Burton, Chairman. Public Health Service Publication No. 1745, pp. 205, 207.

or a kidney transplant if they are not to die. Confronted with these figures, the response is often to appeal to home dialysis, and to the ability of mass production to reduce the cost of these machines. The fact, however, is that less than 20 percent of patients with renal failure are suitable for home dialysis. Many more do not live in homes that are suitable. 1,600 patients are now on in-center dialysis, only 800 in homes. Moreover, a major part of the cost is in the monthly or yearly supplies for the machine. In-center dialysis costs aproximately $15,000 a year. To maintain a patient for 10 years on these machines would cost $150,000. Home dialysis, I am told, now costs about the same for the first year, of which $5,000 is for the equipment. After the first year, $3,000 to $5,000 a year is a good estimate. Ten-year survival on home dialysis might cost as much as $65,000.

A kidney transplant costs $15,000 for the first year, plus $500 each year thereafter for drugs and postoperative care in the uncomplicated case. It is difficult to tell the cost of the heart transplants that have been performed—since this is now borne by various "research" funds and are mixed with other hospital and personnel services. $50,000 is as good an estimate as any. Such a figure is exclusive of the cost of hospital care for the days waiting for a suitable donor to be found. I understand that a capillary kidney may soon be available, units of which are disposable. That would drastically lower the cost of dialysis. But dialysis is poor treatment at best, even if successful in saving lives. Transplants are indicated instead in a great many of the cases.[4] This means that it is impossible to avoid the practical and moral problem of patient selection. The problem could be eased by improvements in the practices surrounding these procedures. Lack of uniformity in the medical criteria used leads to less utility of these sparse resources in the nation as a whole. Lack of agreement and uniformity in the medical criteria also stands in the way of insurance coverage of dialysis.

4. For medical reasons, but also because of the serious psychological and family problems that are developing as home dialysis becomes more common. Lowering costs one way may raise costs in another: in necessary social and psychological services, if life is to be saved by these means. Men and women in their marriages are not meant to be capable of independent existence, but it is an unnatural burden and greater than many can bear to be completely dependent on one another as well as on a machine for existence itself.

In any case, from one costly life-saving remedy to another, the moral question of how to choose among medically acceptable patients is going to remain with us. One avoids this question only by concentrating on one remedy at a time and supposing its maximum distribution. That would be to concentrate the "idea of progress" (plus American know-how and mass production in the solution of problems) on one medical miracle at a time in the conquest of death. With respect to any one or more of the diseases from which, say, one out of every seven of us now dies, it is reasonable to say that the costly life-saving remedy, when discovered, could be funded and the personnel trained to extend the remedy to everyone who needs it. Still the fact remains that research is now going on, at the National Institutes of Health in Bethesda, Maryland, and at other large medical centers, into therapies for the many ills of mankind which, when perfected, are all simply not soon, if ever, going to be budgeted and made available to everyone. Looked at the other way round, if our goal is that the seven out of seven of us who are going to die shall not do so, health needs are by definition infinite. In an age of medical technology, every time one effective remedy follows another the question arises anew: Who shall be allowed to live when not all can be saved?

Let the Better Man Live

The most widely discussed practice of patient selection by an estimation of a patient's social worthiness, or his worth to others, is that of the "public committee" set up by Dr. Belding H. Scribner of the University of Washington at the Swedish Hospital in Seattle.[5] This committee was established when it became evident that the "kidney machine" offered a possible 100 percent effective way of saving the lives of patients suffering total renal failure, and yet it seemed likely that this would be the first such therapy withheld from general use, because of the cost to make it available to all who might benefit. Since then the Veterans Administration has established dialysis programs in VA hospitals. With the VA centers there are

5. For the following account see Shana Alexander's article, "They Decide Who Lives, Who Dies," in *Life* magazine, November 9, 1962, pp. 102–10, 115–28. See also Herbert Lawson's report, "Kidney Machines Save 'Doomed' Lives But Raise Ethical Issues," in *The Wall Street Journal*, August 22, 1963; and Robbins and Robbins, "The Rest Are Simply Left to Die," *Redbook*, November 1967, pp. 80–81.

now an estimated total of 250 centers throughout the country. Of these, 60 are or will shortly be primarily training for home dialysis.

Dr. Willem J. Kolff of the Cleveland Clinic, who pioneered in the invention of the kidney machine during World War II in occupied Holland, deplores the need for any selection at all. "Am I to understand that the richest country in the world cannot afford to take care of its ailing citizens?" he protests. "Lay committees tend to legalize and give a pretext of respectability to a deficiency that should not be condoned." [6] More recently it has been estimated that we could preserve the lives of persons needing kidney dialysis at no more cost per week than formerly was expended on a patient with tuberculosis in a sanitarium, or treating and housing those with mental illness today.[7] Perhaps these analogies show that we could extend dialysis to all who would benefit by dialysis. It may be that morally society should not abandon kidney patients, or force a choice among competing patients, any more than this should have been allowed to happen in cases of tuberculosis or be allowed in mental illness. Still the fact that tuberculosis is contagious and mental patients are burdensome or dangerous to others, while total kidney failure removes its victims quickly by death, is not irrelevant to the questions whether we are *likely* to give top social priority to kidney dialysis or transplants. Moreover, it is worth repeating that today there are many more treatments that are irremediably extraordinary and costly, and a multitude of troubles in our society contending for our attention and resources.

In any case, at any given time and place, the medical profession faces the problem of having to choose who shall live and who shall be allowed to die. Even if we believe that every new remedy can

6. "Letters and Comments," *Annals of Internal Medicine* 61, no. 2 (August 1964): 360.

7. See Henry K. Beecher, "Scarce Resources and Medical Advancement," Ethical Aspects of Experimentation with Human Subjects, *Daedelus*, Spring 1969, p. 290–291, 309. Dr. H. E. deWardener estimates that the present cost of maintaining a tuberculosis patient in a sanitarium in England is the same amount, and that the cost of maintaining mentally deficient children in hospitals in England is one-third to one-half the amount, needed to treat a patient on intermittent kidney dialysis in a hospital. "Some Ethical and Economic Problems Associated with Intermittent Haemodialysis," in G. E. W. Wolstenholme and Maeve O'Connor (eds.), *Ethics in Medical Progress: With Special Reference to Transplantation* (Boston: Little, Brown, 1966), pp. 112–13.

shortly be extended to everyone who needs it, and the same for the next costly remedy after that, etc., medical resources remain sparse at any given time and place, and the problem of patient selection cannot be avoided. The Seattle committee is the prototype of one way to solve this question of how to choose who lives and who dies. When not all can be saved, a choice must be made; it cannot be postponed to some future ideal time when sufficient funds and trained personnel will be available.

When set up, the Seattle public or lay committee made the final selection of the patients to be entered in the dialysis program after a medical panel had made its selection on medical grounds. The committee is now an advisory one; the medical staff makes the final decisions. When the Seattle committee was set up, the medical criteria aimed at selecting good research subjects. The trend is now toward the clarification of medical criteria to be used in a proved therapy. This means that strictly medical criteria are likely in the future to admit a larger number of acceptable patients; and if the trend is also toward medical judgments rather than lay committees, this could simply mean a shift in those responsible for final patient selection. Under conditions of scarcity, this could simply mean that physicians make judgments of social worth, or such judgments hidden among the stated medical criteria. The Seattle committee is therefore still worth examining as a prototype of one way to choose.

Persons suffering with any other systemic disease, e.g., diabetes, are medically unacceptable. There can also be negative psychological indications, e.g., a patient may be judged unlikely to tolerate the regimen of dialysis twice or three times a week, diet control, care of the cannula in his arm, etc. Still, more applicants pass these broad "medical" tests—some of which hide the fact that social judgments, e.g., cooperativeness, are made—than can be accommodated on the machines. When moving from criteria for selecting good research subjects to criteria for selecting acceptable patients, some physicians even believe that "you can dialyze anybody." Then the requirement of a "stable, emotionally mature adult under 45" is already an arbitrary one dictated by the scarcity of the medical means for averting death after total kidney failure. The fact that children may not mature physically on dialysis and will not likely be able to stick to the diet is a sort of medical reason for excluding them, but one hardly commensurate with the consequence of doing so—except on the warrants of a patient-centered ethics of not always intervening to save life, which would be valid even if no one else needed the machines. The fact that children will require an indefintely greater number of years on dialysis is a reason based on medical scarcity, while the fact that only adults have dependents who need them is a reason of comparative worth to others, lending support to the exclusion of children. Extrinsic worth, surely, if the child always loses in this comparison! Still, given these criteria, it is now estimated that there are 8,000 to 10,000 new candidates appearing every year who would be medically acceptable for kidney dialysis in the United States, and all will need to be maintained indefinitely (plus an equal number more the next year, etc.) until they can be given a kidney transplant. The latter, more revitalizing remedy, in turn, requires that "space" be saved for such patients on the kidney machines to save their lives in case the graft is rejected.

These were some of the considerations that moved Dr. Scribner and his colleagues to assemble a lay committee further to winnow the applicants in need of dialysis. In 1962, for example, 30 patients with kidney failure sought the artificial kidney treatment at Swedish Hospital. Seventeen were chosen by the medical panel, and the lay group then had to narrow the selection to 10. Ten should live, they said, seven must die. A seven-member "public" committee makes these final decisions; in 1963 the committee was composed of a lawyer, a clergyman, a housewife, a banker, a labor leader, and two physicians. The group is anonymous to protect it from public pressures. Its first responsibility was to choose how to choose, to decide how to decide such questions of life and death. The committee decided to base its decisions on broad social and economic criteria.

"The Admissions and Policies Committee of the Seattle Artificial Kidney Center at Swedish Hospital" was, in fact, a life-or-death committee. There is nothing wrong with that, since someone tragically has to decide such questions, provided they have rightly chosen how to decide them. The doctors advised them to reject automatically anyone over 45 years of age; and also to reject children. They voted to keep the committee's membership strictly anonymous, and also that they did not want to know the real names of the patients either. They needed to know, in weighing these cases against one another, the following factors: age and sex; marital status and number of dependents; income; net worth; emotional stability, with particular reference to the patient's capacity to accept the treatment; educational background; nature of occupation; past performance and future potential; and the names of people who could serve as references. Excluded from review were any kidney-failure patients who were not residents of the State of Washington—a limitation, we may sadly note, that would not be placed upon the patients to be served in the emergency room of any good hospital.

The decision-making process went something like this. Over a chemist and an accountant competing with three other patients for two places, the debate was whether they should be ruled out on economic grounds because both had substantial net worth, or ruled in because they had the finest educational backgrounds and the greatest potential for service to society of all the five candidates. Concerning a small-businessman with three children, a surgeon on the committee was impressed with the fact that "this man is active in church work," which was for him "an indication of character and moral strength." The housewife observed: "Which certainly would help him conform to the demands of the treatment." Or, countered the lawyer, "help him to endure a lingering death." Whereupon the minister spoke: "Perhaps one man is more active in church work than another because he belongs to a more active church." Both these men having made ample provision for their families, their deaths will not force their families to become a burden on society. But that would be to penalize the very people who have been most provident.

Between a man with three children and a man with an older wife and six children, we must for the sake of the children reckon the surviving widow's opportunity to remarry. In estimating "worth to society", how much chance would an artist or a composer have before this committee in comparison with the needs of a woman with six children? (Of "bourgeois values," more later.)

"What happens when we get two men with the same job, the same number of children, the same income, and so forth?"

"At our committee's first meeting we seriously discussed selecting candidates by drawing straws. We were going to make it easy on ourselves by having a human lottery! Frankly, I was almost ready to vote for the lottery idea myself." So spoke the surgeon, who confessed he slept better nights after these group decisions than after many of his own individual decisions.

Some doctors and references write better than others. How can the committee not be swayed by the writing ability of those who compose the reports or by their capacity to make a good case for an applicant? And if the committee gets its own staff of investigators, would not they have to be anonymous too; and would not the committee still be swayed by the bias of persons intervening between them and the patients? How should anyone weigh these imponderables: the life of a man who, if he is permitted to continue living, can make the greatest contribution to society; against the life of a man who by dying would leave behind the greatest burden on society? Concluded Shana Alexander, the author of the *Life* magazine article from which I have taken these vignettes: "A candidate who plans to come before this committee would seem well-advised to father a great many children, then to throw away all his money. . . ."

Said one of the patients fortunate to have been chosen: "What a dreadful decision! It's like trying to play God. Frankly, I'm surprised the doctors were able to round up seven people who were willing to take the job."

Finally, if a patient is given a place in a kidney dialysis program because he "passed" a comparative evaluation of his worthiness in terms of broad social standards of eligibility, the needs of his dependents, or his potentiality for contribution to humanity, one can ask whether he should be removed from the program when his esteemed character changes. Legally this would be questionable, but to ask this question is one way of clarifying the moral legitimacy or illegitimacy of using such criteria at all. "If you really believe in the right of society to make decisions of medical availability on these criteria," as Dr. George Schreiner said, "you should be logical and say that when a man stops going to church or is divorced or loses his job, he ought to be removed from the programme and somebody else who fulfills these criteria substituted. Obviously no one faces up to this logical consequence." [8]

8. George E. Schreiner, "Problems of Ethics in Relation to Haemodialysis and Transplantation," in Wolstenholme and O'Connor, *Ethics in Medical Progress*, p. 128;

Reviewing all that happens in patient selection by social criteria, David Sanders and Jesse Dukeminier, Jr. find "a disturbing picture of the bourgeoisie sparing the bourgeoisie," and remark that "the Pacific Northwest is no place for a Henry David Thoreau with bad kidneys." They conclude that "justice requires that selection be made by a fairer method than the unbridled consciences, the built-in biases and the fantasies of omnipotence of a secret committee." [9] That may be an extreme judgment, even a pitiless one, upon those anonymous citizens of Seattle who were only trying to do a job assigned them in the most responsible way they knew. Moreover, the Seattle committee has for years been the butt of discussion simply because it is the most celebrated instance of this mode of patient selection. We need to remember that in an estimated 42 percent of the dialysis centers, patients are assayed in terms of their social utility. With or without a lay committee this may be a part of the admissions procedure; physicians themselves can and do employ such nonmedical tests. Therefore, what we are examining is the principle of selection, not a single committee and its practice, except illustratively.

Indeed, Sanders and Dukeminier immediately go on to say that ad hoc comparisons of social worth are "no less objectionable" when delivered by panels of physicians, hospital personnel, and social workers; "medical men are no more qualified to play God . . . than ordinary mortals"; "it may be even more objectionable for the decision to be made by physicians." [10] This is true, I suggest, not only because physicians owe the highest loyalty to a patient's medical care which ought not to be mixed with social assessments having possibly fatal consequences. It can also be argued that a public com-

---

it is customary to assume that the doctor-patient "contract" requires that a patient not be arbitrarily dismissed from treatment. Therefore a man in his early forties will be continued on dialysis past 45 years of age, even at a center where after 45 he would not be acceptable in the first place. This shows the arbitrariness of age itself as a medical criterion! Why should one man be helped to live past 45 and not another? Or why should not both be unassisted? Exclusion on the basis of age may have been reasonable when research was in view; it is not, if we mean to extend treatment to all who need and may benefit from dialysis.

9. David Sanders and Jesse Dukeminier, Jr., "Medical Advance and Legal Lag," p. 378.

10. Ibid., pp. 378–79.

mittee, drawn from various sectors of the population, is likely to
reflect a broader range of the community's values, and changes in
those values, than panels composed of the members of a single profession. The community's values (bourgeois, if you like) will be operating in any case, once we step upon the path of assessing the social
worthiness of patients. But genuine human values lie beneath cultural values; and these, we may judge, are more likely to come into
play through the prism of a public committee's decisions than
through the selections that will be made from estimates of social
worthiness by members of a single profession.

For this reason, the final point to be made in this section has the
utmost importance. The fact is that "social worth considerations as
well as unconscious biases, can secret themselves within a medical
or psychiatric evaluation." [11] If there is a fairer, more just method of
patient selection, it will have to be stringently observed. Procedures
to ensure equality of patients at risk of life or death will cut across
not only schemes that explicitly evaluate them in terms of extrinsic
worth to others. Such procedures must also disclose the social worth
considerations hidden in many a medical and psychiatric judgment.

One psychologist expressed to the present writer the opinion that
he would judge a patient ineligible for admission to a dialysis
program only if he were (1) clearly psychotic or (2) had an established
record of refusal or inability to follow a physician's instruction.
Psychological-medical reasons for exclusion can easily mean far
more than that. They can come to mean an estimate of a potential
patient's "cooperativeness" or his "congeniality" to the staff. These
are hidden social evaluations which, if they should be made at all,
had best be placed in the hands of a committee more representative
of the community at large. The fact is that many a patient has proved
to be able to cooperate in the treatment's regimen, or not to do so,
contrary to all the evidence beforehand. This needs to be noted,
even if we allow that a doctor who is forced to choose who lives, and
who dies, does not act wrongly in proceeding on the optimum statistics.

The School of Public Health of the University of California at
Los Angeles, under sponsorship of the Kidney Disease Control

11. Ibid., p. 379.

Program, conducted a survey in 1967–68 of dialysis centers throughout the country.[12] Response was received from approximately three-fourths of the estimated 120 centers then in operation—small (12 patients a year), medium (21 patients), and large (30 patients). This study is currently being updated (in all respects except patient selection) for an estimated 250 centers now in existence. On the question of patient selection, the present study shows that medical suitability and the absence of other disabling disease is the most frequently used criterion; age, the next most common; psychiatric evaluation and potential for vocational rehabilitation share third place; social welfare evaluation of the patient and his family is next, followed by the patient's willingness to cooperate and his intelligence; financial resources is next; and finally some purely practical considerations, such as distance from the center or the suitability of a patient's house for home dialysis.

12. The following information is based on a personal communication from Dr. Laurence R. Tancredi, of the National Center for Health Services Research and Development, Department of Health, Education, and Welfare. The study mentioned in the text above has now been published; see Albert H. Katz and Donald M. Procter, *Social-Psychological Characteristics of Patients Receiving Hemodialysis Treatment for Chronic Renal Failure*. Kidney Disease Control Program, U.S. Department of Health, Education, and Welfare: Contract No. PH–108–66–95, July 1969. Add to the conclusions drawn from my interview with Dr. Tancredi the following findings: "Patients were predominantly white (91 percent), male (75 percent), married (79 percent) and in age groups 35–54 years (59 percent)," Ibid., p. 3; "The study population originally consisted of 852 cases, 629 males and 223 females," *Ibid.*, p. 11; "The underlying basis of selection appeared to be patients 'most likely to succeed' in medical and social terms. Consequently, it is not possible to estimate statistically from this group what percentages of patients would succeed if all patients were treated, or if patients *were* selected at random," Ibid., p. 14; "A minority of centers (23) administer intelligence, personality or vocational aptitude tests to prospective patients," Ibid., p. 23; "Such factors as the congeniality of the patient as an individual, economic burdens of dependents if patient wasn't selected, 'demonstrated social worth,' 'future social contribution,' which have overtones of moral judgment and middle class bias were considered of minor importance by the majority of centers, although from one-fifth to one-third rated them important," Ibid., p. 24; mental deficiency would definitely exclude selection of a patient in 68% of the centers; poor family environment, in 29%; criminal record, in 25%; indigency, in 21%; poor employment record, in 20%; lack of transportation, in 17% and nonresidency in the State, in 17%, Ibid., p. 25; "Although sex was reported not to be an important criterion, the fact that there were 173 women in a sample of 689 patients points strongly to the contrary," Ibid., p. 26; "The predominance of males was partially due to the 179 patients on dialysis at the Veterans Administration hospitals. Excluding VA patients, the study population was 66 percent male and 34 percent female," Ibid., p. 27.

This ranking of the criteria for patient selection in current use quite evidently contains both explicit and possibly hidden comparative evaluations of patients in terms of social worthiness or extrinsic worth to others, and this has no correlation with whether a center has set up a public committee to do the evaluating. Among 16 possible selection criteria, demonstrated "social worth" of the patient, his potential future social contribution if rehabilitated, and his likelihood of vocational rehabilitation were listed as separate tests. The demonstrated "social worth" of the patient is always taken into account in 8 centers, and this is considered important but not consistently evaluated in 20 other of the reporting centers. Likelihood of vocational rehabilitation (perhaps an acceptable criterion if this includes a possible change of jobs) is always applied by 28 centers, and considered important and usually applied by 37 others. Thus 76 percent of the centers evaluate job rehabilitation potential. In addition 42 percent of the centers go further and evaluate "future social contribution"—a figure which shows that this test means something more than whether a patient can function well enough to return to a job. We have already spoken of how difficult it must be to predict or to remove bias from estimating "stable emotionally mature adult," "demonstrated willingness to cooperate" in a dialysis regimen, or "congeniality" to the staff, which are among the tests used.

Finally, this study showed the centers disclaiming selection on the basis of sex. The mean rank of the patient's sex is on the level of "not used" (0.1) in the selection process. Yet the fact that there were only 169 women on dialysis in this sample of 688 points strongly to the contrary. Kidney failure is hardly correlated with sex to that degree. Prior selection by private physicians cannot be discounted in explaining the actual selection by sex. Still it is evident that referring physicians or the centers (whether or not the physician's judgment is supplemented by that of a public committee) are using broad social evaluations in selecting patients, in this case, self-support and number of dependents. The reader may recall that women figured in the reported deliberations of the Seattle committee largely as "factors" determining the fate of husbands thrown into comparison. There must be a better way to select patients for sparse medical resources that determines who lives and who dies. That alternative will be examined in the next section.

The foregoing description of the actual practice of patient selection shows that, if the alternative is better, it will need to be stringently observed to protect against the propensities of medical and paramedical personnel to make hidden judgments of social worthiness.

A Human Lottery?

In selecting the patients with fatal illness who are to be given treatment that is not available to everyone equally in need of it, the lawyer's norm of equal protection and due process and the moralist's norm of fairness, justice, or equal respect for human lives can be implemented only by one of three methods. Each of these methods is designed to exclude comparisons of the social worth of individuals, or of their extrinsic worth to others.

First, certain rules can be announced in advance which are not discriminatory but based on statistical medical probabilities. Thus we could state certain formal, if somewhat arbitrary, rules that put people in categories while excluding comparative judgments among them individually. If persons over 45 or 50 are to be excluded from hemodialysis, then no one need compare the worthiness of one 55-year-old man with another. If children should be excluded because they likely cannot endure the treatment and will not develop normal puberty, then no one need estimate the intelligence or family background of children, or take account of letters of reference. Even a policy of restricting the services of a given hospital to in-state residents is to be preferred to accepting "notable" out-of-state applicants. These rules would be universalizable de facto standards of selection —a significant improvement over much current practice, but not yet a sufficient or a sufficiently moral principle of selection.

Second, random patient selection can be instituted, either by lottery or by a policy of "first come, first served." The Los Angeles County General Hospital Renal-Dialysis Center, for example, uses a lottery system to select among medically graded applicants on record, while the Detroit Receiving Hospital affords the same equality of opportunity by a policy of "first come, first served." These two procedures are in principle the same, and we will consider them as if they were one. "First come, first served" amounts to an on-going lottery. Moreover, in the use of sparse medical resources there will often in practice be medically suitable patients who have already come to the center among whom selection must be made when there is room for them on the program. We have then only two principles to choose between in choosing how to select patients: randomness among lives presumed to be equally valuable, and comparisons of social worthiness or extrinsic worth to others. I assume that physicians and only physicians are competent to make a prior medical selection; and, indeed, that their experience in an on-going lottery may be sufficient to uphold a judgment that a medically more suitable applicant will come next week for whom room on the program should be held open. This would be to allow maximum latitude to a doctor's distribution of sparse medical resources within the terms of the judgments he, and he alone, is competent to make. Still, randomness would ensure equality of opportunity to live, and not die, to every one of a class of patients, and it would forbid the physician from raising questions of comparative social merit as a means of determining who lives and who dies.

In the search for a more impersonal method of selecting who is to be saved from among the dying, the model is the casting of lots among passengers apparently doomed to die in an overloaded lifeboat, which is the rule in U.S. maritime law. The decision in *United States v. Holmes* [13] accepted lottery in such a desperate lifeboat situation as the procedure which alone would rule out arbitrariness and manifest equal respect for equal rights to life when not all can be saved. An English case, however, rejected a lottery as "grotesque," expressing the same aversion to the idea of a "human lottery" as did one member of the public committee at Seattle's Swedish Hospital. Instead, however, of endorsing judgments of comparative social worthiness to reach decisions concerning life or death, the English court ruled that all must wait and die or be rescued together. [14]

From this decision one might, abstractly, conclude to yet another

13. 26 F. Cas. 360 (No. 15,383) (C.C.E.D. Pa. 1842).

14. *Regina v. Dudley*, 14 Q.B.D. 273 (1884). Justice Benjamin Cardoza approved the English and rejected the American rule of law, saying, "Who shall know when masts and sails of rescue may emerge out of the fog?" ("What Medicine Can Do for Law," in *Selected Writings of Benjamin Nathan Cardoza*, Margaret E. Hale, ed. New York: Fallon, 1947, p. 390). One hears similar statements made in the medical ethical context in support of unending efforts to prolong life, because some new discovery or life-saving remedy may emerge like a sail of rescue out of the fog, but not in support of the proposition that sparse life-sustaining remedies should be withheld while all wait and die until all can be rescued together.

possibility for resolving conflicts of lives when not all can be saved. Overloaded dialysis centers, we might say, are to be compared with overloaded lifeboats. If neither social worthiness nor a "human lottery" should be used in passenger or patient selection, the conclusion to be drawn would seem to be that there is no sound basis for choosing anyone to be saved, because not all can be saved and each one has a right to life equal to any other. This possibility will be discussed, obliquely at least, in the course of our examination of the justification for choosing randomness over social worthiness in patient selection. These remain the two realistic alternatives. Still, it is significant to note that random selection has as its model casting lots in the overloaded lifeboat situation; that from pondering such a procedure sensitive minds like Benjamin Cardoza and Edmond Cahn have been repelled by it; and that—far from going to selection in terms of social worth—they have felt impelled to say that when faced with choosing one life at another's expense no selection can ethically be made.

In analyzing the lifeboat cases in their applicability to the problem of patient selection, David Sanders and Jesse Dukeminier, Jr., seem to me to be mistaken in drawing a distinction between the law and the moral principle governing in cases of jettison and the law and moral principle governing in cases of rescue. These authors seem to believe there is a morally significant distinction between a decision to jettison some of the passengers from a lifeboat made by those who are also imperiled, and a decision to rescue some from the dying made by persons not doomed. "Selection for hemodialysis," they write, "is analogous to a situation where there are thirty persons in a sinking boat and a second boat, with room for five persons, comes by. A committee on land is to decide and advise by radio which five persons will be transferred to the second boat." [15]

Jettison initiated by doomed men and rescue initiated by men who are secure on shore with their well kidneys are, of course, different moral situations. But these situations do not differ in the principle of selection to be used if selection must be made. Sanders and Dukeminier need not have sought for another principle or a principle underlying the rule of equality in shipwreck cases. That rule of equality, and how alone to accord equality, applies to human rescue

15. Sanders and Dukeminier, "Medical Advance and Legal Lag," pp. 374–77.

by third parties as well as to decisions to jettison by men who themselves are among the imperiled. In the Holmes case, the rescuers were aboard: the mate Holmes, who gave the order, and the rest of his crew were needed for rowing. Holmes made the decision to jettison in his official capacity, being the highest ranking officer aboard among the imperiled. The issue in human rescue or in jettison is how to exclude arbitrary decisions in determining who lives and who dies when not all can be saved.

Sanders and Dukeminier cite Professor Paul Freund in his Gay Lecture at Harvard Medical School: "The governing principle is not the merit or need or value of the victim but equality of worth as a human being. The governing principle, it might be said, is that man shall not play God with human lives." [16] I suggest that here Freund proposes two alternative statements of the same governing principle. Perhaps "man shall not play God with human lives" is a principle that underlies or bases the rule of equality in shipwreck cases. If so, it is also a principle that underlies or bases the rule of equality in cases of human rescue. In the case of jettison or of rescue, "the essence of playing God," as Sanders and Dukeminier say, "is to look at A and to look at B, assay them, declare B is worth more than A, and save B." [17] True enough; but this is also the essence of a violation of the principle of equal rights to life in making forced selections either to jettison or to rescue. In both cases, it is "equality of worth as a human being" that comes into competition with that of another human being. This equality of worth as a human being mandates the randomizing of selection if selection is the only way to avoid all perishing. Neither in jettison nor in rescue should worthy lives or lives having unequal worths to others be thrown into comparison. Granting that men are unequal in all sorts of respects, these are not relevant moral features to be reckoned in deciding who lives and who dies.

The moral difference between these two situations is only that, if I am among the doomed, I may be more in need of the constraints of a socially accepted governing principle of the equality of worth of every human being in order for me to be fully willing to place myself

16. Paul A. Freund, "Ethical Problems in Human Experimentation," *New England Journal of Medicine* 273 (1965): 687.

17. "Medical Advance and Legal Lag," *op. cit.* p. 375.

under a casting of lots and to see the justice of its outcome. Still, I allow that for someone safely on shore among the rescuers, "the governing principle that man shall not play God with human lives" by making direct comparisons of the social worth of individuals in deciding questions of life and death may be a salutary expression of, and the ultimate ground and source of, "the governing principle of the incomparable equality of worth which every man has as a human being." How else am I going to be able to restrain my normal human propensity to do good by thinking more highly of some lives than I ought to think? How else am I going to be willing to have blood-washings fall upon the deserving and the undeserving alike, and good blood chemistry shine upon the needy no less than those who are needed?

When the ultimate of life is the value at stake, and when not all lives can be saved, it can reasonably be argued that men should stand aside as far as possible from the choice of who shall live and who shall die. Men should then "play God" in the correct way: he makes his sun rise upon the good and the evil and sends rain upon the just and the unjust alike. This physicians do when in order to ensure equality of opportunity to live they devise a lottery scheme or adopt the practice of "first-come, first-served" to determine who among medically equal patients shall be admitted to a kidney dialysis program or be given an implanted vital organ. The equal right of every human being to live, and not relative personal or social worth, should be the ruling principle. When not all can be saved and all need not die, this ruling principle can be applied only or best by a random choice among equals.

Random selection is preferable not simple because life is a value incommensurate with all others, and so not negotiable by bartering one man's worth against another's. It is sustained also because we have no way of knowing how really and truly to estimate a man's societal worth or his worth to others or to himself in unfocused social situations in the ordinary lives of men in their communities. The equal right of every human being to live ought generally to prevail since men and their communities are organized around a plurality of social goals and many sorts of manifestations of the uniqueness of personal beings. There can be a describable sort of "exception" to this ruling principle (guaranteeing by random selection equal possibility of life when not all can be saved) if and only if a community and its members have (or have been reduced to) a single focus or purpose and goal under some quite extraordinary circumstance.

Professor Paul A. Freund of the Harvard Law School stated the ethical principle governing choice of who shall live and who shall die, and he also stated the sole qualification to be added to this ruling principle. "My own submission," Freund writes, "was that in the matter of choosing life or death, not involving specific wrongdoing, no one should assume the responsibility of judging comparative worthiness to live on the basis of unfocused criteria of virtue or social usefulness, and that either priority in time, or a lottery, or a mechanical selection on the basis of age should be followed." [18] Freund gave an illustration of a community of men reduced to "focused criteria" in which comparative social usefulness can be and should be employed. This was the decision to allocate penicillin, in short supply in 1943 among the U.S. Armed Forces in North Africa,[19] to victims of venereal disease rather than to victims of battle wounds. What could possibly justify giving penicillin to men "wounded in brothels" instead of to men wounded in battle? [20] The justification depended on the special requirements of the practice of medicine on men in battle. The restoration of a larger number of men more quickly to fitness for the limited purpose in which they were engaged was the only—and it was a sufficient—excuse. The particular decision of the Theatre Medical Commander in this case can be generalized into a universalizable stipulation designating the morally relevant features of situations which alone justify deciding questions of life and death in terms of comparative social worthiness. One may act in accord with a morality of social utility in a situation, such as this one, "where objectives were closely defined—maximum fighting power as rapidly as possible."

Two additional illustrations can be given. While in the lifeboat

18. Paul A. Freund, "Introduction to the Issue Ethical Aspects of Experimentation with Human Subjects," *Daedalus*, Spring 1969, p. xiii.

19. The same circumstance of the scarcity of antibiotics in England during the war morally permitted *withholding* them from a "control group" of patients in order finally to prove their greater degree of effectiveness in contrast to established treatments.

20. The expression is Henry K. Beecher's, in agreement with Freund. *Daedalus*, Spring, 1969, p. 280.

situation the ruling principle of equal right to life should be ensured
to the passengers by random selection among them if not all can be
saved, Freund's qualification of this rule applies to a choice between
passengers and the crew if the latter are needed because of special
knowledge and skill in rowing in order for any to be saved. Here
again the objectives of all aboard are closely defined; they have one
purpose: to endure the storm and reach shore or rescue.

The morality of triage in disaster medicine is the second illustration. In the case of natural or man-made disasters, victims most in
need of help—on whom normally we would lavish resources—must
simply be set aside, and nothing be done for them. First priority must
be given to victims who can quickly be restored to functioning. They
are needed to bury the dead to prevent epidemic. They can serve as
amateur medics or nurses with a little instruction—as the triage
officer directs the community's remaining medical resources to a middle group of the seriously but not-so-seriously injured majority. Even
among these, I suppose a physician should first be treated. It is not
enough to say that "those casualties whose immediate therapy offers
most hope for the conservation of the common good should receive
first priority." [21] We must go on to say that first priority should be
given to those casualties whose immediate therapy offers most hope
for the conservation of a quite specific, minimal common good, i.e.,
mere survival and the restoration of the conditions of there being
any good or a good in common or a common good in any higher
sense. When it comes to that, who can say who most matters? Or who
should say who matters most when the consequence of doing so
determines life and death? The good is not common that does not
flow back upon all alike. How one participates and for what just
rewards may vary or be debated in a society, but participation itself
—life in the human community—cannot rightfully be made contingent upon quality of contribution. Triage decisions are all a function
of the narrowly defined, exceptional purposes to which a community
of men may have been reduced. In these terms, comparative social
worthiness can be measured.

But, as Freund says, "life is rarely so circumscribed in its goals."
No one can tell the worth of an old man sitting on the porch watch-

21. Thomas J. O'Donnell, S.J., "The Morality of Triage," *Georgetown Medical Bulletin* 14, no. 1 (August 1960): 70.

ing a sunset, or ponder imponderables like the relative moral worth of comparative genetic inheritances, or say whether a disturbed or seemingly undisturbed child should be saved. When tragically not all can be saved the rule of practice must be the equality of one life with every other life, which in such a case can be implemented only by randomizing the choice that necessarily must be made among them. To begin to estimate comparative worthiness to live on the basis of unfocused criteria of virtue or social worthiness would be to presume to make a (nearly) total estimate of a man's life. "The more nearly total is the estimate to be made of an individual, and the more nearly the consequence determines life and death, the more unfit the judgment becomes for human reckoning. . . ." The more nearly total is the estimate made of an individual, the nearer we would be to presuming "to act as gods on the Day of Judgment." [22]

Here we see the important and informative distinction between a practice that "plays God" and a practice that is fit for the reckoning of men who imitate rather God's care (before the Judgment Day!) alike for the good and the bad, the profitable and the unprofitable, the deserving and the undeserving, and seeks to serve those who are only needy no less than those who are needed. In allocating sparse medical resources among equally needy persons, an extension of God's indiscriminate care into human affairs requires random selection and forbids god-like judgments that one man is worth more than another.

All Should Die When Not All Can Be Saved

The case of *United States* v. *Holmes* and the imaginative discussion of this case by the late Edmond Cahn,[23] Professor of Jurisprudence at New York University Law School, opens up another and an

22. Paul A. Freund, in *Daedalus*, pp. xiii–xiv. The same point was made by David Sanders and Jesse Dukeminier, Jr., "Medical Advance and Legal Lag: Hemodialysis and Kidney Transplantation," Reflections on the New Biology, *U.C.L.A. Law Review* 15, no. 2 (February 1868): 376–77: "Opinions of social worth are infinitely more diverse than opinions concerning the design of a belfry. . . . Ad hockery is not the stuff from which constitutional guaranties of equal protection and due process are made."

23. 22 Fed. Cas. 360 (C.C.E.D. Pa. 1842); Edmond Cahn, *The Moral Decision: Right and Wrong in the Light of American Law* (Bloomington: Indiana University Press, 1955), pp. 61–71. The reader may want to refer to my discussion of the Holmes case and of Cahn's philosophy of law generally, in *Nine Modern Moralists* (Englewood Cliffs, N.J.: Prentice-Hall, 1962), Chapters 8 and 9.

abysmal possibility. When not all can be saved, no one should be selected from among the doomed or the dying, since each has equal worth as a human being. Such would be a conscientious judgment that is not altogether unreasonable when men stand before the ultimate of life or death—even though Professor Cahn would never have proposed this as a solution of the problem of the distribution of sparse medical resources under "normal" conditions, but only for the overloaded lifeboat case, and even though the medical profession would not give the suggestion a moment's thought.

We need to examine this admittedly abstract possibility—abstract if proposed as an alternative to either randomizing choice or choosing by some standard of extrinsic worthiness—for two reasons. (1) Professor Cahn's sensitive reflections on the Holmes case excellently expresses the revulsion of many people against the idea of instituting a "human lottery." (2) Paradoxically, it is our sense of the ultimate, "congeneric" covenant among men and of the incomparable equality among men when they face starkly the option of living on only because another man must die which holds the consciences of men back from life-and-death decisions by standards of social worthiness. A religious sense of righteousness among men who are equal before God, which Cahn possessed in such fine degree, is the same outlook which sustains randomizing any choice men must make among the dying. This is the bearing, I shall argue contra Cahn, of an ultimate covenant among men in the human community upon choosing how to choose who lives and who dies, both in overloaded lifeboats and in the case of overloaded life-saving therapies.

Holmes was one of nine seamen in an overloaded and leaky lifeboat who gave the orders as the mate—all members of the crew deemed necessary for rowing in the storm—to throw overboard fourteen male passengers to lighten the boat. The judge, in charging the jury as to the law, said that if no seaman could possibly be dispensed with, then the victims should have been chosen from among the passengers by casting lots, provided—as in this case—there was time enough to do so. Acting under these instructions, the jury found Holmes guilty of manslaughter, but he was given a suspended sentence because of the jury's recommendation of mercy.

Cahn wants rather to "judge Holmes' judge than Holmes" [24]—for

24. This and subsequent quotations concerning this case are taken from *The Moral Decision*, pp. 70–71.

his ruling that lots should have been cast. In drawing this conclusion Cahn imports the righteousness of mankind's ultimate covenant directly and unrefracted into the arena of legal decision and established societal practices and expectations. The dimensions of that crucial moral situation seem to him utterly incommensurate with the arrangement the judge suggested: "the crisis involves stakes too high for gambling and responsibilities too deep for destiny." From what Cahn understands to be the absolute requirements of righteousness when men face such options, he is driven to conclude that none can "be saved separately from the others" and that "if none sacrifice themselves of free will to spare the others," "they must all wait and die together." I cannot myself believe that any such thing can be the meaning of the justice which the law ought to endeavor to exact. Instead of fixing our attention upon "gambling" as the solution—with all the frivolous and often corrupt associations the word raises in our minds—we should think rather of equality of opportunity as the ethical substance of the relations of these individuals to one another that might have been guarded and expressed by casting lots. Then we will see that the judge spoke for the good in law. In many other matters, the courts undertake to impose social control and corrective justice by means that might seem to be incommensurate with the human relations involved, e.g., when they assess money damage for loss of life or limb. Likewise, the judge in requiring lottery spoke for the principle of the equal worth of human beings when any must be selected from among the doomed or dying.

On the other hand, Cahn speaks admirably of the good that may be beyond all law and human contrivance, but whose relation to the latter we shall have to examine. Yet at this level also one may question whether his analysis of the final covenant among men is quite right. Cahn's reflections on this case actually show much of the imprint of biblical righteousness, although he mistakenly insists that his is an "anthropocentric" view of the law. The lifeboat situation, he writes, brings into full force the "morals of the last days." This means that all the established relationships in which an individual usually stands are stripped away; all his distinguishing features and all the special bonds of responsibility that pertain to normal human existence in its fixed orders and institutional framework are now gone. This leaves him "a generic creature only," responsible only but fully to the *genus* in every man in the boat and not to their

specific particularities which are defined by continuing social relationships. "Every person in the boat embodies the entire genus. Whoever saves one, saves the whole human race; whoever kills one, kills
mankind." "For where all have become congeners, pure and simple,
no one can save himself by killing another. . . . He has no moral
individuality left to save. Under the terms of the moral constitution,
it will be *wholly* his self that he kills in his vain effort to preserve
himself."

It should be pointed out in passing that these people in their
desperate plight were not wholly stripped to congeneric relationships. Two married men and a little boy were spared; and two
women—sisters of one of the victims—voluntarily leaped to join
their brother in his death. And the mate selected the males only, and
not women or children, for inclusion among those to be forcibly
ejected. Should he perhaps have thrown overboard a 300-pound
woman, if she had been aboard, for the sake of saving two 150-pound
men? It is, of course, to forestall such dilemmas arising (in which any
solution which suggests itself is so obviously incommensurate with
what is at stake in the collision of life with life) that Cahn attempts
to abstract from every specific particularity of the situation. Casting
lots would have satisfied that requirement. Instead, Cahn departs
from the idea of a lottery in exactly the opposite direction from the
proposal that men should evaluate social worth in making passenger
selection. He allows none to be saved, mistakenly identifying any
selection with "saving oneself."

It is more important to indicate, however, that in his reflection
upon this situation Cahn transgresses the limits of his own "anthropocentric" view of the good in law and of the moral covenant beyond all law and beyond all schemes for selection among the dying.
He speaks, of course, of people becoming "mere congeners" under
circumstances in which the "morals of the last days" prevail. In spite
of this terminology, however, it seems clear to me that no interpretation of merely generic responsibility provides adequate basis for, or
is the actual source of, the conclusions he draws, apart from the cor-
rectness or incorrectness of the judgments he makes in defining the
justice possible at law or in shipwreck cases (or in patient selection).
I think it is clear that these are the requirements not of a natural
"moral constitution" but of human life-in-community constituted

by the covenant-righteousness of men together, nakedly equal before God.

Thinkers in the past who have put forward theories fundamentally like that of Cahn have not ordinarily drawn such extreme conclusions merely from a morality of generic responsibility. Kant's categorical imperative was: "Act so that in your person as well as in the person of every other you are treating mankind also as an end, never merely as a means"; [25] but it is doubtful whether he would suppose that fidelity to "mankind" as an end would itself go the length of all waiting and dying together. For John Locke, men in a state of nature —where all are congeners—suffer the inconvenience of having to judge in their own case; yet as such they have the right and the duty to preserve mankind in general. But in saying that it is the law of nature and of reason for man also to preserve the rights of others as his own, Locke inserts this qualification: "when his own preservation comes not in competition, ought he, as much as he can, to preserve the rest of mankind." [26] Surely this is the extent of obligation that can be "anthropocentrically" based on nature and reason or on the "moral constitution"; and this was enacted, surely to the maximum requirement, by the judge's ruling that lots should have been drawn. Generic duty gives equal primacy to self-preservation while setting it in the context of any arrangement which makes this most compatible with the preservation of mankind generally. Who knows, perhaps if the male passengers had not been thrown violently overboard at what must have seemed to them the arbitrary command of the mate, if instead they had been called upon to share in lots as the means of securing general and equal application of what had to be done to and upon all alike, they might not have resisted so wretchedly—they might have evidenced their agreement with the general will arising from all and not only from the mate's command. To such height "conscience's generic commands" [27] and rules of law may rise. But hardly to the level of requiring that men should all wait and die together rather than that the lives of some be saved.

Cahn is actually voicing a moral judgment that roots in the bibli-

---

25. *The Fundamental Principles of the Metaphysic of Ethics* (New York: Appleton-Century-Crofts, 1938), p. 47.

26. *Concerning Civil Government,* ch. 2.

27. *The Moral Decision,* p. 243.

cal tradition which measures fidelity in terms of a higher righteousness. It is significant that he writes: "The crisis in the longboat was
apocalyptic in character, the kind of crisis in which, as Jesus saw,
family ties, earthly possessions, and distinctions of every conceivable
kind become null and void." It is only the immediate presence of
the claims of the righteousness of God between man and man, and
not any sense of generic injustice, which asks of men that on occasion
they be unwilling to save their own lives at the unavoidable cost of
another, and which enables them on occasion to have such faith that
their own lives are securely in God's hands as to be able actually to
make the sacrifice.

Still these "morals of the last days" always impinges upon the administration of justice and upon contrivances for passenger or patient selection. "This planet we live on is not entirely unlike the
longboat of the *William Brown*." Overloaded life-saving therapies
are also much like the longboat. It is not enough to say that this is
only a metaphor. It is not enough to say that an awareness of the
"morals of the last days" or of the righteousness of God between
every man in the longboat of the social order provides us "only a
moral attitude or an answer, not a moral decision." For at every
moment we are making decisions as men ultimately before the righteousness of God, either to throw our lives away or to keep them for
a possible better accounting, even if only for a better opportunity for
meaningful sacrifice. As men whose actual generic situation has been
revealed under God to contain possibilities and duties we would
never have suspected, we must decide whether to preserve the genus
in ourselves, or the genus in others, or else we settle for some feasible
arrangement for doing either with equity and justice.

We might conclude from all this that no one should let himself be
saved at the expense of another who loses in the casting of the dice.
He can declare himself willing to die when not all can be saved, and
lighten the longboat or the dialysis center of his weight. He might
affirm of himself that it is better for one man to die than for a
whole people to perish. This is a safe and honorable doctrine on the
lips of Jesus, who applied it to himself. But it is quite another thing
for action in accord with these words to come from a Caiaphas, who
forthwith applied them to someone not himself. So a prostitute
might say it is better for her to die, or a banker that it is better for

him to die, than for everyone or for a laboring man with five children to perish. But on the lips of another, a panel of physicians or of laymen representative of the community, these become the words of Caiaphas calculating social utility or a prostitute's unworthiness, while perhaps saving some man who made his contribution, among other things, to her profession.[28]

Perhaps Sanders and Dukeminier apprehended the possible venture of self-sacrifice in the forced choice of who lives and who dies when they made a distinction between jettison as a decision made by the imperiled, and rescue as a decision made by men who are not among the doomed. In any case, Cahn's ruling that in "the morality of the last days" all should wait and die together must be regarded as the introjection of the self-sacrificial spirit of charity into the structures of decision-making, which then as a rule of law (of the fundamental law, no less) is impervious to the creative possibility of saving some by means of any fair arrangement which a wise charity might devise.

The foregoing should constrain us to say that one among the doomed or dying may elect to jettison himself, because of any judgment of the worth of another that he may have in mind. That he at least should be willing to have his worth count for no more than that of any other human being. That he should accept a procedure of passenger or patient selection which has generality of application and whose fatality may then come equally as well to him as to anyone else. That, claiming no exception for himself because of special merit measured by some scale of human worthiness or worth to others, he rightfully may claim that any demerit he may have in these terms be not counted to jettison him or to warrant failure to rescue. The immediate translation of a covenant of righteousness and faithfulness among men cannot be either that all must wait and die or be rescued together or that some are to be saved according to inequalities of their social worth. Instead, the translation of fidelity among men must surely be into the principle that every person in the longboat of hospital practice has equal worth as a human being. When these worths are in competition for sparse medical resources, when not everyone can be saved who needs a particular life-saving

28. A remark of Paul A. Freund on patient selection in the panel discussion at the American Medical Association's Second Congress on Medical Ethics, Chicago, 1968.

remedy, random patient selection would seem to be the only way to acknowledge and adhere to the inherent worth every man has as a man among men.

How Shall Sparse Medical Resources Be Distributed Justly?

Dr. Warren J. Warwick of the University of Minnesota Medical School has written an article on organ transplantation which bore the subtitle "A Modest Proposal." [29] That was a reference to Swift's biting and satirical suggestion that the inhabitants of Ireland might increase the food supply by eating their children. Only the subtitle indicated that Dr. Warwick was not entirely serious in putting forward his proposals, except for the bizarre nature of some of them— bizarre to the public and the medical profession, but not so much so when set down beside many of the things the revolutionary biologists are willing to contemplate.

Cadres of ambulance chasers with consent forms and "accident watching clubs" should at once be formed among the populace, equipped with helicopters. (This will, somewhat unfortunately, have the "spinoff value" that the victims' chances of recovery may be improved.) If this is not enough to secure an ample supply of organs, some further simple measures can be taken. "Prohibition of seat belts and other safety devices, cancellation of speed limits and removal of road warning signs would make driving a greater risk and pleasure to our thrill-seeking youth and would increase the number of accidents," especially head injuries. If anyone objects that this would be a policy deliberately designed to kill people, let him reflect that American know-how can surely master the logistics of using several of the organs of a simple victim, thus saving five or six lives in place of one. That would satisfy the cardinal moral principle to which all enlightened men subscribe, namely, the greatest happiness of the greatest number, and the view that in prudent pursuit of this goal men should not be so absolutistic as ever to say "never."

We need not only a new definition of death so that more organs can be salvaged, writes Dr. Warwick, but a totally new philosophy of the body as well. Society should have the right to tax a man's body by claiming its organs, since social resources have maintained his

29. Warren J. Warwick, "Organ Transplantation: A Modest Proposal," *Medical Opinion and Review* 4, no. 6 (June 1968): 20–25.

health—just as we tax his estate on the grounds that the common prosperity had something to do with the wealth a man earns. If necessary this socialization of the body could be further extended: "A dollar value would be calculated for each transplantable organ, and when the state's services to the body equals the organ's worth, the state would collect for its services by transplanting the organs to deserving recipients"—or at least to recipients not in arrears. Women desiring abortions could be persuaded instead to allow the fetuses to be born and used as suppliers of organs. In our society it at first would be necessary to induce in these fetuses some congenital malformation; then surely some women would be willing to make a career of bearing these short-lived monsters and selling their organs. "Since the organs would be used to restore infants with other congenital abnormalities to normal productive lives, the mothers performing this service would become revered members of society."

Dr. Warwick concludes his article with the plea that, since organ transplantation is clearly a predictable winner of the public's support, physicians must not again back "proved losers," such as the archaic notion that preventive medicine and presymptomatic treatment are better than later treatment. Funds to learn more about the care of the heart or the prevention and cure of kidney or liver disease and to support the education of the public in health care are simply not going to be forthcoming in amounts at all comparable to funds for spectacular replacement of hearts and other organs. Instead we are going to squander precious resources on persons who have squandered their own. Whatever first-year and second-year medical students may think about preventive medicine, the profession as a whole must get where the action is. This is definitely not in preventive medicine or presymptomatic treatment. Loose livers will simply get new ones. [30] The American Way of Not Dying is bound to win out. Doctors had better not bank on preventive treatments.

I decided to begin the final section of this chapter with a reference to Dr. Warwick's article largely for the fun of it, but also because his final, satirical thrust favoring preventive medicine and presymp-

30. Besides, to raise the question, as did Dr. Leon Kass, "A Caveat on Transplants," *The Washington Post*, January 14, 1968, whether we should replace the lungs of smokers or the cirrhotic livers of alcoholics comes dangerously close to the outmoded religious dogma that the wages of irresponsible living is death.

tomatic treatment over organ transplantation breaks wide open the most incorrigible social and ethical question that I know concerning modern medical practice, and indeed concerning social policy at large. This is the matter of ordering our medical priorities and ordering our overall social priorities, including medical needs, in some more rational way. What should be the medical priorities? Indeed, who shall say or how do we go about deciding what sorts of medical services should be given priority over others, and how much of a nation's resources should be spent on medical care in comparison to other claims and needs?

We Americans commonly believe that we can do anything money can buy. We take that to mean that everything can be done that science or men generally know to do. In this we are like the patriotic speaker at a commencement assuring 400 seniors that every one of them could become President. The speaker ought rather to have said that any one of them, or at most several in their generation, could become President; that no one fulfilling the legal requirements was barred from this accomplishment. So no one medical accomplishment is beyond our grasp, or quite a number from among all that research funds can buy, plus vast sums for the social distribution of proved therapies. But not everything can be done in the provision of medical services that human ingenuity devises and money can buy, or men need, even if there were no other human claims and social needs calling for expenditure of the nation's resources.

To say that we can do anything we decide to do is (if it is not an expression of hubris) simply to say that we have the opportunity and the forced necessity of choosing what shall be done from among the many things that are possible, but not all possible together. This is the question of setting priorities, which—tragically, perhaps—must be faced and thought through by the medical profession and by society in general. It is a question that is almost if not altogether incorrigible to rational determination. Therefore, we generally order our priorities by not ordering them; decisions of great import for the lives of men and the future of mankind are made by not deciding them. This issue must at least be lifted up to view, since there can be no good reasons and no good moral reasons for decision by indecision, for allowing medical priorities and social priorities to be determined by who has the most spectacular therapy or the loudest voice in the land.

Symbolic and symptomatic of this issue within the practice of medicine—indeed, within surgery alone—is the fact that, when Great Britain's first heart transplant was performed on Mr. Frederick West, so limited were the facilities at the National Heart Hospital that the operation caused a dozen operations to be postponed, simply because the only place sterile enough initially for Mr. West's postoperative care was the operating room in which he received his new heart.[31] Let us not dismiss this problem by saying that the London hospital, or England as a whole, had sparse medical resources, and that the United States can do better. That may be true, but it is not to the point. Let us rather use this case as a prism through which we can comprehend the fact that when measured against the human need any nation, and mankind as a whole, possesses only what must be called sparse medical resources, and sparse social resources for meeting the other human needs as well. The blunt truth is that this is permanently the human condition—especially perhaps in modern times when "the fear of death appears to have become ubiquitous with secularism," [32] when death is regarded as an unmitigated disaster, and men hope to be saved from illness and death by scientific and medical technology in a measure that true religion never cared to promise.

If we can do any one or a number of things, we cannot do everything in the service of human health. This means that we are forced (and have the opportunity) to decide among the needs and the procedures for serving them. This in turn means that—before we get to such fascinating questions as deciding who shall live and who shall die, because kidney machines and organs for transplant are and are likely to remain in short supply—there is a more fundamental ethical and social question to be raised about the medical priority to be given to these procedures themselves. Behind that is the question how the medical profession and society generally decide such questions, and the probable immorality of letting them decide themselves by professional and social indecision.

I am told that, with less funds for research and for extending medical care than is spent on kidney dialysis, it is reasonable to

31. *Sunday Times*, London, May 12, 1968; and "New Hearts for Old," Herder Correspondence, August 1968, p. 242.

32. Charles D. Aring, "Intimations of Mortality: An Appreciation of Death and Dying," *Annals of Internal Medicine* 69, no. 1 (July 1968): 138.

hope that we could soon eradicate at least one or two of those kidney diseases with the (for me) unpronounceable names which cause total renal failure that today may put people on the machines or else kill them. (Acute and chronic glomerulonephritis are not obviously corrigible to preventive medicine.) Why not do both? is the normal reply; but, seeing that it would take a large budget to provide kidney dialysis for the medically acceptable patients needing permanent dialysis or facing death who are accumulating at the rate of 7,000 to 8,000 new "ideal" patients a year (or 50,000 new end-stage kidney patients, not so "ideal," who are equally in need), the reply is rather like saying that almost everyone could become President.[33] In recognition of this problem, one dialysis specialist tells me he is thinking of writing a paper on "What is money?" He envisions persons with total renal failure dialyzing one another; presumably, some at work making the machines, others producing the supplies which are a large, irreducible, and recurring cost, etc. Then he will have to figure how much it will *cost* to train people to do these tasks, and establish the logistics of an internal "barter" economy among all the people who must die if they do not get blood washings twice or thrice weekly. He will soon discover that "money" is precisely the best known means of overcoming the deficiencies of a barter economy.

The issue grows and grows and the question resounds louder and louder throughout medical practice and our society generally as we move from dialysis to kidney transplants and as the transplantation of other vital organs may be expected to become a proved therapy. The present writer has heard heart transplantation defended because the "spinoff" would be that we will learn more about the heart and its care. This sounds like defending our costly manned space program because of its indirect benefits to the American economy. Why not give these things the top priority? I repeat there is a question that is reached sooner than the choice of who shall live and who

33. The bill introduced in Congress by 64 House members and 26 Senators, June 28, 1969, to set up a national program to provide artificial kidney treatments was limited to the 8,000 ideal patients, i.e., patients who would have made good research subjects in the early stages of the development of this treatment. The bill would authorize expenditure of $74 million by 1974 to build and equip centers, training of technicians, etc. See the *Washington Post,* June 29, 1969. That figure is far too low, like funding one ABM.

shall die when not all can be saved by a given, costly, and scarce procedure.

This sooner question is: What priority should be given to the development and use of earlier therapies? Should medical specialists in last-ditch remedies continue their unspoken and undeliberate "conspiracy" with the American Way of Not Dying to give these remedies the greater prominence and a powerful claim upon our overall sparse medical and social resources? Behind that is the question: How does the medical profession decide such questions and help the nation to decide? There is cause for some disturbance when the same day's newspapers can carry the report that Dr. Cooley is "upset" over the lag in heart donors and also a statement of the World Health Organization urging more research into the cause, prevention, and cure of coronary ills.[34] The latter praised the "spectacular and stimulating results" that have been obtained by the active intensive care, rehabilitation, and surveillance of victims of heart failure, while yet saying that we know little of the cause and prevention of this illness, which may be "associated with the present mode of living" and which is reaching "enormous proportions," with younger people being stricken in increasing numbers. It looks as if somebody's medical priority is showing!

So far we have been speaking of research, preventive medicine, presymptomatic treatment, and earlier curative treatments that fall within the same range of illness or failure of function for which transplantation is proffered as an end-term remedy. "Too often we buy apples without considering the oranges thereby foregone." [35] The question I am raising can be enlarged, still within the range of medical priorities. We are rightly filled with amazement and admiration by the transfer of the heart, liver, both kidneys, and a cornea from a single donor into five different recipients at Memorial and New York Hospitals, in operations supervised by Dr. C. Walton Lillehei. This involved twelve teams of surgeons and the logistics of doctors racing with the heart through the tunnel connecting the two hospitals. The first interhospital transplantation of a heart was heralded as a practice that "inevitably" must become common practice

34. *New York Times,* February 28, 1969.
35. David L. Bazelon, "Medical Progress and the Legal Process," *The Pharos,* April 1969, p. 35.

in the use of organs, since it is technically possible for one donor to give life to as many as 17 people who certainly will not happen to be together in the same hospital. On the same day this event was reported, the *New York Times* editorialized that the numbers "can ultimately be raised to the millions; it is not too soon to begin preparing to take full advantage of these hopeful new perspectives." [36] Neither is it too soon to ask ourselves the question: How ought we to esteem this astonishing performance in a city whose hospitals and general health services are in decay? Where the infant mortality rate creeps steadily upward? Where there is great need for better medical care for the poor?

Finally, we have to locate our medical priorities (whatever these should be, and however who says what they should be) in the larger context of social priorities. To what extent ought medical needs be served in comparison to eradicating poverty, stopping the decay of our cities, depolluting our atmosphere and streams, defending the nation, and aiding underdeveloped peoples? Again, it is quite clear that while all things are possible, all things are not compossible, as Leibniz said. In any case, we ought not to dignify a "decision" by indecision favoring spectacular interhospital transplantations in the millions by simply saying this "inevitably must become common practice" since every potential donor has 17 organs that can be used. On the other hand, it is not much of a solution to say that the nation's first order of business is its cities because people are liable to riot, while there will only be private grief and no picketing when one by one thousands die for want of an organ or when a patient having diabetes or over a certain age or from another state or who won't "contribute" much to "society" is excluded from renal dialysis.

I do not know the answer to these questions, nor how to go about finding the answer.

> It has been estimated that early detection of cancer of the cervix through Pap tests might save 9,000 lives a year. If funds are limited, we could and should compare the costs of such a detection and treatment program for cancer with the cost of combatting renal disease by transplants or dialysis. The comparison becomes more difficult when an alternative program

36. February 21, 1969.

will not save lives but will instead, say, prevent blindness by detecting and treating glaucoma. Other health programs promise even less dramatic benefits. But a program of preventive dental care would promote the comfort and well-being of millions of Americans at a fraction the cost of saving a few thousand lives through hospital dialysis. . . .

But no test will ever tell us whether our choice between a dialysis program and an equally expensive program of preventive medicine was right or wrong. Individuals will differ in their evaluations. If one man believes that a hundred healthy children are a better investment than keeping one oldster alive on dialysis, his colleague who disagrees cannot claim his friend is wrong. They could, of course, agree to settle their dispute by attempting to measure the community consensus. But who then can say the community consensus is right or wrong? [37]

A significant beginning on some of these programs could be made with the money spent to keep Astromonkey Bonny in orbit for twelve days in July 1969. But then the space program seems connected with our sense of national well-being. We need not recite all the other causes that compete with medicine for funds.

In any case, in a culture that deems death always a disaster, medical resources must necessarily be limited. Then perhaps we ought to acknowledge bluntly and boldly that triage is among the rules governing normal medical practice. In disaster medicine—in the event of a nuclear attack upon a city, or in the case of the typhoons that struck the gulf coast of Texas a few years ago—death is accepted and the worst cases, who would require teams of surgeons for long hours, are set aside while the medical resources that.are plainly unequal to the need are devoted to saving the many who can be saved more quickly. Disease and death are like the typhoon or the bomb in their attack—in this age when the National Institutes of Health are researching more therapies than can possibly be funded. Where medical resources are irremediably sparse when measured by the need, we may have to learn not always to give the advantage to spectacular and costly treatments in ordering our priorities, if medical resources are ever to be distributed justly. This would be a form of triage,

37. David L. Bazelon, "Medical Progress and Legal Process," p. 35.

accepting the death of some of the most desperate sorts of cases in order to give first attention to many more whose medical needs are urgent, to be sure, but who are not yet at the end-stage of some fatal illness. Prevention may be worth pounds of cure. Under conditions of poverty of medical resources relative to need, when not everything can be done that ideally should be done, it does not necessarily follow that the maximum research and personally and socially costly medical care should be expended upon the most desperate cases first. And under conditions of poverty, it does not necessarily follow that medical care ranks first among our national goals. We may have to learn again an ancient wisdom concerning the acceptable death of all flesh.

Yet in suggesting that something like triage may have a role to play in preplanning the distribution of medical research and services, I am acutely aware that a "leveller" policy of egalitarianism which would first do the simple things or first meet the most fundamental human needs before going on to virtuoso medical performances would not be a very helpful principle to apply in ordering our priorities. A civilization consists of many different qualities and levels of activities, as does medical practice. In the recovery of Europe after World War II, opera houses were rebuilt along with housing for the homeless. Men did not wait until everyone was well sheltered before turning to music. Life would now be poorer had they done so. It may be that the development of organ transplantation should be compared with building opera houses while there is need for medical clinics and general practitioners among the teeming masses of the poor in our cities; and that medical practice would be poorer if we first did the simple things before going on to virtuoso performances in medical practice. Conditional values should not always be first served. Still this does not alter the fact that not everything can be done that is worth doing, and we must determine the relative human and social importance of doing this, that or/and the other things that medical science makes possible.

It would be good to hear the medical profession debate thoroughly and in public the question of the ordering of medical priorities and how this ordering should be determined. That may be too much to expect, but if it could happen we the people might learn not only the direction in which to throw tax money for medical research and the distribution of medical services, but also how as a people we should go about deciding the nation's priorities in general.

We have now come full circle. A society is not a machine. Neither is it an organization having neatly tiered priorities. A society is an unfocused organization of many diverse, often conflicting, interests and pursuits. There are communities within communities pursuing a common good, and many ways in which the uniqueness and welfare of their members are manifest. Each of us may have a clear idea of what we think the priorities should be, but none can speak for the whole or persuade his neighbor. There is need, as we have said, for more mutual thought to be given to the setting of medical and social priorities generally, but the expectation that this can be achieved is finally totalitarian, or else can only have a leveling or reductionist effect on the practice of medicine and on the whole human enterprise. We may perhaps know when priorities are decidedly out of joint; but no one knows exactly where are the joints. Civilization is simply not an arrangement of human activities in a set hierarchical order. A society is largely an unfocused meshing of human pursuits.

For this reason, triage or selecting patients by standards of worth to the group can be justified in only the exceptional case of communities of men who have (or have been reduced to) a focused social purpose. For this reason, when a sparse life-saving remedy is extended to any who need it, it should be made available to all equally. Patient selection in a society having many unfocused goals should not be made a means to achieve other goals than saving life. Patient selection should not be made an occasion for the enhancement of other values than saving the life of any who have worth as human beings— certainly not when no one knows a neatly tiered arrangement of the "contributions" mankind needs.

Index

Alexander, Leo, 25–26, 164n
Alexandre, G. P. J., 76–77n
American Medical Association, 2, 19–26, 220
Anglo-American law: ethical substance of law of assault, 37–39; legal burial traditions, 204–05
Aring, Charles D., 3n, 134–35, 269n
Aristotle, 41n
Assault and battery, 37–39
Augustine, Saint, 209

Barnard, Christiaan, 228
Barth, Karl, 60, 154–56
Batt, John, 193n
Beecher, Henry K., 13n, 21n, 39, 39n, 89, 90n, 92, 97n, 104n, 106–07, 107n, 117, 119n, 243n
Bentley, G. B., 183n, 191n
Berger, Peter, 136, 136n
Bickel, H., 27
Biörck, Gunnar, 63n, 87
Brain death, 60–68 passim, 76–79, 82, 84–87; clinical criteria for, 89–92; criticized as death declaration, 91–94, 96–98. See also Harvard Report
Brain test: of brain death, 64–66, 76, 78–79, 82, 85–87, 89–90
Brain transplants, 65n
Braunwald, Eugene, 13n
Burger, Warren E., 38

Cadaver organs, use of: compared with blood donation, 212–13; sale of, 213–15; giving vs. taking, 209–10; legal burial traditions, 204–05; view of Jehovah's Witnesses, 210; Jewish views of, 210; objections to, 200–02; routine salvage of, 198–99. See also Uniform Anatomical Gift Act
Cahn, Edmond, 254, 259–65
Calne, R. Y., 77n, 105n, 203, 203n

Cameron, D. C. S., 147
Canon of loyalty, 2, 5, 35, 185; to dying, 112, 129, 131, 160, 164; from parent to child, 25, 57; between physician and patient, 36, 222, 227; violated in heart transplants, 222
Captive population: of children in institutions, 41, 44–45, 54–55; as protected under Food, Drug and Cosmetic Act, 44–45; as applied by New York State Civil Rights Bill, 55; of prisoners, 41–43. See also Proxy consent
Cardoza, Benjamin, 253n, 254
Cartesian dualism, 187, 193, 209. See also Christian ethics
Cavanagh, John R., 134, 149n
Cellular life, 59, 83, 88n
Chamberlain, Geoffrey, 17–18
Christian ethics: Karl Barth, 154–57; exceptional situations, 160–61n, 163–64; imperative life saving, 141; principle of totality, 166–70, 178–81; Protestant and Catholic views compared on organ donation, 165–70, 177
Christian ethics, Protestant, 176–77: Cartesian dualism, 187–88, 193, 209; on organ donation, 185–87. See also Organ donation
Christian ethics, Roman Catholic: on dying process, 81n, 96, 98–99, 152, 157, 158n; on medical ethics, 119n, 188; on physicalism, 180–81; and principle of totality, 178–81. See also Organ donation
Clinical death. See Death, clinical
Clinical Investigations Using Human Beings as Subject by U.S. Public Health Service, 47n
Coadventurers. See Partnership, patient and doctor
Consequence ethics, 2
Coma, 86–87, 90n, 91, 97, 106, 115, 117n, 132–33, 140n: irreversible, 89, 161–64

277